Observed Brain Dynamics

Observed Brain Dynamics

Partha P. Mitra
Hemant Bokil

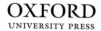

OXFORD
UNIVERSITY PRESS

2008

OXFORD
UNIVERSITY PRESS

Oxford University Press, Inc., publishes works that further
Oxford University's objective of excellence
in research, scholarship, and education.

Oxford   New York
Auckland   Cape Town   Dar es Salaam   Hong Kong   Karachi
Kuala Lumpur   Madrid   Melbourne   Mexico City   Nairobi
New Delhi   Shanghai   Taipei   Toronto

With offices in
Argentina   Austria   Brazil   Chile   Czech Republic   France   Greece
Guatemala   Hungary   Italy   Japan   Poland   Portugal   Singapore
South Korea   Switzerland   Thailand   Turkey   Ukraine   Vietnam

Published by Oxford University Press, Inc.
198 Madison Avenue, New York, New York 10016

www.oup.com

Oxford is a registered trademark of Oxford University Press

XIR71570
Detail of the Mona Lisa, c. 1503-06 (panel) (see 3179)
by Vinci, Leonardo da (1452–1519)
Louvre, Paris, France / The Bridgeman Art Library
Nationality / copyright status: Italian / out of copyright

Library of Congress Cataloging-in-Publication Data

Mitra, Partha.
Observed brain dynamics / Partha Mitra, Hemant Bokil.
    p. ; cm.
Includes bibliographical references and index.
ISBN 978-0-19-517808-1   1. Brain—Mathematical models.   2. Brain—Physiology.
3. Neural networks (Neurobiology)   4. Electroencephalography.
[DNLM: 1. Brain—physiology.   2. Mathematics.   3. Neural Conduction—physiology.
WL 300 M687v 2008]   I. Bokil, Hemant.   II. Title.
QP376.M5828 2008
612.8'2—dc22   2007019012

9 8 7 6 5 4 3 2 1

Printed in the United States of America
on acid-free paper

To our parents

Preface

As you read these words, a dynamic, rapidly fluctuating pattern of electrical activity in your brain forms the basic substrate of your conscious perception, thoughts, and feelings. Technical advances in contemporary neuroscience enabling measurements and visualization of neuronal activity have led to the following widespread sentiment, whether expressed colorfully by journalists or more soberly by academics: problems that have plagued philosophers since antiquity are approaching resolution.

A closer examination reveals, however, that major challenges remain to be overcome. Despite the volumes of data generated by increasingly sophisticated techniques, we still have only limited ability to directly measure neural activity under fully physiological or naturalistic conditions. Equally importantly, we do not yet know how to quantify measured activity in ways that yield the most meaningful insights into the relationship between the activity patterns and nervous system function. A microscope and a staining technique provide a reasonable starting point for studying neuroanatomy, where visual examination alone can lead to progress in understanding; visually examining multichannel recordings of electrical activity or brain image sequences is less effective as a means to understand the dynamical behavior of the nervous system.

Even the simplest study of nervous system dynamics calls for an extra level of quantification. In effect, in addition to the primary measurement device— electrode, microscope, or an magnetic resonance imaging scanner—the investigator must employ a second, theoretical instrument. Such instruments for analyzing neural signals are the subject of this book.

The application of quantitative measures to neural activity has a fairly short history in contrast with similar quantification of phenomena relating to the physical sciences. Recordings of trains of action potentials were initially displayed visually, along with time markers, and a simple but crucial advance occurred with their quantification through the use of spike rates (number of action potentials per second). Similarly, electroencephalographic (EEG) recordings were also initially displayed as raw traces, and quantitative characterization emerged with evaluations of the EEG spectrum. These two measures allowing for time dependence still account for most of the quantifications of neuronal dynamics in current studies.

A variety of more complex methods have been introduced more recently, due largely to the availability of adequate computational power. Our emphasis will be on simpler classical measures for the following reasons. First, given the complexities inherent in studying neuroscientific phenomena, there is incentive to use the simplest analysis method adequate for a particular task. The typical neuroscientist with many demands on his or her time cannot afford to spend years learning technical material involved in the more complicated analysis techniques. Second, the multiplication of esoteric methods to analyze and quantify data makes sharing and communicating scientific results virtually impossible; it is easier for experimentalists to find common ground in the more classical measures.

There is a substantial amount of theoretical work involved, some of which still remains to be done. The problems of estimating even simple measures of dynamics from small amounts of neural signals, and performing appropriate statistical inference, require sophisticated theoretical apparatus. Analogy may be made with an optical microscope: the difference between an inexpensive and an expensive microscope lies in optics that are free of aberrations and capable of approaching fundamental resolution limits. A similar example from signal processing is that whereas simple spectral estimates are relatively easy to construct, estimators that reach resolution limits while minimizing estimation variance require more work. In addition, there are substantial computational challenges: the size and complexity of the data sets requires the involvement of computer scientists for the development of the necessary data management and visualization tools, as well as computer clusters to speed up the data processing.

This book is written for a broad range of readers. We begin with a set of philosophical essays that should be accessible to a general audience. We hope that physical scientists and neuroscientists will find these chapters useful as a broad survey of ideas and concepts, which are ultimately critical to understanding the subject matter of the book, but that often remain unstated. Some of the material is original and intentionally provocative, which we hope will energize the reader to rethink established dogma in the field.

The second and longest part of the book is a crash course in mathematics and statistics, starting from elementary material and leading up to advanced topics such as stochastic process theory and time series analysis. The first two chapters in this section contain tutorial problems meant to be an integral part of the text, and readers wishing to use these chapters for self-pedagogy should work through the exercises. Determined readers with knowledge of basic algebra and calculus should gain enough understanding in the second part of the book to be well equipped to use the specific techniques presented in later sections.

In the third part of the book, we present the application of signal processing or time series analysis methods to a variety of neurobiological time series data, including electrophysiological recordings made with microelectrodes, EEG and magnetoencephalographic recordings, functional magnetic resonance imaging measurements, and dynamic optical images of neural activity. The fourth and final part of the book contains two chapters on special topics, which will be most useful to the investigator interested in analyzing real data sets, but which also provide some tutorial material to the non-neuroscientist wishing to enter the field from the physical or mathematical sciences.

Our attempt to make the book self-contained, by including preliminaries and tutorials with advanced applications, may indeed be foolhardy, because this material could normally cover several courses. Nevertheless, we saw an urgent need for selected pedagogical material to fill the lacuna in the mathematical and statistical training of the average neuroscientist or biomedical scientist. We have been involved for many years in teaching data analysis methods to neuroscience trainees, and the major problem we encounter in our students is a lack of necessary basic knowledge in mathematics or statistics, whether forgotten due to disuse or never encountered in previous training. For biomedical scientists and trainees without the luxury to read a shelf full of textbooks, it is our sincere hope that the second part of the book will serve as a refresher course in background material often taken for granted in theoretical and computational neuroscience textbooks. Indeed, it may be useful quite generally as a refresher course in mathematics, statistics, and signal processing for biologists.

The problems discussed in this book reflect an ongoing evolution in theoretical neuroscience. As data sets grow larger and more complicated, theoretical methods to analyze and interpret these data have gained in importance. The methods we present generate statistical models and summaries of data, which provide the necessary bridge between empirical, experimental work and abstract modeling. It is often impractical and not always useful to publish full sets of raw data in neuroscience, yet theoretical models in neuroscience are not often sufficiently general to allow useful reporting of data only in terms of these models. The intermediate measures we describe are a way of communicating summaries of data sets that are relatively independent of interpretation: these summaries can be expected to remain valid even if a particular theoretical interpretation is invalidated by later experiments. Conversely, matching

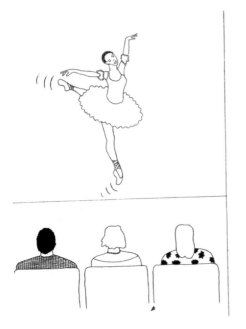
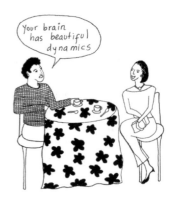

Ana Marie Velasco
may 2005

theoretical models to these intermediate summaries could give the theorist enough abstraction so as not to overfit details of the experiments while also retaining a rich description of the data set without reducing it to a few parameters.

Over the past several years, we have built the methods described in the third and fourth parts of the book into algorithms and software that should be of practical use for analyzing neurobiological time series data and for more general scientific signal processing applications. These efforts have culminated in the Chronux data analysis platform, which is freely available from *http://chronux.org*. We hope that access to these methods will enable neuroscientists to report standardized measures of dynamics, using classical signal processing measures, along with uncertainty estimates.

Neuroscience is a broad and flourishing discipline with many conflicting perspectives. Of necessity, this book presents a particular point of view, and we have made no attempt to provide a comprehensive survey of the relevant material. In the fall of 2006 there were about 340 neuroscience journals, and more than 14,000 abstracts were presented at the annual meeting of the Society for Neuroscience. Even within the narrow field of neurobiological time series analysis, there are many threads that we could not cover in this volume. Omissions should not, however, imply disrespect. Rather, we hope that the presentation of a coherent perspective will help the reader make sense of a large, active, and somewhat fragmented field of research. Currently in many neuroscience laboratories, significantly more time is spent struggling with issues of data analysis than with actual data gathering. Above all, we hope that this book will aid the process of analyzing and thinking about neurobiological time series data and as a result bring us closer to unraveling mysteries of how the brain works.

Acknowledgments

P.P.M. wrote the first two parts of this book, whereas the third and fourth parts reflect joint authorship between H.B. and P.P.M., with H.B. bearing primary responsibility. We are very grateful to a number of colleagues who contributed their efforts toward four of the chapters in the later parts of the book. The book would have taken a lot longer to write if we had undertaken all the material ourselves, but we also wished to retain the unity of an authored volume as compared to an edited one. We therefore chose a middle course, where most of the chapters were written by us, but we invited the following colleagues participate on some chapters. The chapter titled "Spike Sorting" was largely written by Samar Mehta with help from David Kleinfeld and Dan Hill, the chapter titled "PET and fMRI" is a shortened version of a draft prepared by Jason Bohland, the chapter titled "Optical Imaging" was condensed from a version prepared by Andrew Sornborger, and the chapter titled "Entropy and Mutual Information" contains material from a longer draft prepared by Jonathan Victor. In addition, we are grateful to Emery Brown, Uri Eden, Bijan Pesaran, and Wayne M. King for help with some of the figures in the book, including the use of appropriate data sets. We accept full responsibility for any inaccuracies we may have introduced. We also thank Rohit Parikh, Richard Murray, Daniel Valente, and Keith Purpura for reading portions of the book and offering corrections and comments, as well as Cara Allen for extensive editing.

PPM benefited greatly from a decade at Bell Laboratories, in an atmosphere that was intellectually stimulating and challenging. Much of the material presented in the third part of the book was developed during this period through collaborative efforts with several colleagues, including David Kleinfeld and Seiji Ogawa. It was a privilege to be able to simply walk across the Bell Laboratories building at Murray Hill, NJ, and consult leading experts in many disciplines. The book owes a particular debt to the work of David J. Thomson, who educated us in thinking about time series data and developed the multitaper method of spectral analysis that plays an important role in the book, and also to Catherine Loader for educating us in local regression and likelihood methods, as well as for providing the Locfit software package. P.P.M. would like to gratefully acknowledge several colleagues for fruitful collaborative interactions that led to papers from which we have drawn material for the book, including Bijan Pesaran, Richard Andersen, Rodolfo Llinas, Ofer Tchernichovski, Nicholas Schiff, Keith Purpura, Jonathan Victor, Larry Cohen, and many others. The material presented here was shaped during the summer workshop on Analysis of Neural Data (1997–2001) and the Neuroinformatics course (2002–2006) at the Marine Biological Laboratories through many interactions with both student and faculty participants at the workshop and the course.

The line drawings found in the initial chapters are original artwork by Ana Maria Velasco and are the results of a collaborative effort between her and one of the authors (P.P.M.). P.P.M. envisioned the design for the cover, which Cara Allen prepared. She also collected the photographs reprinted in the book and secured copyright permissions. The description of the cover image is based on a reference supplied by Eliza Watt.

We are grateful for the support of Cold Spring Harbor Laboratory, which has been the home institution for both authors during the later stages of the book. P.P.M. has received generous support from the NIH (grants MH062528 and MH071744, the latter being the principal source of support for the Chronux software platform (http://chronux.org) that encapsulates the methods covered in the book in a publicly available form), the McKnight Foundation, the Keck Foundation, the Sloan-Swartz Foundation, and Landon and Lavinia Clay.

This book would not be possible without the extraordinary patience and gracious encouragement of the editors at the Oxford University Press, including Fiona Stevens who initiated the process and saw the book through its early days, and Craig Allen Panner who later took up the reins following a transitional period with Joan Bossert. Given the four years since this book's inception, we would have almost certainly given up without the editors' faith in our ability to complete the task. Finally, to our family, friends and colleagues who have been so patient during periods when the book consumed our time and efforts, we remain very much indebted. I, H.B., would particularly like to thank Aylin Cimenser for help and support.

Cover Illustration: "Moti Mentali" or Motions of the Mind

The word *emotion* comes from the same Latin root as the word *motion*, hinting at the intimate relation between dynamics and mental states. This connecting thread runs through classical art forms, from the formal classification of emotions and the corresponding gestures in Sanskrit drama to the theories of emotional expression in Renaissance painting and sculpture. Leonardo da Vinci had a particular interest in how *moti mentali*, the motions of the mind, should be depicted in a portrait. It is speculated [139] that he may have written a manuscript on the subject, which is now lost. The following quote from notes thought to be copied from Leonardo's work by Francesco Melzi[1] is evocative:

> Various are the expressions of the face due to emotions, of which the first are: laughter, weeping, shouting, singing in high or low tones, admiration, anger, joy, melancholy, fear . . . All this will be discussed in the proper place, that is, the variety of appearances which the face, as well as the hands, and the whole person assumes with each of these emotions, and these you, painter, must of necessity know, and if you do not, your art will truly show bodies that are twice dead.

Our cover illustration is a tribute to this artistic idea, which is also sensible in modern neuroscientific terms, that facial expressions reflect the dynamics of mental states. It is, after all, what makes Mona Lisa's smile so enigmatic. We observe the dynamics of her brain obscurely, as it were, through her smile, and wonder what she was thinking.

---

1. From the Codex Urbinas 107–108, c. 1492, as cited by Kwakkelstein [139]. Quote has been abbreviated as denoted by the ellipses.

Contents

PART I

CONCEPTUAL BACKGROUND

1

Why Study Brain Dynamics?

nityam anityam[1]

In this chapter, we treat a number of general questions regarding the dynamics of the nervous system. First, we address why we are interested in dynamics at all: in this context, we examine active and passive views of the brain. Second, we consider some basic questions regarding the quantification of nervous system dynamics, including the importance of shared metrics. Third, we consider some basic questions relating to the arrow of time in physics and in biology.

1.1 Why Dynamics? An Active Perspective

Why study the dynamics of the brain? Although there are many compelling reasons, perhaps the most profound is that the dynamical pattern of electrical activity in neurons almost certainly forms the basic substrate of subjective, conscious awareness, as illustrated vividly by the phenomenon of absence seizures, where subtle alterations of these dynamical patterns lead to a transient and reversible loss of consciousness. Similar changes occur during sleep; the "statics" of the nervous system, namely the anatomy, are left the same, while the patterns of dynamics of the neural activity are altered, as is evident from alterations of the electroencephalogram (EEG). The key to unraveling the mysteries of subjective awareness in terms of underlying physical phenomena

1. Sanskrit aphorism that may be translated as *only change is permanent.*

3

probably lies in a careful study of the dynamics of different parts of the brain on a fairly rapid timescale.

Apart from long-standing questions of philosophical significance, there are of course a host of pragmatic reasons for studying nervous system dynamics. Also, it is not just the rapid electrical dynamics that are of interest: somewhat slower neurochemical dynamics, including that of neuromodulators and hormones, short- and long-term plasticity in the nervous system, the longer developmental dynamics, and the much longer evolutionary dynamics are important topics of study.

However, one conceptual distinction we would like to discuss at the outset perhaps characterizes a properly dynamical perspective. This is the distinction between "active" and "passive" views of the brain, a dividing line that runs through both experimental and conceptual approaches in neuroscience, and it appears in different guises in other areas of biology as well. This is related to, but not the same as, the distinction drawn between sensory and motor systems; rather, it is the difference in emphasis placed on the spontaneous activity of the nervous system as opposed to externally driven activity. Interestingly, there is a close analogy with a well-known conceptual shift in the history of physics: the active/passive divide is in some sense the difference between Aristotle's view of dynamics and Galileo's and Newton's views. To understand this analogy, we turn to how Aristotle conceptualized motion and how that concept was changed in Newtonian mechanics.

In simple terms, in Aristotle's physics, everything that moved was ultimately being moved by an external driving force, originating from a "prime mover." Aristotle's prime mover was somewhat abstract, but was given a perhaps more concrete and picturesque form by St. Thomas of Aquinas, who envisaged angels pushing the planets in their orbits (fig. 1.1).

Aristotle's view was consistent with the everyday experience that if an object is not subjected to a motive force, it eventually comes to a halt. However, extrapolating from careful studies of smooth spheres rolling down inclined planes of diminishing slope, Galileo came to the radically different perspective that bodies could continue to move indefinitely without an applied force. This was codified in Newton's first law of motion, and the angels were released from their duties of pushing planets and asteroids around in their orbits. An external agency was no longer required to explain uniform motion. In Newtonian mechanics, external forces were necessary only to explain departures from this uniform motion.

An Aristotelian conception of causation permeates a fair fraction of contemporary neuroscience. One has the stimulus-response theory of behavior, which holds that all behavior may be explained in terms of responses to external (driving) stimuli, whether in the form of immediate reflex actions or conditioned reflexes containing the memory of past stimuli; similarly, behavior

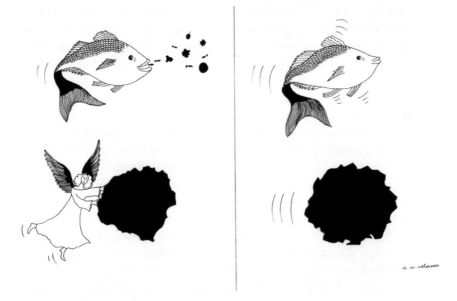

Figure 1.1: In Aristotelian physics, all motion needs an external mover, whereas Galilean mechanics allows for the possibility of spontaneous motion without needing a driving force. The stimulus-response theories of behavior, or explanations of behavior in terms of rewards, bear similarity to Aristotelian dynamics, whereas spontaneous or endogenous behaviors have a Galilean or Newtonian flavor.

is seen as being driven by "reward." We will discuss these theoretical perspectives in more detail in the next chapter. Here we want to note only that this view is not properly dynamic, in the sense that the motion of the system is explained in terms of external forces. It is easy to understand why this point of view would naturally give more weight to the sensory systems, as is the case in neuroscience research, because those are the entry points of external influences into the brain. This also leads to a view of the brain as an "information processing device" or a "computer." A computer, conceptualized rigorously as a Turing machine, is a general purpose function evaluator (i.e., an "input-output" device), the dynamics of which is essentially of an Aristotelian nature (a function evaluator is effectively driven by its inputs).

We will contrast this "static" perspective with an "active" point of view, emphasizing that the nervous system has its own dynamics, which is perturbed by the external influences. The active perspective has traditionally been adopted by ethologists, focuses on instinctive behaviors, and is rooted in an evolutionary approach. The idea that the nervous system is spontaneously active is of course well known: for example, consider the following quote from

Adrian [3]:[2] "There are cell mechanisms in the brain which are set so that a periodic discharge is bound to take place. The moment at which it occurs can be greatly altered by afferent influences, but it cannot be postponed indefinitely." However, a largely passive approach, as characterized above, might treat the spontaneous activity of the system simply as noise corrupting a particular experimental manipulation (which is more often than not in a stimulus-response mode). Alternatively, the natural behavior of the system may be given a more central place in the investigation. In other words, from a passive perspective, dynamics can be an afterthought, but if one adopts an active perspective, issues relating to dynamics gains primary importance.

In physics, Aristotelian dynamics is a discarded theory; the subtext of our example is the obvious one, that the stimulus-response view of the brain should follow suit. However, we would like to add some nuances to this message. We recognize that both the active and passive points of view have utility. Indeed, the stimulus-response method has provided great insight into the workings of the brain and the methods discussed in the later parts of this book are useful both from active and passive points of view. In fact, given that the stimulus-response point of view dominates in neuroscience, we have had no alternative but to give more room to the corresponding methods for function estimation and regression that relate neural activity to external stimuli. However, we maintain that the active perspective is the better one, and this is in large measure why we have chosen to emphasize the study of dynamics through a careful understanding of stochastic process theory and time series analysis methods. Hopefully, future work on the subject will emphasize the active perspective and more room can be given to the corresponding techniques in the books that wait to be written on the subject.

1.2 Quantifying Dynamics: Shared Theoretical Instruments

Once it is recognized that studying neural dynamics is an important scientific problem, the question immediately arises about how to characterize and quantify the dynamics. This is the content of the technical sections of this book. Here we discuss an example which illustrates that quantitative measurements of dynamics are neither mysterious nor inaccessible.

At some level, the idea of having quantitative measures seems problematic: how can something as ephemeral as dynamics be usefully quantified? However, such quantifications are actually widely used by the lay public, and are even written into the legal code. Take for example measurements of sound intensity levels, which can be easily obtained by buying a sound pressure level

2. Cited in Hebb, "The Organization of Behavior."

(SPL) meter. Sound pressure levels are defined by integrating the spectrum of pressure fluctuations in the air over the audio frequency range, and as we will discuss later in the book, the spectrum is one of the basic ways of quantifying dynamics for a time series. Therefore, a statement that the sound levels in a discotheque are above 100 dB SPL is really a quantitative statement about the dynamics of ambient sound waves.

This example not only illustrates that dynamics can be meaningfully quantified, but that such measurements can be made very useful through a shared standard and the availability of instruments to make the measurements. Neuroscience could benefit from similar standardization of dynamics, which is currently lacking. Even the quantification of EEG dynamics, perhaps the most widely used neural measurement in a biomedical setting, lags far behind consumer audio technology in this respect. Outside of a small community of quantitative EEG researchers, there are no set conventions for reporting the levels of EEG spectra, although the problem is precisely analogous to the problem of reporting SPLs. One might be concerned about setting absolute baseline levels in the EEG case, but such problems do not arise when dealing with relative levels or changes. In fact, general adoption of the decibel scale for spectra, used widely in the engineering literature, might be a big step forward.

Science is a social enterprise, and shared quantifications form the common currency or language in which transactions of knowledge take place; absent such shared measures, or theoretical instruments, the growing edifice of neuroscientific understanding is bound to suffer the fate of the mythical Tower of Babel (fig. 1.2).

1.3 "Newtonian and Bergsonian Time"

The first chapter of Norbert Wiener's (fig. 1.3) classic *Cybernetics* [246] is entitled "Newtonian and Bergsonian Time." In this chapter, Wiener discusses a dichotomy that is at least as profound as the one that separates the active and passive perspectives discussed above. In contrast to Newton, Henri Bergson (1859–1941) was a proponent of vitalism, the doctrine that holds that a nonphysical driving force is necessary to explain life. The dichotomy to which Wiener refers is the *apparent* difference between the dynamics of physical systems on the one hand, and biological and human engineered systems on the other. We say apparent difference, because biological systems or human-engineered systems are certainly physical systems and subject to the laws of (mostly classical) physics. The distinction being drawn is between two sorts of physical systems, but we use "physical" and "biological" as convenient shorthands (rather than refer to, say, "those physical systems which are conventionally referred to as biological systems"). Newtonian dynamics prevailed over

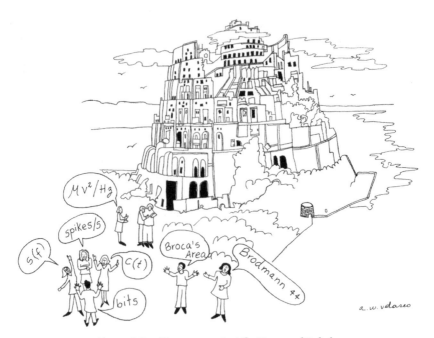

Figure 1.2: The neuroscientific Tower of Babel.

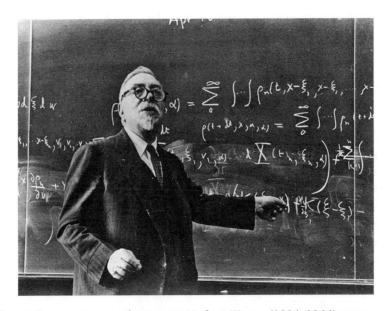

Figure 1.3: American mathematician Norbert Wiener (1894–1964) was a founder of the subject of cybernetics, a term he coined for the application of the theories of communication and control to machines and animals.

Bergsonian vitalism, but Wiener points out that in some ways this was a Pyrrhic victory, as we will discuss further.

There are in fact three different dichotomies that Wiener discusses in this chapter of *Cybernetics*. Two of these are familiar: reversible versus irreversible dynamics (the so-called thermodynamic "arrow of time"), and deterministic versus random behavior. These two dichotomies run through several centuries of research in the physical sciences, in particular in understanding how reversible microscopic dynamics and irreversible macroscopic dynamics may be reconciled. However, Wiener also hints at a third dichotomy, namely the seeming distinction between the thermodynamic "arrow of time," and the "arrow of time" in engineering and biology. We will discuss all three dichotomies because they play important conceptual roles in thinking about the dynamics of the nervous system.

1.3.1   Reversible and Irreversible Dynamics; Entropy

First let us consider reversible microscopic dynamics and irreversible macroscopic dynamics observed in physical systems. Microscopic physical laws relevant to understanding biology and our everyday experience are time reversible; Newton's equations do not have a privileged direction in which time flows.[3] The coordinates and velocities of the planets at any given point of time determine where they are going to be in the future; but so do they determine where they had been in the past. Instead of an explanation of the sort "the moon is at this location now because it was at location X moving with velocity V yesterday night," we could equally say "the moon is at this location now because it needs to be at location Y moving with velocity U tomorrow night." We chose a planetary example for illustration, but time reversal works equally well of course in the microscopic domain of atoms and molecules relevant to biological systems. Although we typically do not advance explanations of the second sort, they are actually perfectly valid because Newton's equations do not distinguish between them. We may feel uncomfortable about the second kind of explanation because it violates our common sense notion of "causality," but that is a statement about our psychological makeup rather than about the laws that govern motion.

However, as our common sense notion may indicate, irreversible phenomena are all around us in our macroscopic, everyday experience. Thanks to Boltzmann, Gibbs, and others, we now have an understanding of how systems with reversible microscopic dynamics come to exhibit irreversible macroscopic behavior seen in thermodynamics. The understanding can be summarized by

---

3. Weak interactions break time reversal invariance, but these departures are small and have no bearing on the "low energy" physics regime, both classical and quantum, that is relevant for the understanding of biological phenomena.

saying that "the entropy of a closed, macroscopic system undergoing spontaneous change always increases." This is a complicated subject, and a detailed discussion is outside the scope of this book; however, the essential idea may be stated quite simply. Apart from the relevance to understanding irreversible dynamics, we include this discussion here because a number of investigators have invoked the concept of entropy in analyzing neural time series data (which we evaluate critically later in the book). Readers interested in the subject should gain a basic understanding of the concept of entropy in a physical system and why entropy increases during spontaneous change. Our discussion follows that of Lebowitz [141].

Origins of Irreversible Behavior in Physics

To do this, we need to introduce the idea of phase space or configuration space. For a collection of N classical particles in a three-dimensional volume, this is a 6N dimensional space, where each point in the phase space specifies a unique assignment of a three-dimensional position and a three-dimensional momentum to each of N particles. Therefore, each point in phase space can be thought of as an "initial condition" of the system, and a volume in phase space is a collection of such initial conditions.

The microstate of the system corresponding to individual points in phase space is not amenable to direct observation. Instead, experimental observations and control deal with macroscopic degrees of freedom (such as pressure or density for a gas). A "macroscopic" state of the system is described by the volume in phase space for which the microstates are consistent with the given values of the macroscopic degrees of freedom. Note that phase space volume is distinct from the volume in three-dimensional space occupied by the particles.

A thermodynamic description of the system is in terms of these macroscopic state variables. The essence of irreversible behavior is that during spontaneous change in a closed system (not driven by external factors), the macrostate variables cannot change arbitrarily. Rather, they always proceed in a direction that is consistent with the increase of certain quantity called the thermodynamic entropy of the system. The concept of thermodynamic entropy was developed by Clausius and others through a study of the efficiency of heat engines. Boltzmann had the crucial insight that related this macroscopic, thermodynamic irreversibility to the reversible microscopic dynamics.

The argument is as follow: it is difficult to "aim" a trajectory of the microstate starting from a large phase space volume and ending in a small phase space volume, but easy to aim at a large volume starting from a small volume. Pictorially, consider a small and a large patch of grass. If one stood at a random location on the small patch and tossed a ball, it is more likely to end up somewhere on the large patch than the converse (tossing from the larger patch and the ball landing on the smaller patch). There is a simple but inherent asymmetry to the problem that does not originate in the dynamical system per se (the person pitching the balls) but in the volumes of phase space corresponding to the initial conditions and the available final conditions. Suppose we initially observe the system in a macrostate M_0 that corresponds to the microstate being in a small phase space volume. Now consider that a different macrostate M_1 is "available" to the system, in that there are no dynamical constraints to prevent the system from starting in a microstate consistent with M_0 and ending up in M_1. Let the corresponding phase space volumes be $\Gamma(M_0)$ and $\Gamma(M_1)$. The "aiming" argument given above would imply that if $\Gamma(M_0) < \Gamma(M_1)$, then the system is more likely to end up in M_1 starting from M_0 rather than the reverse. Because the phase space volume corresponding to a macrostate for a thermodynamic system is very large, the ratio $\Gamma(M_1)/\Gamma(M_0)$ is huge and this likelihood is almost a certainty. Therefore, if a system is observed undergoing a change in the macroscopic state variables, the corresponding phase space volume is almost certain to grow rather than shrink.[4] The logarithm of the phase space volume consistent with a fixed set of macroscopic conditions is known as the Boltzmann entropy:

$$S = k \ln \Gamma \qquad (1.1)$$

The argument outlined above indicates why the Boltzmann entropy is expected to increase during spontaneous change in the system. Boltzmann associated this mathematical quantity with thermodynamic entropy (obtained, for example, by integrating the specific heat of the system). This identification provides the bridge from microscopic dynamics to macroscopic thermodynamics and forms the basis of statistical mechanics.

According to this argument due to Boltzmann, the arrow of time that we observe in the physical world around us has to do with special initial conditions. The universe started out in a low entropy state and is spontaneously evolving to a higher entropy state, thus specifying the direction of time. A universe at thermal equilibrium would have no such arrow of time.

We have discussed Boltzmann's notion of entropy, which does not necessarily involve any probability theory because it is defined in terms of phase space volumes consistent with macroscopic conditions. Later, we will encounter Gibbs or Shannon entropy, which is a conceptually distinct quantity defined for arbitrary, discrete probability distributions. In the context of thermodynamics, there is a relationship between the two quantities. For large system size, the Boltzmann entropy can be shown to be equivalent to the Gibbs-Shannon

---

4. The knowledgeable reader will point out that Hamiltonian dynamics with holonomic constraints conserve phase space volume. The idea then is that the smaller original phase space volume is smeared over the larger volume through a process of stretching and folding. The picturesque analogy that has been given is that of a lump of dough being kneaded by a baker; a small drop of oil placed initially in the dough will eventually be uniformly spread throughout the larger volume through the process of kneading.

entropy of a specific probability distribution defined over phase space (the so-called Boltzmann distribution).

The relation between the two entropies has been the source of conceptual confusion and has led to attempts to generalize the laws of thermodynamics to arbitrary settings where they do not apply. The Gibbs-Shannon entropy can be defined quite generally for probability distributions that have no relationship to a physical dynamical system close to thermodynamic equilibrium. In those contexts, the corresponding "entropies" are abstract mathematical constructs, and one should not expect to discover underlying thermodynamic laws in the system simply because such entropies can be mathematically defined. Thermodynamic laws are empirically falsifiable scientific laws grounded in real physical phenomena, not the result of the ability define a mathematical quantity.

1.3.2 Deterministic Versus Random Motion

The motion of the planets follows laws that are not only time-reversal symmetric, but also orderly; this regular, deterministic dynamics is perhaps the most important of the phenomena that led to the development of modern science through the Newtonian laws of motion. However, if one zooms in on an atom or molecule making up the macroscopic systems described above, the motion one observes appears to be far from orderly. How such seemingly disorderly motion arises out of orderly and deterministic laws of motion is now also well understood. If one knew all the forces impinging on the atom or molecule as a function of time, then one could apply purely deterministic laws of motion and figure out its trajectory; absent such knowledge, it is more convenient and parsimonious to model the dynamics of the particle as a random walk, a stochastic process with suitable properties. Use of stochastic process based modeling is ubiquitous in biology and will play a central role in this book.

1.3.3 Biological Arrows of Time?

The orderly and reversible laws of Newtonian dynamics contain the seeds of the irreversible and stochastic behavior that we observe in the physical world close to us, and the origins of this behavior are now fairly well understood. However, there is a further, "biological" arrow of time that is not quite the same as thermodynamic irreversibility, although it is contingent on irreversible thermodynamic processes in the environment supplying "food" to biological systems. This is the process of evolution, which may be characterized as the *retention of accidentally found solutions*. If the challenges that an organism encounters in trying to survive in an uncertain environment are viewed as *problems*, then the natural selection process generates *solutions* to these problems, and these solutions are retained in the genetic code of the lineage. Over evolutionary timescales, there has been an accumulations of these problem-solution pairs as reflected in the growing diversity of the phylogenetic tree.

Instead of becoming more and more homogeneous through the process of equalizing macroscopic thermodynamic gradients, systems have become more intricately structured over time.[5] Similarly, an arrow of time may be seen in the life cycle of an organism, or even in the locomotor behavior of animals. The same development of increasingly intricate structure is seen in the history of human-engineered systems, driven perhaps by an analogous mechanism of "keeping found solutions." There are a number of interesting things to be said about the dynamics of a biological system from this perspective, within the lifetime of the organism or across evolutionary time scales.

However, perhaps the most interesting thing of all has to do with an *explanatory* arrow of time in the reverse direction. Apart from explaining observed biological phenomenon in terms of the past, we also have explanations that in a sense point backwards from the future. Explanations or accounts that relate to the function performed by a biological system are of this sort; these explanations are of the form that "we observe phenomenon X in the organism, because this enables the organism to do Y."

Teleological explanations of this nature have a particularly bad history, because they have been the source of circular explanations and loose thinking. However, this does not prevent biologists from offering such explanations, and understanding function remains a key issue in biology. Indeed, there is nothing unsound about constructing a theory of system design in terms of its function; this is precisely what is done in engineering courses taught in universities, ranging from feedback control theory to the theories of communication systems and of computation. We will have more to say about this later, but in the context of the present discussion it is of interest to note that it is yet another instance where our thinking about biological systems runs counter to the style of explanations for Newtonian dynamics, where function does not play a role. The physical laws of motion of course universally apply, but somehow seem to not address some essential aspects of the phenomena. We are still looking for better conceptual-mathematical frameworks to describe and understand biological dynamics and biological "arrows of time"; hence, a fortiori, our interest in studying brain dynamics.

---

5. No violation of the second law is needed or implied, because biological systems are open systems in contact with the larger environment, the *total* entropy of the biosphere and the rest of the environment has increased.

2

Theoretical Accounts of the Nervous System

It is a popular turn of the phrase that nervous systems are the most complicated objects that scientists study. There is an element of hyperbole to this; if nervous systems are complex objects, then collections of nervous systems considered together (i.e., societies or ecosystems) could be considered even more complicated, if one had to keep track of every detail. However, there undoubtedly is some truth to the statement about nervous system complexity, whether measured in macroscopic terms through the diversity of animal behavior enabled by nervous systems; in microscopic terms by counting the number of cell types or numbers of genes expressed in the brain; or in terms of the intricate connectivity patterns of the nervous system, which remain to be unraveled in all but the simplest of organisms.

Given the complexity of nervous systems, it is perhaps no surprise that the landscape of theories about the nervous system is confusing, reminiscent of the parable about the blind men and the elephant (fig. 2.1). Unlike in molecular cellular biology, there is no shared "central dogma" about nervous system organization and function. Only experts in liver function hold strong opinions about how the liver works, but almost anybody is capable of introspection and psychological insight and has pet notions about how the brain works. There may well be as many neuroscientific theories as there are neuroscientists. The exponential growth of the number of subfields and associated journals only exacerbates the problem.

The list of relevant theoretical accounts of the nervous system is long and difficult to arrange in a logical order: psychophysics, behaviorism, ethology, psychology with various prefixes, sociobiology, cognitive neuroscience, affective neuroscience, neuronal biophysics and computational neuroscience, molecular neurobiology, and so on. This does not even mention fields such as economics

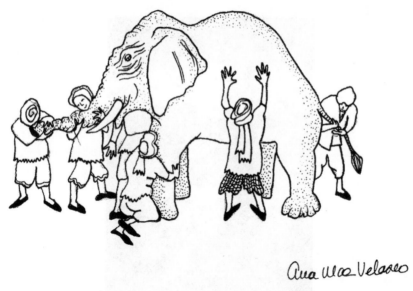

Figure 2.1: The blind men and the elephant.

or linguistics that deal with neuroscientific phenomena without falling into neuroscience proper. In some sense, because all human activity ultimately originates in neural activity in human brains, each discipline that involves human behavior can be expected to give rise to an interdisciplinary branch of neuroscience, be it in association with the arts or literature or the law. Therefore, there seems to be little hope for a unified theoretical account of nervous system dynamics with broad scope any time soon. This is all the more poignant given that the nervous system itself is the integrator, par excellence, of complex phenomena across levels of organization, as pointed out famously by Sherrington (fig. 2.2).

2.1 Three Axes in the Space of Theories

One way to grapple with the almost zoological diversity presented by the large number of theoretical accounts of the nervous system and of animal behavior, would be to understand the principle dimensions along which the theories differ, a set of *axes*, as it were, for the "space" of theories (fig. 2.3). An alternative is a hierarchical taxonomy. These are not completely different approaches—one can imagine having only one or two "values" along these axes, thus leading to a number of discrete categories. We present below three "axes" that seem to capture some of the major distinctions between classes of theories: level of organization, direction of causal explanations, and instrumental approach. We explain below the intended meaning of these labels.

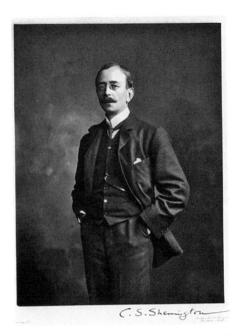

Figure 2.2: British physician and scientist Sir Charles Scott Sherrington (1857–1952) is best remembered for his study of reflexes and spinal cord circuitry. He shared the 1932 Nobel Prize in Physiology or Medicine with Edgar Douglas Adrian for their work on "the function of neurons."

This kind of metatheoretic speculation may be dismissed as a useless philosophical exercise. It is of interest to note, however, that with the advent of the Internet, there has been a resurgence of interest in taxonomies and hierarchical organization of knowledge to grapple with the same kind of issue in a number of different contexts; this can be seen with the development of the so

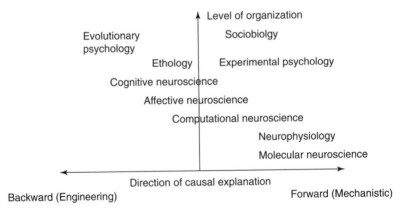

Figure 2.3: The space of theories.

called semantic web technologies. There may indeed be some need for a "theory of theories" as developed in this chapter.

Because we have set out to categorize theories, a few words are in order about what we mean by a *theory* for the purposes of this discussion. We will not get into the morass of trying to define a theory but proceed from examples. That said, most of the "theories" consist of the conglomeration of the set of phenomena to be described, background assumptions, and a conceptual framework that ideally is formalized in mathematical language, although this is not always a good thing in the context of biological phenomena. We advisedly do not use the word "model" because this seems to have a finer granularity than the word "theory," which might contain a collection of models.

One final note should be emphasized; the theories that we are trying to categorize are meant to be different descriptions of a single underlying reality, observed at different scales and described in different ways. This epistemic versus ontological distinction is important to keep in mind. The multiplicity of theories dealing with the nervous system of an animal is a matter of convenience but does not of course imply that there are many different nervous systems. Ascribing reality to a partial description of the system is a form of the so-called mereological fallacy, which confuses a part for the whole. This is not to say that the phenomena described by a given theory are not real, only that it should be recognized that the theory provides a certain level of description of the phenomena in question.

2.1.1   Level of Organization

This axis deals with the distinction that one has in mind when talking about microscopic or macroscopic theories. We could have also referred to spatial or temporal scale; indeed, it is a commonplace that the nervous system in particular and biological systems in general span many space and time scales. Not surprisingly, theories are also distinguished by the spatial or temporal scales to which they apply. Evolutionary theories, for example, apply at longer time scales compared with theories about nervous system development. Theories dealing with development apply to longer time scales compared with neural network theories that treat electrophysiological phenomena. Similarly, molecular cellular theories are finer grained in space than neural network theories, which are in turn finer grained than psychological theories of behavior.

However, we refer to the *level of organization* instead of *scale*, although the two could be synonymous under some circumstances. The idea is that a given theory may apply at a particular level of organizational complexity rather than to a specific spatial scale. The theoretical framework that deals with the biomechanical aspects of locomotor behavior applies to animals of very different physical sizes, yet essentially has the same content at substantially different physical scales. However, this is a theory that applies to the same level of organization, at a macroscopic level compared to a theory of macromolecular dynamics. In contrast, a theoretical framework dealing with the movement of herds, shoals, and flocks treats yet a higher level of organization.

How useful is this axis in arranging the different theoretical accounts we have listed in the beginning? For example, theoretical accounts of cellular biochemical networks, neural network theories, cognitive and affective psychology, as well as sociobiology apply at increasing levels of organization. Some theories may deal with the same level of organization but may be differentiated along different axes; for example, ethology and experimental psychology deal with the same level of organization of the nervous system (namely the level of behavior of the whole organism) but differ along the axis to be discussed below, of instrumental approach.

Rather than regard the level of organization as a continuous axis, one may define a set of major levels of organization for the nervous system: intracellular networks; intercellular networks, which may be further divided into micro and macro circuits; the whole organism and its behavior; societies; and ecosystems. One may also want to group theories into the temporal scales of the corresponding phenomena: fast electrical activity, slower neuromodulatory and hormonal activity, cell division and developmental time scales, and finally evolutionary time scales. Thus one might want to define separate axes for levels of organization that are primarily spatial in nature or primarily temporal in nature. We have grouped these together for simplicity, but a more refined scheme could separate them.

Levels of Organization in Physics and Engineering

Level of organization is a relevant axis in physical and engineering theories as well. In physics, theories form a rough ladder spanning levels of organization from subatomic particles (particle physics), atoms and molecules (chemistry), fluids and solids (condensed matter physics), and so on. The more macroscopic phenomena (and the corresponding theoretical accounts) are typically simultaneously at larger spatial scales and slower temporal scales, so it does not become necessary to develop separate spatial and temporal axes. In engineering, one encounters the concept of *layering*; the Internet, for example, consists of a number of layers or levels of organization, the so-called physical layer, TCP/IP, and application layers being three of the major ones. The analogy is not perfect, because these "layers" share physical infrastructure at the macroscopic scale, but the temporal granularity does show a progression, from the rapid modulation of the signal in the physical layer, longer time scales for the IP "packets," and yet longer time scales associated with files in the application layer.

Bridging Across Levels

As emphasized earlier, we break up the same reality into multiple levels of description for purposes of convenience; the multiplicity of levels of organization is epistemological rather than ontological. The question therefore naturally arises as to how to link together phenomena at these different levels. It is instructive to see how this happens in the physical sciences and in engineering, and to compare and contrast the two.

Integrating out high-frequency degrees of freedom: In physics, there are two important principles that bridge scales. The first is performing averages over rapidly varying, *microscopic* degrees of freedom, to leave the more slowly varying, *macroscopic* ones. The rapid variations could be in space or in time, and the averaging procedure relies on the law of large numbers. At the microscopic level, one has several replicas of some microscopic subsystem, such as atoms in a gas, with local interactions that are relatively homogeneous. The locality of the interactions permits the averaging procedure governed by the law of large numbers.

The macroscopic degrees of freedom can be thought of as *emerging* from the averaging process from microscopic degrees of freedom, and are often referred to as *emergent phenomena*, although *emergent descriptions* would perhaps be a better phrase, keeping in mind the epistemological/ontological distinction. One case of bridging across scales that has generated much interest both in physics and in the lay literature corresponds to when the phenomena at different levels resemble each other, a situation referred to as scale invariance.

In contrast, in complex engineering systems with multiple levels, whereas the macroscopic systems are made up of microscopic components, these components are usually not identical copies of some basic subsystem. One does not find lots of little cars inside a car, or lots of little copies of any given component for that matter (fig. 2.4). In addition, the interactions between parts are not necessarily local or homogeneous. Therefore, the law of large number style averaging that plays an important role in physics plays less of a role in engineering. Although averaging over identical components does occasionally allow an engineering system to gain robustness against component failure, engineering function depends more often on different components doing different things in a coordinated manner. This coordination is achieved using a combination of distributed, local control laws as well as hierarchically directed top-down control.

As we will argue in the following section as well as in the next chapter, the organization of biological systems resembles that of complex engineering systems. It is therefore to be expected that the law of averages is not in general a good way of bridging across biological levels of organization. The nervous system is a case in point: even though it is made of many neurons, the connectivity patterns of the neurons are not in general local or homogeneous,

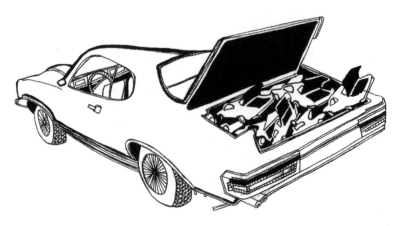

Figure 2.4: Cars are not made of little cars (or some other collection of identical parts).

and the behavior of the organism does not reflect a simple arithmetic averaging across the properties of the neurons in the brain. Such averaging probably does play an important role in local neural circuits but less of a role beyond the microcircuit level.

Symmetry principles: A second, and perhaps more important way in which the different levels are connected in the context of physical theory, is through the existence of symmetry principles.[1] The simple existence of a symmetry principle or invariance dictates the form of the laws of physics at a given level of organization of matter. Rather than starting with the atomic or molecular degrees of freedom and integrating out the high-frequency components, one can directly write down the laws of fluid motion based on invariance under translations in space and time, conservation of mass, and so on. This leaves some undetermined parameters, which can be empirically measured or deduced from microscopic theory via an integration procedure. The symmetry principles bridge different scales, and when present in the system, are the most basic physical principles.

Symmetry principles do not directly offer a similarly powerful way to bridge across levels in either engineering or biology. What, then, should take its place? We argue here and in the next chapter that there are engineering principles, laws of design, as it were, that apply across levels in both engineering and biological systems, and help bridge the levels together. An example that we will repeat for

---

1. A system has a symmetry when some property of the system is left unchanged by applications of elements of the corresponding symmetry group. For example, the laws of classical nonrelativistic mechanics are left unchanged under translation, rotation and uniform motion.

emphasis is the usage of measurement-based feedback control to maintain a fixed level, or *homeostasis*. Such homeostatic mechanisms exist at different levels of organization in biological systems ranging from intracellular networks, to neural networks, to organ systems, and so on. These engineering principles have a similar flavor of generality as do the symmetry principles in physics.

In an abstract sense, there is perhaps some relation between engineering principles and the symmetry principles in the sense of *invariance*. Just as some aspect of the physical system is left unchanged by applications of elements from the symmetry group, *function* in an engineering sense also implies a kind of invariance. In fact, one can talk about two kinds of invariance associated with engineering function. First, the same engineering function may be implemented using different physico-chemical substrates. This relates to the computationalist view that algorithms implemented on Turing machines composed of neurons[2] should have the same status as algorithms implemented by semiconductor based Turing machines. Second, specification of a function in an engineering sense is often the specification of an *interface:* this is the so-called black box approach, where the function of a device is given by its input-output relationships rather than what is inside it.

Simplicity and Complexity

In *Science and Hypothesis*,[3] Poincare pointed out that when going across levels of organization, one can encounter relations in both directions between the simple and the complex. Simplicity can be hidden below superficial complexity. It is now well understood that simple rules can give rise to superficially complex behavior. This is demonstrated by simple cellular automata that can give rise to seemingly complicated patterns and simple dynamical systems that exhibit seemingly complex chaotic dynamics.

Conversely, complexity can be hidden below superficial simplicity: whether in physics, where the law of averages hides the microscopic complexity from macroscopic observations, or in engineering where the microscopic complexity of the constituent parts (of a car, for example) is not evident from the seemingly simple behavior of the whole.

Both of these directions are also evident in bridging levels of organization in biological systems. The microscopic complexity of the nervous system is not necessarily evident from the seemingly simpler behavioral level, although the complexity of the nervous system is itself a result of putting together simple parts using simple rules. This shows that levels of organization, and

---

2. Whether such "neural Turing machines" are a good way of thinking about some part of the brain is of course a matter of debate.

3. A. N. Kolmogorov, Chapter X1, p. 230, in *Mathematics: Its contents, Methods and Meaning*. Edited by A. D. Alexandrov, A. N. Kolmogorov, M. A. Lavrent'ev. Mineola, NY, Dover, 1999.

therefore the corresponding theoretical framework, may alternate between simple and complex.[4]

2.1.2 Direction of Causal Explanations

The second axis for organizing theories that we will discuss is the *direction of causal explanation* in the theory. At the outset, it is important to emphasize that we are talking about causal *explanations,* and no implication is being made that causes *exist* in reality; this is the epistemological/ontological distinction we have emphasized earlier in the general discussion about theories. It may be convenient within a theory to use a causal explanatory framework, but this does not mean such causal links concretely exist. Following David Hume, we lean towards the point of view that only correlations are observed, and "causes" cannot strictly speaking be inferred from such correlations, no matter what inferential procedure is used.[5] In the following discussion, it should be understood that when we speak of causation it is in the "as if" sense: a statement such as "X causes Y in this theory" is simply shorthand for the longer but more cumbersome statement that "the relation between X and Y in this theory is as if X causes Y."

The distinction along this axis is between theories with *forward* causation and *reverse* causation—also designated as the distinction between proximate and ultimate causes. As we will see below, this distinction between theories deals with mechanistic explanations of *how* questions and engineering explanations of *why* questions.

By forward causation, we refer to theoretical frameworks where an event is explained in terms of a chain of past events or a macroscopic phenomenon is reduced to its underlying microscopic constituents. This is the way physical theories are typically used to explain biological phenomena,[6] a research program sometimes referred to as reductionist. Mechanistic grounding of neuroscientific phenomena in the laws of physics, as championed famously by Helmholtz (fig. 2.5), as well as the gradual demise of vitalism and dualism, marks the birth of modern neuroscience.

In contrast, engineering style explanations reverse the direction of causal explanation. Consider an example of such an explanation: the lens of the eye

---

4. A similar alternation takes place between the analog and digital architectures at different levels: individual neurons exhibit digital behavior when firing action potentials, but averaging over many neurons or over time provides an analog firing rate. At the next level, however, the animal may exhibit discrete behaviors that again has a digital flavor.

5. Despite Hume's reservations, attempts to "infer" causal explanations from correlations continue unabated.

6. As discussed in the first chapter, with the exception of weak violations of time reversal invariance at subatomic levels that do not appear to be directly relevant to biological phenomena, the microscopic physical theories relevant for biology are time reversal invariant and are indifferent to explaining the present in terms of the past or the future.

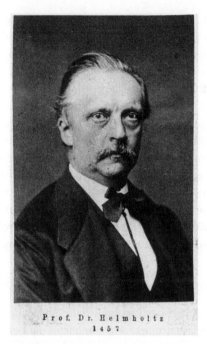

Prof. Dr. Helmholtz
1 4 5 7

Figure 2.5:   German physiologist and physicist Hermann Helmholtz (1821–1894) noted the conservation of energy in biological processes and was the first to measure the speed of impulse propagation along a nerve. His research in sensory physiology and perception led to empirical theories on spatial and color vision, motion perception, and the sensation of tone.

has a convex shape so that it can refract light and focus it on to the retina. It is this desired function that provides the backward or ultimate cause for the shape of the lens. Such explanation is grounded in evolutionary thinking: the idea is that the shape of the lens has evolved over many generations, with the *biological function* (in this case focusing light) acting as a selective filter, leading ultimately to eyes that perform the function well.

There is of course also a mechanistic explanation for the shape of the lens in a particular animal eye in terms of the developmental genetic program that leads to the formation of the proper lens shape and material transparency of the lens. These two styles of explanation go hand in hand, and both are indispensable in understanding biological systems. This contrasts, with say, trying to explain weather patterns; these are physical phenomena with almost biological levels of complexity in behavior. Nevertheless, there is no meaningful sense in which weather patterns perform a function that can be analyzed using engineering theories.

Theories of the nervous system that emphasize function and backward causation are sometimes referred to as computationalist accounts, although from our discussion in the next chapter it should become clear that is might be better to adopt a broader taxonomy of engineering theories, in which the theory of computation is one out of several that apply to understanding nervous system function.

Of course, theories may be purely descriptive and not imply causation in any direction. Ethology provides a descriptive theoretical framework at the behavioral level of description that does not really have a causal component either of a mechanistic or engineering nature.[7] Therefore, if the axes of *direction of causal explanations* were to be replaced by discrete categories, one could adopt the three categories of forward causation, backward causation, and no causation in the explanatory framework. This third category is important because it is relatively free of theoretical constructions and focuses more on a systematic description of the phenomena involved. This leads us naturally to a discussion of the third axis, that of instrumental approach.

2.1.3   Instrumental Approach

Theories cannot be constructed without data, and data cannot be gathered without using specific instruments. The mode of data gathering can have a strong effect on the theories constructed to explain them, and in extreme cases theories can become specialized to specific instruments or measurement methods. There are of course too many measurement techniques applicable to the nervous system to categorize theories according to instruments. This would lead to categories that do not have any particular meaning or generality beyond the specifics of the measurement technique.

However, there is one broad distinction in the way measurements are made that does perhaps deserve a separate axis, and this is the distinction between the empirical and the controlled experimental method. Ethology and experimental psychology are examples of fields that are distinguished along this axis. The purely empirical approach is one of observation only, as exemplified in physics by the field of astronomy: the laws of gravitation were discovered by studying the motion of the planets and the moon, not subjected to experimental control. One weakness of the empirical method is that it is difficult to distinguish between correlations between two variables that are not based on any mechanistic linkages, and correlations that do arise from mechanistic linkage.

On the other end of this axis is the so-called method of controlled experiments, where one of the quantities (the independent variable) is changed in a controlled manner, and the other quantity (the dependent variable) is measured. After accounting for chance variation, this method reveals mechanistic

---

7. One could argue that ethological descriptions lean towards evolutionary and functional styles of explanations and therefore toward backward causation.

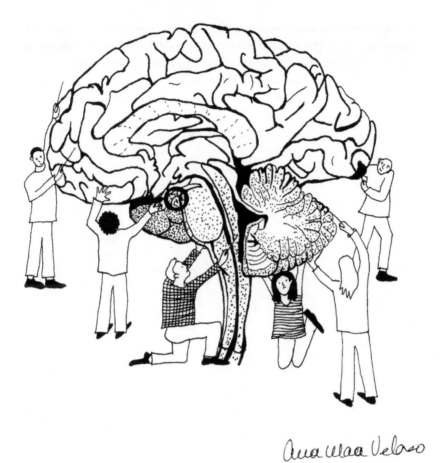

Ana Maa Velaso

Figure 2.6: Partial views of the brain.

linkage between the two variables. The two methods are not simple binary categories, but there are gradations between them, and one can be closer to one or the other end of the spectrum. For example, cognitive neuroscience tends to make more use of the method of controlled experiments, whereas affective neuroscience is closer to empiricism of the ethological approach, although neither is strictly experimental or empirical in approach. In studying evolution as in studying astronomy, there is little choice for the most part other than to employ the empirical method.

2.1.4 Conclusion

What can we gain from this discussion of a taxonomy of theories about the nervous system? One way to proceed would be to label a theoretical exercise by its position along the three axes described above; this would ameliorate the multiplication of theoretical accounts about the nervous system. The approach also provides a way of contextualizing the existing theories, and understanding their interrelations. Finally, when asking questions about nervous system function or dynamics, one can situate the query in the space described above, and therefore gain an understanding of what principle questions remain to be asked and answered.

3

Engineering Theories and Nervous System Function

In this chapter we present a very brief résumé of the major components of engineering theory in the context of the nervous system. We do not provide a detailed account of nervous system biophysics because there are multiple up-to-date textbooks on the subject, and we also briefly cover the biophysical material relevant to specific measurement techniques in individual chapters in the third section of the book.

The treatment of engineering theories is included because these are essential to thinking about brain function, yet it is difficult to find a suitably elementary account of these theories in a condensed form. We attempt to clarify concepts such as *information* and *computation* that have become common currency in discussing the nervous system and have influenced the signal processing methods used to analyze neurobiological signals. Throughout this discussion we hope to place these concepts in context to help judge proper and improper usage of the associated techniques. More generally, however, we hope that this short tutorial will excite the reader's interest in a fuller exploration of the many aspects of theoretical engineering and its applicability to the study of the nervous system.

3.1 What Do Brains Do?

As emphasized in the previous chapter, one may study the nervous system from a mechanistic perspective, to understand how its macroscopic behavior arises from the microscopic constituents, or from an engineering perspective, to understand what its functions are and how well it performs these functions. The mechanistic route is by now well established, starting with the biophysics

27

of individual neurons and proceeding through layers of neural network modeling. A lot remains to be done in empirical terms to gather enough information to constrain such models and in the development of appropriate analytical and computational tools to deal with the increasingly complex models. However, at least in basic conceptual terms, there is some idea as to how one should proceed. The same cannot be said about engineering theories of brain function, where the outlines of the research program is less clear.

When studying the physiology of the body, one can fairly unambiguously identify specific bodily functions, such as locomotion, ingestion of food, respiration, circulation of blood, and so on. It is also possible to identify the organ systems associated with such functions, namely the musculoskeletal system, the feeding apparatus, the lungs, and the heart. When it comes to the brain or the nervous system, the overall function seems to be more abstract. Textbooks in neuroscience usually contain a statement of two about how the broad function of the brain is to perform "information processing." It is a picturesque analogy—lungs process respiratory gases, hearts pump blood, stomachs process food, and brains process information.[1] Unfortunately, such a statement is too abstract; it does not immediately lead to a detailed understanding of brain functions or whether the brain can be thought of in terms of appropriate functional subsystems in order to break the problem down into smaller parts.

Cognitive psychology does adopt a black box, modular view of the brain and attributes specific functionality to the component boxes. However, these models are to a large extent results of fitting behavioral data from constrained tasks and are tenuously connected with actual neuronal circuits inside the brain. Moreover, when such tasks are applied to nonhuman animals, there is a strong anthropomorphic bias; animals in their ecological habitats do not usually perform "two alternative forced choice" tasks or other simple tasks from the repertoire of the cognitive psychologist.

However, any systematic attempt to study animal behavior in an ethologically relevant manner clearly shows the existence of elementary classes of behavior. The three major behavioral categories may be labeled nutritive, reproductive, and defensive behaviors; each major category may be further subdivided. In particular, the first two behaviors necessarily include locomotor behaviors in animals; whereas plants can make their own food, animals must move in order to find nutrition. Perhaps the most fundamental function of the nervous system is to enable such movement: in an uncertain environment, the moving organism must constantly avoid obstacles and otherwise adjust its

---

1. Such usage is reminiscent of the "humors" of the ancient Greeks. In an article on the philosophy of science [196] p. 490, Gian Carlo Rota and Jeffery Thomas Crants write: "Modern chemistry was founded by discarding the commonsense notions of earth, air, fire, and water. Such mantras as *consciousness*, *creativity*, *information*, and even *time* are the earth, air, fire, and water of our day. Only a trenchant critique of the vague assumptions that lie behind these words will lead to a foundation, and hence to the success, of the newer sciences."

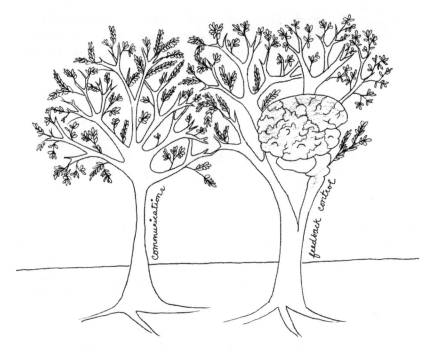

Figure 3.1: "Brain fruit" growing on "engineering theory trees."

motion through a feedback process involving sensory organs. Control theory is therefore implicated early on in studying nervous system function. Animal communications arise naturally in the context of social behaviors of groups of organisms; whenever the nutritional, reproductive, or defensive function involves more than one animal, and coordination between two animals requires the usage of a communication system. Concepts from communication theory such as coding and filtering are of relevance in trying to understand such systems. Algorithmic problem-solving procedures as implemented on digital computers are less easy to demonstrate in animal behavior, so paradoxically it is the theory of computation that seems to have the least direct bearing on nervous system function.

3.2 Engineering Theories

It is premature to look for a grand unified theory of engineering or design principles in biological systems. Also, while it is tempting to commence on a de novo discovery process for such principles, it seems efficient to start with some of the important branches of existing engineering theory (controls, communication, computation)[2] and to examine whether these apply to biological systems, and if not, what modifications are in order. In turn, such a study may enable cross-disciplinary interactions between engineering theories and the discovery of new engineering principles, perhaps leading to a entirely different taxonomy for the subject matter.

Superficial analogies to engineering concepts are sometimes made without a proper demonstration of a good match between the biological phenomenon in question and the engineering theory. The exhortations of Shannon and Peter Elias in a pair of famous editorials in the Transactions on Information Theory (reprinted in this volume) should be kept in mind. Therefore, there is need for greater clarity and conceptual rigor before engineering principles can be elevated to the rank of explanatory scientific theories in biology. In particular, the identification of function for many biological systems remains problematic. To make progress, one needs clear exemplars of biological systems where there is a relatively unambiguous identification of a relevant engineering theory.

The theory of evolution is the ultimate bridge between biological phenomena and any considerations regarding engineering principles. In this context, two ideas have a close bearing on the topic of discussion in this chapter. The first concept is Krogh's principle in comparative animal physiology. We have argued above that rather than pick an arbitrary biological system and look for an appropriate engineering theory, a better strategy might be to pick a well-understood engineering theory and look for an exemplary biological systems that shows a good match. This is similar in spirit to Krogh's principle, which holds that one should find an organism that specializes in a specific task to study the organ system associated with that task or function. The relation to evolution is that such an organism has probably derived selective advantages from its specialty. If selection pressures have acted strongly enough on the corresponding trait, then the limits of the performance may have been tested, and the outlines of the solution may be clearer.

The second relevant idea is that of convergent evolution. An engineering principle may be regarded as a "problem-solution" pair. If two animals have found the same "solution" to a given survival problem, then this either reflects common origin through shared ancestry, or convergent evolution, where the trait evolved separately during two different evolutionary events. In the latter case, there is increased likelihood that there is an underlying engineering principle, which constrains the solutions to be similar. More generally, a systematic study of the range of solutions found by animal nervous systems to the

---

2. We do not wish to imply that this is all that is taught in an engineering department. In particular, subjects drawn from the physical sciences, including mechanics, thermodynamics, electromagnetism, and so on, play a central role in the typical engineering curriculum and are of course essential to building airplanes and power grids. We have drawn a formal distinction between physical and engineering theories to emphasize the notion of function in the latter case.

common set of survival challenges is central to the future study of engineering principles of nervous system function.

3.2.1   Control Theory

The usage of feedback control, in the form of water clocks and other regulators, dates back to antiquity. The engineering discipline of control [62, 78, 79] is significantly more modern and has grown rapidly in the twentieth century, during the war as well as postwar periods. A principle focus in control theory is the design of dynamics in the presence of uncertainty. One starts with a system that may not have the desired behavior and then engineers the system so that it does. Perhaps the simplest behavior is homeostasis—maintaining a constant level of some variable (such as body temperature)—but other more complex behaviors can also be designed.

There are limitations to such design; physical or mathematical constraints may mean that some behaviors cannot be achieved. Elucidating these limits is an important aspect of the theory. It is also important that the design be robust to uncertainty in knowledge about the system, components used to engineer the system, as well as uncertainty about external disturbances. A central idea for achieving such robustness is to use feedback. For example, in the simplest case of homeostasis, if external perturbations cannot be predicted, they can be measured if an appropriate sensor is available. If there is also an appropriate actuator that can influence the dynamics of the system in question, then the sensor measurements can be fed back to restore the system to the desired constant level.

Although sensor actuator pairs forming univariate control systems are widely familiar and do not necessarily require sophisticated mathematical apparatus, multivariate systems are more complicated in their behaviors and require more care. Multivariate systems that possess some degree of locality in space (such as the power grid) are the subject of study of distributed control. The related theory of games deals with multiple interacting systems with some degree of autonomy but with multiple objective functions.

To the student, it may initially be difficult to distinguish control theory from the mathematical theory of dynamical systems. These are of course closely related; however, it is useful to bear in mind that the difference between a simple study of the differential equations underlying the dynamics of a system and a control theoretic study of the same system is the distinction between a mechanistic and an engineering theory. In the latter case, the notion of function is important: one is typically trying to get the system to do something useful. In the former case, one asks whether the existing behavior of a system can explained by writing down an appropriate dynamical system ("analysis"). In the latter case, we want to know how we can design the system to have a desired behavior ("synthesis").

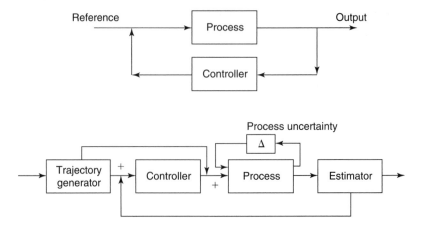

Figure 3.2: Classical and modern views of control system design. In the simplest case, the output of the process or plant is fed back to the input of the plant through a controller. From the modern perspective, the input reference signal is replaced by a trajectory generator, the sensed signals are subjected to statistical estimation to determine the underlying state of the plant, and uncertainties in the plant parameters are explicitly taken into account.

Of course, in the case of a designed dynamical system to which control engineering has already been applied, these distinctions are blurred. However, keeping in mind the evolutionary process through which a human-engineered (or biological) system came to be in its current form, such a distinction is still a useful one. If one can identify the sensors, actuators, a plant to which these are added, and an appropriate control objective for the system, then one can apply control theoretic ideas to "reverse engineer" the final product.

3.2.2 Communication Theory

A principal concern of communication theory is the establishment of protocols that allow one or more senders to effectively communicate with one or more receivers over a noisy medium or channel. The elegant and well-known model of single-user communications due to Claude Shannon [203] (fig. 3.3) consists of a data source, an encoder that prepares the data for transmission over the communication channel, and a decoder that recovers the data from the noisy received signal. The encoder is further broken up into a source encoder, a channel encoder and a modulator, as well as a similar decomposition holds for the decoder.

The encoding and decoding process provides robustness to noise in the channel, and enables noise-free transmission up to a limiting rate designated the channel capacity, which is given in terms of the maximum mutual information between the channel inputs and outputs. Although the original signal,

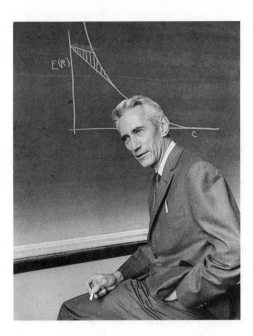

Figure 3.3: American electrical engineer and mathematician Claude Shannon (1916–2001) founded the mathematical theory of communication. Shannon, perhaps more than anyone else, epitomized the theoretical engineer in the twentieth century, combining deep mathematical insights with profound breakthroughs in engineering design and elegantly simple presentations of these results.

and the signal in the physical channel are themselves analog, the output of the source encoder and the input to the channel encoder are a digital data stream. The robustness to noise originates in part due to this intermediate discrete representation and in part through the usage of error correcting channel codes. This entire theory was already well developed in Shannon's first two papers on the subject [203].

Much of the effort in single-user communication theory is directed toward the design of source codes and error correction channel codes that efficiently achieve transmission rates approaching the limiting capacity. Closely related is the subject of cryptography, where a shared protocol is developed between a sender and a receiver that prevents an eavesdropper listening to the channel deciphering the message being sent. This theory was also worked out by Shannon at the same time that he developed the mathematical theory of communication. These fundamental advances in theoretical engineering principles have not been paralleled since Shannon's time, although the pace of progress has remained consistently high [230] and has received a recent boost from the growth of modern communication networks. Note that we have used the narrower phrase *communication theory* rather than the more broadly defined *information theory* [50] to emphasize the application to communication systems.

While single-user communication theory is highly developed, the same cannot be said of multiuser communication theory where there are multiple senders or receivers, with some degree of interference between the different signals and some degree of autonomy between different senders or receivers. Note that if all senders and all receivers were completely coordinated with full knowledge of other senders or receivers, one is back to the case of single-user communications with vector inputs and outputs.

Multiuser communication systems are widespread, for example in cellular telephony where a wireless base station has to receive signals from multiple cell phones at any given time. One way to accommodate multiple users over a single communication channel is to divide up the available resources, or multiplexing. Time, frequency, and code division multiplexing of the wireless communication channel are all in current use and may be compared with similar strategies adopted by animals communicating over a shared acoustic channel.

One of the signatures of the limitations of multiuser communication theory is that it has not played a large role in network communications over the Internet, where a simple feedback mechanism is used rather than elaborate error correcting codes. This points to the need for further developments in communication theory for understanding biological communication systems that rarely correspond to single pairs of senders and receivers.

Communication Theory and Neuroscience

One place where single user communication theory has been invoked in neuroscience, is in the treatment of sensory organs of the nervous system to estimate channel capacities. There are some conceptual difficulties with this, however. It is difficult to see who the sender is in the outside world with whom a receiving element of the nervous system has established a communication protocol. "Information" is often spoken about without due attention to delineating a sender-receiver pair. Without such a delineation, it is difficult to justify the application of the concept of a communication channel to a sensory system.

Moreover, there is the important question of time delays (fig. 3.4). Single-user communication theory in its basic form does not take time delays into account. Error free transmission only occurs in the limit of infinitely long time delays caused by the encoding process.[3] Because sensory organs are typically used by the animal nervous system in a closed loop feedback system, such delays are detrimental to system function, and it is not clear to what extent the system can afford error correcting codes interposed in the sensory communication channels. Without such coding, the application of the concept of channel

---

3. However, practical benefits can be obtained for finite delays since the error decreases exponentially with the delay.

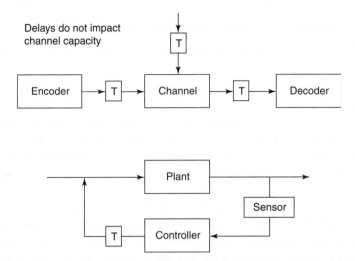

Figure 3.4: Introduction of time delays has no impact on the capacity of a single-user communication channel because the channel capacity is strictly speaking obtained in the limit of infinite coding delays. However, the introduction of time delays in even the simplest control system can have deleterious consequences. Delays impact control system performance and generate instabilities. This shows the difficulties with using single-user communication theory to describe sensory systems, which are embedded in a control loop (e.g., with the musculoskeletal, system as plant) and are therefore sensitive to delays.

capacity is open to question. In contrast to channel coding, a different context in which mutual information–based measures appear in communication engineering is that of rate distortion theory. As pointed out by Berger [25], this may have a closer bearing on nervous system function.

A different way to resolve the conundrum is to note the distinction between delay and bandwidth. The spatial or temporal bandwidths of sensory channels are indeed meaningful quantities that make sense in communication theory, and they may be experimentally measured and theoretically analyzed. The "signal to noise ratio" or SNR of such channels is also a meaningful quantity to study. For additive gaussian noise channels, the channel capacity is given by the product of the bandwidth and the logarithm of the SNR. Because the bandwidth and noise properties of the sensory channel can be separately measured, one strategy would be to study these quantities separately without taking their products and formally constructing a channel capacity, which is problematic due to the reasons outlined above. The *delay* of the channel can be studied in addition to the bandwidth and is conceptually a distinct quantity; a sensory channel with high bandwidth could have long or short delays. A short delay is inconsistent with the presence of any elaborate coding scheme.

One may adopt the position that "information" or entropy is simply a statistical measure of uncertainty, like variance, and mutual information a measure of statistical association, like covariance, without attributing any functional significance to these measures. This is a legitimate use of the concepts of entropy and mutual information (although the word entropy is better suited for the first usage than the word information[4]). Unfortunately, this does not automatically establish any relation to the engineering notions underlying communication theory and therefore removes these measures from their original and powerful context.

It can be noted separately that the pragmatic value of entropic or informational measures of uncertainty may be limited by difficulties in estimation. Moreover, these measures are quantitative but not necessarily very informative. For example, in studying the functional relationship between a discrete input and a discrete output, it is customary to capture the uncertainties in the relationship using a confusion matrix of the conditional probabilities of outputs given inputs. The mutual information is a single number that elegantly summarizes this confusion matrix. However, in understanding the functioning of the system it may be important to examine the detailed structure of the confusion matrix—for example to see if it has a block structure separating sets of inputs that are more frequently conflated. Therefore, usage of entropy or mutual information measures for purposes of characterizing statistical variance and association needs to be supplemented by more detailed quantification.

3.2.3   Computation

The theory of computation [206, 225] ranges from abstract logical issues in meta-mathematics, to concrete issues relating to computer hardware and software to solve real life problems. The theory arose from attempts to formalize and automate mathematics, which initially gave rise to the formal models of computation. The most celebrated and useful of these models is due to Turing (fig. 3.5), which in its original form deals with integer arithmetic. Although models have also been proposed more recently for real arithmetic [30], these are of more limited value because such models cannot be implemented in practice (as opposed to the Turing model, which forms the conceptual basis of modern day computers). Other models such as quantum computation [74] are

---

4. In an interesting interview cited in [8] (see http://mit.edu/6.933/www/Fall2001/Shannon2.pdf), R. Fano is quoted as follows: "I didn't like the term Information Theory. Claude did not like it either. You see, the term "information theory" suggests that it is a theory about information—but it's not. It's the *transmission* of information, not information. Lots of people just didn't understand this . . . I coined the term "mutual information" to avoid such nonsense: making the point that information is always *about* something. It is information provided by something, about something."

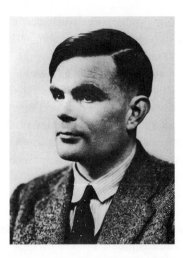

Figure 3.5: British mathematician Alan Turing (1912–1953) was a theoretical founder of modern computer science. In formalizing his model of computation, Turing drew motivation from his reflections on the human thought process.

of great theoretical and experimental interest and may someday lead to practical breakthroughs, but they have little conceivable relation to biological systems and will not be discussed here.

One may adopt a broad or narrow view of what computation is. Because the theory of computation is associated with the formalization of mathematics, according to the broadest point of view, a computational theory is simply a formal mathematical theory. According to this point of view, any dynamical system described mathematically is a computer. We feel that this is too broad a definition to be useful. Also, mathematical formalism is basic to all quantitative sciences, and it is not clear anything is gained by attaching the word *computation* anything that can be mathematically described. This kind of loose usage leads to much conceptual confusion among practicing biologists, and in our opinion should be avoided. We feel that the words *computer* and *computation* should be used in more precise ways, with a narrower domain of definition that does not attempt to include everything. One way to do this is to focus on computers as devices that solve a particular type of engineering problem.

To think of computers from an engineering perspective, one needs to understand the kind of problems that computers solve. Turing machines can be thought of as formally addressing the "decision problem" relating to set membership: namely, providing a yes/no answer to the question of whether something belongs to a given set. Not all decision problems can be effectively solved by Turing machines. Those problems that do not have effective solution procedures are called undecidable. If a problem can in principle be solved by a Turing machine, one still needs to know how difficult that solution is. This is the subject of computational complexity, which gives rise to the notion of complexity classes such as the celebrated P (polynomial time complexity) and NP (non-polynomial time complexity).

Formally, a Turing machine consists of a finite state automaton that reads symbols belonging to a finite set from an infinite tape and performs an action (consisting of writing a symbol on the tape and moving left or right), based jointly on the symbol read and the original state of the machine. This cycle repeats until a "halt" symbol is read. The tape starts in an initial configuration, and if the procedure terminates, the tape is in a final configuration, which is the output of the machine. Thus, a computer, regarded as a deterministic Turing machine, can be thought of as a function evaluator. Although the theory of computation tells us what functions can be computed and how long it might take, from a conceptual perspective a computer is still a function evaluator, or a flexible input-output relationship.

Defined in this narrow way, a computer is a useful concept in understanding biological function, but one that can also be disambiguated from, say, a communication system, which consists of a sender, a receiver, and a channel. In engineering practice, of course, the sender and the receiver may each employ embedded computers, which in turn may employ embedded protocols for communication across subcomponents. However, at each level, one is able to draw a useful connection between some level of organization of the system and its function, with a canonical engineering theory.

A set of concepts central to the theory of computation that are also biologically relevant are the ideas relating to formal languages and syntax. Rather than develop the theory of computation in terms of automata or machines, one can carry out the development in terms of the strings of symbols that are read by these machines. The corresponding decision problem is to determine whether a given string (a sentence) belongs to a designated set (a language). One way of specifying a language is by the means of a generative grammar, a formal procedure using symbols and rewriting rules that can in principle give rise to all sentences in a grammar.

The Chomsky hierarchy arranges languages in nested groups of progressive complexity. The lowest level of the hierarchy contains languages that are recognized by a finite state automaton, whereas the highest level contains languages recognized by a Turing machine. One might conceptualize the brain of a speaker of an English sentence to contain an instantiation of the corresponding generative grammar, whereas the brain of the listener who can determine the grammaticality of the sentence might be conceptualized as holding an instantiation of the corresponding automaton that recognizes that language. Chomsky hypothesized that human languages cannot be properly modeled at the lowest level of the hierarchy (finite state grammars), and require a grammar from a higher level. For example, nested English sentences that are easy to

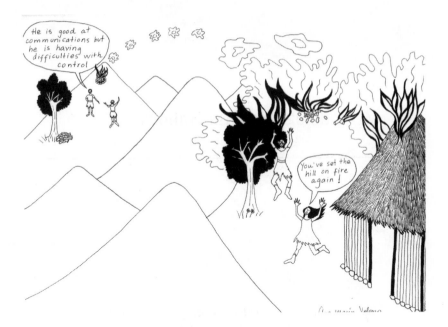

Figure 3.6: The consequences of disconnect between engineering theories.

judge as grammatical have long-range dependencies that are succinctly captured by context free grammars but not by finite state grammars. This is an application of a computational concept to a biological communication system and illustrates the overlap between the subjects even though they have been compartmentalized for convenience.

4

Methodological Considerations

Though this be madness, yet there is method in 't.
—Polonius, in *Hamlet*, Act II, Scene 2, by William Shakespeare

Practicing neuroscientists often view philosophical or conceptual considerations with suspicion, as exemplified by Santiago Ramon y Cajal's vigorous
exhortations[1] about the sterility of abstract rules in his *Advice for a Young Investigator* [189]. The importance of laboratory experiments, as emphasized by
Cajal, is certainly not to be belittled; to date, neuroscience remains a primarily
experimental discipline. However, no amount of empirical or experimental
work will necessarily undo a conceptual confusion or error in reasoning.

In fact, such conceptual confusions are perhaps a significant hindrance
to progress in contemporary neuroscience, as argued by Bennett and Hacker
[23]. In this chapter, we make some comments about avoiding conceptual
pitfalls and general methodological considerations. This could raise the ire of
readers who would rather see concrete results than philosophizing, but one
should remember the following remark made by Einstein in this context:

A knowledge of the historic and philosophical background gives that kind of
independence from prejudices of his generation from which most scientists
are suffering. This independence created by philosophical insight is—in my

---

1. Some of it rises to the level of diatribe (e.g., a chapter entitled "Diseases of the Will" with headings
"Contemplators" and "Megalomaniacs").

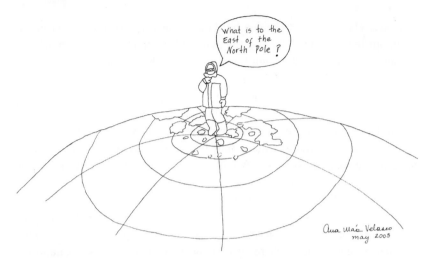

Figure 4.1: The importance of conceptual clarity: questions may be so ill formed that they do not make any sense and are best left unaddressed. The question "What is to the East of the North Pole?" is ill formed because the directions East and West are not defined at the North Pole. This illustration is inspired by Wittgenstein's "East Pole" example ([247], lecture VI) cited in [23].

opinion—the mark of distinction between a mere artisan or specialist and a real seeker after the truth.[2]

4.1 Conceptual Clarity and Valid Reasoning

The content of this section can be formalized in mathematical terms. Such formalization is of practical importance today due to computational tools that allow for automation of reasoning procedures. However, we will not attempt to provide any details of such formalism here. Rather, we would like to point to some of the concepts. There are two basic ideas: the first is that statements should be well formed; this is the subject of study of syntax. The second is understanding the rules of consequence, namely what follows and what does not follow from a well formed statement. This is the domain of logic.

4.1.1 Syntax: Well-Formed Statements

To the nonmathematician, the concept of syntax is familiar in the form of the grammar of a given human language. Different human languages have different

---

2. From an unpublished letter from A. Einstein to R. A. Thornton, as cited in [121].

syntaxes. The sentence "The dog bit the man" is syntactically correct in English, but the sentence "The dog the man bit" is not. On the other hand, the former sentence (with the English words replaced by Bengali words) is grammatically incorrect in Bengali, whereas the second form is correct. Formal grammars (as familiar in computer science) constitute a mathematically precise formulation of the idea of such grammars. We have briefly discussed the hierarchy of grammars in the previous chapter, in the section on the theory of computation. Note that a sentence may be syntactically correct but not mean anything, as illustrated by the famous example "colorless green ideas sleep furiously" constructed by Noam Chomsky.

Neuroscientific concepts are formulated in informal language. This allows for conceptual confusions in the form of ill-formed statements, not necessarily in grammatical terms but in terms of the concepts involved. It is not clear that it is either possible or desirable to devise a formal language to discuss neuroscientific concepts. However, one area where there is significant interest in formalization, is in the area of nomenclature or so called "controlled vocabularies." If one does not even have an agreed upon set of terms to refer to the objects in the domain of discussion, it is difficult to achieve conceptual clarity. Although such formal nomenclatures might be difficult to imagine currently for subject areas such as cognitive psychology, one might think that the situation is better in more concrete areas such as neuroanatomy. Unfortunately, even this has proven to be elusive, and is the subject of current research.

4.1.2 Logic: Consequence

Once the syntactical rules have been determined, we can judge whether or not a statement is well formed. The next step is to understand the rules by which one statement may be deduced from one or several other statements. This allows for correct deductive reasoning, which makes sure that valid conclusions are drawn from valid premises. An invalid reasoning procedure leads to a logical fallacy.

As with syntax, logical inference has also been mathematically formalized. Again, such inferential tools do not, as of yet, play an important role in neuroscience. However, assembling a large array of neuroscientific facts into a set of statements to which formal reasoning may be applied is an interesting area for future research.

4.2 Nature of Scientific Method

Paul Feyerabend argued eloquently against too much emphasis on scientific method [73], and it is undoubtedly true that "even a law-and-order science will succeed only if anarchistic moves are occasionally allowed to take place."

Nevertheless, a few things are worth pointing out in this context because they relate quite directly to the basic approaches to data analysis pursued in this book.

4.2.1 Empirical and Controlled Experimental Methods

In attempting to categorize neuroscientific theories in the second chapter, we have already discussed the distinction between the empirical and controlled experimental methods of enquiry. In the former case one proceeds from careful observations without interfering with the source of the phenomena. There is a close correspondence between the empirical approach and the exploratory method of data analysis, or in more modern terms, unsupervised learning. Functional relationships may also be derived between two observed quantities; however, as neuroscientists will be quick to point out, these observed correlations may not arise from underlying "causal" links between the quantities in question. The empirical approach is sometimes put down as "fishing expeditions," but it is worthwhile to keep in mind that some of the greatest scientific theories of all time have followed from purely empirical observations—these include the theory of gravity from astronomical observations and the theory of evolution from careful analysis of existing phylogenetic diversity.

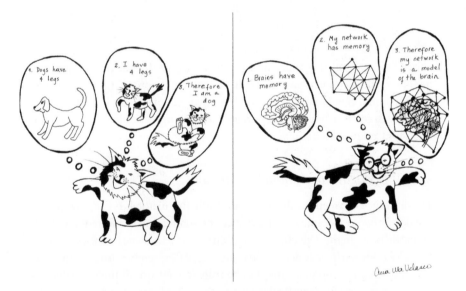

Figure 4.2:   An artist's rendering of a logical fallacy known as the affirmation of the consequent. If A has the attribute B, and C also has the attribute B, it does not follow that A is the same as B. The form of the fallacy illustrated on the left may seem humorous, but the similar argument presented on the right should provide some food for thought.

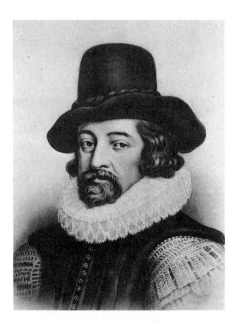

Figure 4.3: English philosopher Sir Francis Bacon (1561–1626) was a proponent of both the empirical and experimental methods of scientific enquiry as opposed to armchair theorizing. He also emphasized the importance of the inductive approach, where generalized conclusions are drawn from particular observations.

In the latter case (method of controlled experiments), some quantities are varied in a controlled manner (independent variables) while other quantities are observed (dependent variables). The usual way to proceed is to determine the functional relationship between these two sets of variables, and not surprisingly, statistical model fitting or regression (or supervised learning) plays an important role in this context.

4.2.2   Deductive and Inductive Methods

The difference between the deductive and inductive methods is roughly the distinction between axiomatic mathematical reasoning and the formation of scientific theories. In the deductive method, one starts with some premises and uses the rules of formal logic to derive consequences. If the premises are true, then the consequences are also guaranteed to be true. In contrast, in the inductive approach, one starts from particular observations and forms theories that generalize these observations. There are no logical guarantees that these theories are true, and the theories cannot be "verified" by adding further observations as is sometimes colloquially stated. The reason is of course that one may later come across an observation that does not fit the theory, and there is no guarantee that a theory will stand up to future evidence. According to Popper, one should therefore try to *falsify* theories rather than try to *verify* them.[3]

These may seem abstract issues but are of practical relevance to some of the questions discussed in the book, particularly in the context of fitting probability models or likelihood models to high-dimensional data, including stochastic process data. The inductive method corresponds to the estimation of an underlying model or probability distribution. In contrast with physics, one does not expect simple mathematical laws to provide accurate fits to the diversity and complexity of biological phenomena. It may be tempting to model a neural time series in terms of a deterministic or stochastic differential equation, but such models can be expected to be context dependent and are not expected to have the same degree of generality and validity as, say, the laws of mechanics in describing planetary motion. One usually has one of two choices: to make simple models and to ignore the lack of detailed fits to the data, or to make detailed statistical models with many degrees of freedom that are closer to phenomenological descriptions than to physics style models. Both approaches have utility, but there is little hope of the kind of inductive procedure that led, say, to Maxwell's equations of electromagnetic phenomena.[4]

The difficulty with trying to infer high-dimensional probability distributions (as necessary for modeling stochastic processes) is known as the curse of dimensionality. The basic idea is simple: if one thinks of probability distributions as histograms, then one needs enough data points in each histogram bin. Suppose we have one-dimensional data and want to distinguish ten levels, then one requires 10 bins. For a two-dimensional histogram, if the same level of resolution is maintained in each dimension, then $10 \times 10 = 100$ bins are required. More generally, in D-dimensional space, one requires $10 \times 10 \times \cdots \times 10 = 10^D$ bins, so the number of required histogram bins grows exponentially with the number of dimensions. Soon, one reaches astronomical numbers of bins, and there is no hope of filling these bins with data in any reasonable period of time. Therefore, trying to do high-dimensional density estimation without strong prior constraints is hopeless. On the other hand, putting strong prior assumptions in place is in conflict with Popper's falsification dictum, because such prior assumptions are tantamount to fixing a very large number of degrees of freedom and cannot be falsified without requiring the same astronomical level of data

---

3. The incentive structure in science currently militates against Popper's dictum because there is little reward for publishing negative results. Nevertheless, efforts to falsify existing theories are important for the health of good scientific enquiry and should be encouraged.

4. One could argue that biological complexity does sometimes yield to simple macroscopic laws, as in economics and in sociology, and it is sometimes suggested that these macroscopic laws resemble the laws of thermodynamics. However, unlike gases and liquids to which the laws of thermodynamics apply, societies and economies are much more heterogeneous and there is no consensus among economists about what the laws of macroeconomics are or whether they are predictive. In comparison, the laws of thermodynamics are precise, predictive, and agreed upon, and it is doubtful that one can make a meaningful comparison between thermodynamic laws and aggregate laws of biological phenomena.

gathering as would fill the original histogram bins. Importantly, the prior assumptions may often be stated in simple terms (for example, smoothness constraints) but still correspond to a large number of effective constraints.

One way out of this conundrum is to adopt a pragmatic approach; note that one is often interested in taking a certain action based on the available data. The high dimensional probability distribution only forms an intermediate to such a procedure (because the actions may live in a low-dimensional space). Such actions might be to choose between a list of potential experiments to do, or to disambiguate two or more prior hypotheses. Therefore, one could proceed by trying to directly build a decision procedure that goes from the data to the actions in question. This is a problem in regression, or *supervised learning*, and has been studied extensively in recent decades. This methodology has been advocated by Vapnik [228], and has been labeled the *transductive* procedure to distinguish it from an inductive procedure of inferring the underlying model or probability distribution.

4.2.3 Causation and Correlation

Biologists in general and neuroscientists in particular are concerned with the conceptual issues surrounding causation and correlation. It is understood that one should not draw causal inferences based on observed correlations. In fact, this is one of the standard criticisms of the empirical or strictly observational method. The idea is that if two variables A and B are observed in constant conjunction (i.e., are correlated), it does not follow that there is a "causal" relationship between the two variables. The usual proposed solution is that of controlled experimentation, varying one of the variables in a *controlled* manner while observing the second variable to see if there is a predictable change. In addition, there are repeated attempts to "infer" causal relationships based on correlation patterns, particularly from multivariate time series data, using fits to underlying models that have some causal property. Although the correlations cannot be used to establish causal relationships, the idea is that they can be used to generate hypothesis about such relationships which can be further tested empirically.

This discourse suffers from imprecision in its definition of what exactly is meant by causation. Arguably, thinking in terms of "causes" was abandoned in post-Newtonian physics. One might colloquially say for example that the sun's gravitational force "causes" the earth to be in its orbit, but such a description is not necessary once the equations describing the dynamics of gravitationally interacting particles are given. The notion of "causation" is replaced by the agency-free idea of "interaction." If two variables interact in a dynamical system, then varying one of them in a controlled manner will cause predictable changes in the other variable, but this does not give one of the variables a special status as "cause" and the other as "effect."

To remove some of the conceptual confusions surrounding the notion of causation, it is also useful to understand the following distinctions.

Fixed Temporal Relationship Is Not Causation

If two events always happen in a fixed temporal order, it is tempting to infer that they are causally related or that they interact. This is in fact the premise behind statistical methods that purport to infer causal relationships from observed correlations. For example, the statistical correlations between two time series may be fit using a causal model, which constrains one variable to affect another only in the future. If such a fit succeeds, it could be declared that evidence has been obtained in the favor of the first variable being related causally to the second variable.

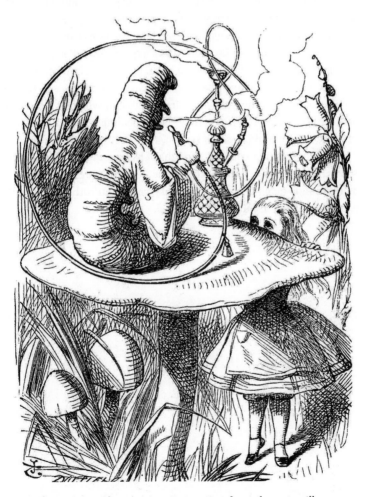

Figure 4.4:   Alice receives instruction from the caterpillar.

This procedure suffers from two defects. First, a fixed temporal relationship does not imply any interactions. Two clocks that keep time properly, one of them being delayed with respect to the other, will maintain a fixed time delay without there being any mechanical linkage between the two. Second, there is the issue of common sources—a third unobserved source may send a disturbance to each of the two measured variables, also with a fixed time delay between the two. Even if the two observed variables have no interactions, according to the above procedure they will appear to bear a causal relationship to one another. Due to both these reasons, statistical procedures for inference of "causal models" should be treated with caution.

Real and Explanatory Causation

A second distinction is between real and explanatory causation. Even if there is no real interaction between two variables, it may be convenient in theoretical or explanatory terms to pretend that such interactions exist, depending on what one is proposing to do with such causal explanations. For example, if the goal is to predict the future behavior of a given time series, in terms of a second series, then a causal model may be used to relate the first series to the second for purposes of making the prediction, irrespective of whether there is a real link between the series. More generally, when dealing with multiple levels of theoretical description of the same system, the effective variables at a macroscopic level of description could be thought of as having interactions between themselves, whereas the "real" interactions lie at a more microscopic level. Here again one is dealing with explanatory causation rather than real causation, but it is still a useful way to proceed.

PART II

TUTORIALS

5

Mathematical Preliminaries

...oh dear, how puzzling it all is! I'll try if I know all the things I used to know. Let me see: four times five is twelve, and four times six is thirteen, and four times seven is—oh dear! I shall never get to twenty at that rate! However, the Multiplication Table does not signify: let's try Geography.

—Alice, in *Alice in Wonderland* by Charles Ludwig Dodgson

In this chapter we briefly review a broad range of mathematical topics relevant to the rest of the book. Readers interested in this book are likely to have a working knowledge of calculus, linear algebra, probability theory and statistics. Therefore, depending on the level of prior mathematical knowledge, some or all of this material can be skipped. However, for the mathematically challenged reader, the material presented in this and the following section provides a crash course. With some diligence in working out the problems, such readers can gain enough acquaintance with the relevant concepts to assimilate the subsequent material in the applications sections.

A brief discussion of real and complex numbers and elementary real and complex functions is followed by a summary of linear algebra, with special attention paid to matrix decomposition techniques. We discuss Fourier analysis in some detail because this is a topic of central importance to time series analysis. After a brief review of probability theory, we come to the core set of topics for this chapter, dealing with stochastic process theory. This includes a discussion of point as well as continuous processes.

Although the coverage of material in the chapter is superficial (because the content of the chapter could easily be extended to several courses), we try to review some of the important concepts and provide pointers to the reader who needs a more detailed treatment of the material. Also, rigorous mathematical definitions and theorems would be entirely out of place here, and we do not make any attempts at maintaining formal mathematical rigor. However, we have tried not to sacrifice conceptual subtlety where it is necessary to deal with a matter of practical importance. The choice of material is idiosyncratic but reflects the author's experience in teaching this material to an audience with a mixed mathematical background.

5.1 Scalars: Real and Complex Variables; Elementary Functions

A distinction between "vector" and "scalar" quantities recurs throughout our discussion. By a scalar we are typically referring to a real or a complex number. Most readers will probably have a clear understanding of what a real number is, although the same might not be true of complex numbers, so they bear some discussion. Complex numbers generalize real numbers, in particular to solve algebraic equations of the sort

$$x^2 + 1 = 0 \tag{5.1}$$

This equation can not have a solution which is a real number, thus necessitating the introduction of the "imaginary" number i which has a negative square, $i^2 = -1$. Although the idea of such numbers is fairly old, the subject was mathematically clarified only during the renaissance, and the notation i for a number whose square is -1 is due to Euler. Complex numbers are of the form $a + ib$, where a and b are real numbers, and can also be thought of as a pair of real numbers (a, b), or a two-dimensional vector; complex numbers are therefore depicted as points on a (two-dimensional) complex plane.

Although complex numbers are clearly abstractions (as opposed to real numbers which have a direct correspondence to our physical intuition), they are nevertheless quite useful abstractions. A well-known example in neuroscience is that the representation of a visual hemifield (the left or right half of the field of view seen by an eye) in the primary visual cortex of a primate can be approximated by a simple relationship involving complex numbers. If (x_1, x_2) are the coordinates of a point in the hemifield, and (y_1, y_2) are the corresponding coordinates in the primary visual cortex (appropriately oriented and centered), then the relationship between the two coordinates turns out to be approximately given by the relationship

$$y_1 + iy_2 = \log(x_1 + ix_2) \tag{5.2}$$

This relationship could also be given in a more complicated form using real numbers

$$y_1 = \log \sqrt{x_1^2 + x_2^2} \qquad (5.3)$$

$$y_2 = \tan^{-1}\left(\frac{x_2}{x_1}\right) \qquad (5.4)$$

Clearly the complex notation allows for a more compact representation in this neurobiologically relevant instance.

An important property of complex numbers is that any polynomial equation with real or complex coefficients is guaranteed to have a complex solution (although in general a real solution does not exist). This means that any polynomial can be written in factorized form

$$x^n + a_{n-1}x^n + a_{n-2}x^{n-2} + \cdots + a_0 = (x - x_1)(x - x_2)\cdots(x - x_n) \qquad (5.5)$$

Finding the roots x_i (or zeros) of a polynomial given its coefficients a_i is a classical problem. Apart from special cases, the roots x_i can be written down only in closed form in terms of the coefficients a_i for only $n \leq 4$. For $n \geq 5$, numerical methods are needed in the general case to find the roots. Instead of specifying a polynomial in terms of its coefficients, it may alternatively be characterized by specifying its roots. Low-order polynomials are used in regression of one variable versus another; spline functions, useful for regression and smoothing, consist of pieces of polynomial functions joined together at isolated points. Finding the roots of polynomials plays a central role in solving ordinary differential equations with constant coefficients, and in problems involving matrices, as we will see below.

Complex numbers play an important role in time series analysis, because they are basic to Fourier transformations. Because complex numbers are equivalent to pairs of real numbers, all operations with complex numbers can be carried out with pairs of real numbers, but this is too cumbersome for practice. This is an example of a useful mathematical abstraction. Even though complex numbers are implemented as pairs of real numbers in low-level computer programs (the C language does not even have a complex variable type), most high-level languages or software in which numerical work is done includes an elementary variable type which for complex numbers. Such abstractions also greatly simplify symbolic manipulations.

A scalar function (i.e., real or complex functions defined on some set), is a rule that associates a unique real or complex number to every element of the set. We are mostly going to be interested in real (or complex) functions of real (or complex) variables. Functions are input-output relationships where for any given input, an output is uniquely specified.[1] By abuse of notation, one sometimes talks about a multi-valued function; strictly speaking, there is no such thing, and one ought not be talking about an input-output relationship where multiple outputs are possible for a given input as a "function." In practice, when thinking about input-output relationships, one has to deal with the possibility that the output is not unique, and may be related to the input only in a stochastic sense. In this case, the mathematical notion better suited to describe the relationship is a conditional probability distribution, as we will see later.

An analytical understanding of a large number of classical functions used to be part of the repertoire of any quantitative scientist until the middle of the twentieth century; with the widespread use of symbolic and numerical software, such knowledge has become the exception rather than the rule. Finite polynomials and ratios of finite polynomials are still part of the broader repertoire.

5.1.1 Exponential Functions

One special function that perhaps transcends boundaries and is well known in elementary form even to the lay public (in the form of compound interest and other growth laws) is the exponential. The exponential of a real or complex number x (or for that matter, a square matrix, or even an operator) is defined by the equation

$$e^x = \sum_{n=0}^{\infty} \frac{x^n}{n!} \tag{5.6}$$

It follows that $e^0 = 1$. The basic properties of the exponential function may be explored through a set of simple exercises (based on Rudin[2]):

- Multiply the series for e^x and e^y, and by rearranging terms show that $e^x e^y = e^{x+y}$. (Will this also work for matrices?)
- Show therefore that $\frac{de^x}{dx} = e^x$.
- Setting $y = -x$, show that e^x is nonzero for all x.
- Defining $\sin(x)$ and $\cos(x)$ by setting $e^{ix} = \cos(x) + i\sin(x)$, work out the series expansions for $\cos(x)$ and $\sin(x)$. Show that the definition implies that $\cos(x)^2 + \sin(x)^2 = 1$.
- By considering the first few terms of the series expansion of $\sin(x)$ and $\cos(x)$, show that there is a real number x_0 between 0 and 2 for which $\cos(x_0) = 0$ and $\sin(x_0) = 1$. Define $\pi = 2x_0$, and show that $e^{i\pi/2} = i$ (and therefore that $e^{i\pi} = -1$, and $e^{2\pi i} = 1$).

---

1. Given a set A, the domain of a function, and a set B, the range, a function f is formally defined as a set of pairs (a, b), where $a \in A$ and $b \in B$. One usually writes this in the form $b = f(a)$. Two conditions have to be satisfied: $f(a)$ should be defined for all a, and b should be uniquely defined given a (although multiple values of a may correspond to the same value of b).

2. W. Rudin. *Real and Complex Analysis*. Third Edition. McGraw-Hill Science/Engineering/Math, 1986.

- Show therefore that for integer values of n, $e^{i(x + 2n\pi)} = e^{ix}$, and that $\cos(x)$ and $\sin(x)$ are periodic functions of x with period 2π.
- Explore the consequences for the above exercises for the function $\ln(x)$, defined as the inverse of the exponential function (i.e., $y = \ln(x)$ is such that $e^x = y$).

Functions of the form $f(t) = e^{\lambda t}$, where λ is a complex number, are called complex exponentials (for example, $f(t) = e^{i\omega t} = \cos(\omega t) + i \sin(\omega t)$). These play a central role in time series analysis, as do sines and cosines. Sometimes, attention is drawn to the fact that these functions extend over the entire real line (in contrast with time localized functions such as wavelet basis functions on a compact intervals), which is supposed to make them unsuitable for processing of real life signals. Nevertheless, they remain fundamental to the analysis of stochastic processes both in theory and in practice. Sinusoids play a basic role in analyzing rhythmic behavior, as is obvious from their periodicity; however, they also provide a way of analyzing a much larger class of functions through Fourier analysis to be discussed later.

Complex exponentials also are basic to the study of ordinary differential equations (ODEs) with constant coefficients. These are equations of the form

$$\frac{d^n x(t)}{dt^n} + a_{n-1}\frac{d^{n-1}x(t)}{dt^{n-1}} + a_{n-2}\frac{d^{n-2}x(t)}{dt^{n-2}} \cdots + a_0 x(t) = f(t) \qquad (5.7)$$

where $f(t)$ is called a forcing function, and a function $x(t)$ satisfying the equation is called a solution to the ODE. Some elementary properties of an ODE may be explored through the following simple exercises, which illustrate the utility of exponential functions for studying differential equations:

- By substituting $x(t) = e^{\lambda t}$ into the equation with $f(t) = 0$ (the homogeneous equation), show that $e^{\lambda t}$ is a solution if λ is a root of the polynomial equation:

$$\lambda^n + a_{n-1}\lambda^{n-1} + a_{n-2}\lambda^{n-2} + \cdots + a_0 = 0 \qquad (5.8)$$

- Denote the n roots of the equation by λ_i, $i = 1 \ldots n$, which we will assume to be distinct for now. Show that $x(t) = \sum_i c_i e^{\lambda_i t}$ is a solution of the homogeneous equation for any choice of constants c_i. It can be shown that all solutions to the homogeneous equation are of this form, and the constants c_i may be determined from "boundary conditions," namely conditions imposed on $x(t)$ or its derivatives at one or more time points. Because there are n unknowns, n conditions are needed in general to obtain a unique solution.
- Consider the case $n = 1$, and find the value of λ_1. By substitution, show that $x(0)e^{\lambda_1 t} + \int_0^t e^{\lambda_1(t - t')}f(t')dt'$ is a solution to the inhomogeneous equation.

5.1.2 Miscellaneous Remarks

We will have occasion to use the so called "delta function," $\delta(x)$, which has the property that for a function $f(x)$ that is continuous at $x = 0$, $\int dx \delta(x) f(x) = f(0)$, where the integral is taken over an interval containing $x = 0$. Although $\delta(x)$ is not really a function in the ordinary sense, it should be thought of as the limiting case of a sharply peaked function with vanishing width whose integral is equal to one. As long as some care is exercised (such as not multiplying together two delta functions with the same argument), delta functions provide a convenient shorthand. For example, a spike train (a sequence of action potentials measured from a neuron) may be thought of as a series of delta functions (as long as one is not interested in time scales comparable to the size of the spike), and one may encounter expressions of the form $\rho(t) = \sum_i \delta(t - t_i)$ where t_i are the times of occurrence of action potentials.

We will assume the reader is comfortable with basic operations on functions of a real variable such as differentiation and integration. We also make widespread use of *basis expansions*, which leads us to the next topic, namely linear algebra. A function of a real or complex variable may be thought of as a vector in a high dimensional (or even infinite dimensional) space. This way of thinking is central to our treatment of time series data (which are nothing other than functions of time) because it gives a geometrical way of conceptualizing problems in time series analysis.

We will confine our attention largely to finite dimensional vector spaces. Formally, the functions and processes that we will be dealing with might be thought of as belonging to infinite dimensional spaces. A number of subtleties must be taken into account when dealing with such infinite dimensional spaces, and these are treated in the branch of mathematics referred to as analysis. However, for all practical purposes, a judicious truncation of the spaces to finite dimensionality will suffice. Experimental measurements are of course finite in number, so although such formal nuances may lead to mathematical elegance, they have little bearing on practical data analysis questions if sufficient care is taken in formulating the problem in finite terms, along with appropriate limiting procedures. Similar remarks apply to measure theory and other mathematical notions that make the formal treatment of stochastic processes rather abstruse. These can be avoided by using simpler tools that are adequate for our present purposes.

5.2 Vectors and Matrices: Linear Algebra

Concepts and methods from linear algebra are part of the core mathematical basis of this book. One important aspect of linear algebra is that it takes a number of intuitive geometrical concepts, such as points in space, angles, distances, areas and volumes, being parallel or perpendicular, and reformulates them in algebraic terms. Because this formalization can be done for arbitrary dimensionality of space, this allows the geometrical intuition we have in two and three dimensional space to be extended to higher dimensional spaces.

This transfer of intuition from everyday geometrical concepts to abstract manipulations in high-dimensional vector spaces is very helpful for two reasons. First, as is discussed in greater detail elsewhere, time series data are high dimensional by nature, and may be though of in terms of points in a high-dimensional space. Therefore, concepts relevant to the numerical and statistical analysis of time series data directly relate to geometrical notions in high-dimensional space. Second, a related reason is that a number of the relevant algorithms, such as solving a set of linear equations simultaneously (e.g., in linear inverse problems, multivariate regression, algorithms involving matrix factorizations, manipulations involving graphs, and spectral analysis) may then be brought within the purview of intuitive geometrical understanding. Drawing on geometric intuition to help understand the formalism of linear algebra, while on the other hand using the formalism to prevent incorrect conclusions being drawn from naive geometry, forms a powerful strategy.

5.2.1 Vectors as Points in a High-Dimensional Space

An n-dimensional vector $\mathbf{x}$ may be thought of simply as a list of n numbers

$$\mathbf{x} \equiv (x_1, x_2, x_3, \ldots, x_n)$$

The component numbers x_i may be real or complex. One also says that $\mathbf{x}$ is a point in n dimensional space. It is easier to visualize n-dimensional real space, which we will do below; with some care, the same geometric intuitions apply to n-dimensional complex space.

Because we perceive three spatial dimensions, we can easily visualize two or three dimensional real vectors as the locations of points in a two- or three-dimensional coordinate system, pictorially depicted by arrows joining the coordinate origin to these points. Such a visualization provides important geometric intuition that is quite valuable; for example, perpendicular or orthogonal vectors may be visualized as arrows at right angles to each other. Higher dimensional vectors seem to be rather abstract entities; however, thought of as lists of numbers, they are quite concrete and useful (fig. 5.1). In particular, we will make use of n-dimensional vectors to represent n successive samples of a time series, $[x(\Delta t), x(2\Delta t), \cdots, x(n\delta t)]$. The geometric intuition derived from low-dimensional spaces continues to be useful in higher dimensional spaces with appropriate caveats.

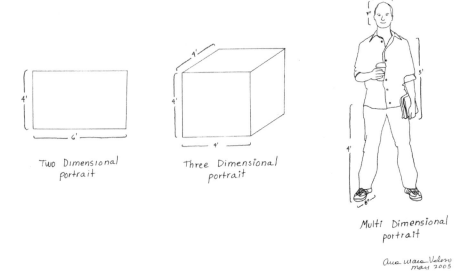

Two Dimensional
portrait

Three Dimensional
portrait

Multi Dimensional
portrait

Ana Maria Valero
may 2005

Figure 5.1: Multidimensional space with dimensionality greater than three is an abstraction that may be initially difficult to grasp if one is limited by two and three dimensional intuition. A starting point to developing such intuition is that a multidimensional vector is simply a list of numbers, which may be used, for example, to quantify multiple attributes of some object.

Vectors can be added, subtracted and multiplied by scalars to give other vectors. These operations are defined by elementwise on the components of the vector, for example

$$(x_1, x_2, x_3, \ldots, x_n) + (y_1, y_2, y_3, \ldots, y_n)$$
$$= (x_1 + y_1, x_2 + y_2, x_3 + y_3, \ldots, x_n + y_n) \tag{5.9}$$

In this way, they are like ordinary numbers; unlike numbers, however, they cannot in general be multiplied or divided. We will usually denote vectors using boldface type, $\mathbf{x} = (x_1, x_2, x_3, \ldots, x_n)$.

5.2.2 Angles, Distances, and Volumes

The length of a vector in two or three dimensions can be generalized to the notion of a "norm" of a vector in higher dimensional space. Different such generalizations are possible; the one that corresponds to the so called Euclidean norm (appropriate for Euclidean geometry) is given by

$$||\mathbf{x}||^2 = \sqrt{|x_1|^2 + |x_2|^2 + \cdots + |x_n|^2} \tag{5.10}$$

From Euclidean geometry, the triangle inequality is satisfied, so that for any two vectors **x** and **y** we have

$$||\mathbf{x}+\mathbf{y}|| \leq ||\mathbf{x}||+||\mathbf{y}|| \tag{5.11}$$

The notion of angle also generalizes from low dimensions, and is given in terms of the "inner product" or "dot product" between two vectors, defined as

$$(\mathbf{x}, \mathbf{y}) = \sum_i x_i^* y_i \tag{5.12}$$

Note that for a complex number $x = a + i\,b$ the complex conjugate x^* is defined as $x^* = a - i\,b$, where a and b are real. It follows from the definitions that

$$||\mathbf{x}||^2 = |(\mathbf{x}, \mathbf{x})|^2 \tag{5.13}$$

The dot product satisfies the Cauchy-Schwartz inequality,

$$|(\mathbf{x}, \mathbf{y})| \leq ||x||\,||y|| \tag{5.14}$$

This inequality permits the definition of the angle between two vectors as

$$\cos(\theta) = \frac{|(\mathbf{x}, \mathbf{y})|}{||x||\,||y||} \tag{5.15}$$

If the dot product is zero, then the vectors are said to be orthogonal or perpendicular. If the orthogonal vectors are also of unit length, they are said to be orthonormal. Note that the idea of vector space as defined abstractly in mathematics is more general than our intuitive notion of three-dimensional space, and not all vector spaces admit a notion of angles or inner products. Those that do, are also called inner product spaces. We will ignore these technical complexities because we will not be dealing with vector spaces that are not also inner product spaces.

- By considering the two- and three-dimensional examples, show that the definitions of length and angle are consistent with the corresponding Euclidean geometric notions.
- Show that the Cauchy-Schwartz inequality implies the triangle inequality.

Other norms (i.e., formalizations of the concept of length of a vector) than the Euclidean norm are possible, and a family of norms of particular interest is given by the so-called p-norms ($p \geq 1$),

$$||\mathbf{x}||_p = (|x_1|^p + |x_2|^p + \cdots + |x_n|^p)^{\frac{1}{p}} \tag{5.16}$$

Note that the Euclidean norm is also the 2-norm. The 1-norm is another norm that will be used later in the book, and the $\infty - norm$ is given by the largest absolute value of the individual coordinates. However, note that the

Euclidean norm is the one that has most widespread use, and appears in the definition of angles between vectors. The inequalities given above generalize to the Minkowski inequality

$$||\mathbf{x}+\mathbf{y}||_p \leq ||\mathbf{x}||_p + ||\mathbf{y}||_p \tag{5.17}$$

and the Holder inequality ($p \geq 1, 1/p + 1/q = 1$)

$$|(\mathbf{x}, \mathbf{y})| \leq ||x||_p ||y||_q \tag{5.18}$$

Given two vectors, one can form a parallelogram with these vectors as the sides. If the lengths of the vectors are a and b and the angle between them is θ, then from elementary geometry it follows that the area of the parallelogram is given by $A = ab \sin(\theta)$. This can be re-expressed in coordinate form using the formulas above for the lengths and angles

$$A^2 = a^2 b^2 (1 - \cos(\theta)^2) = ||\mathbf{a}||^2 ||\mathbf{b}||^2 - |(\mathbf{a}, \mathbf{b})|^2 \tag{5.19}$$

$$A^2 = \sum_{i,j} (a_i^* a_i b_j^* b_j - a_i^* b_i b_j^* a_j) \tag{5.20}$$

$$A^2 = \sum_{i<j} |a_i b_j - a_j b_i|^2 \tag{5.21}$$

In two dimensions, there is only one term in the sum, and the equation simplifies to $A = |a_1 b_2 - a_2 b_1|$. An alternative way of writing this formula is $A = |\det[\mathbf{a}, \mathbf{b}]|$, namely the area is given by the determinant of the two by two matrix formed by taking the vectors $\mathbf{a}$ and $\mathbf{b}$ as columns (or rows). The corresponding formula in three-dimensions relates the volume of the parallelepiped formed by three vectors $\mathbf{a}$, $\mathbf{b}$, $\mathbf{c}$ to the determinant of the matrix with rows (or columns) given by the three vectors, $V = \det[\mathbf{a}, \mathbf{b}, \mathbf{c}]$.[3]

- Compute the angle between the two 4-vectors (1,0,1,0) and (1,1,1,1).
- Compute the area of the parallelepiped spanned by these two vectors.

In n-dimensional space, the volume of the n-dimensional parallelepiped formed by the vectors $\mathbf{a}_1, \mathbf{a}_2 \ldots, \mathbf{a}_n$ is given by $V = \det[\mathbf{a}_1, \mathbf{a}_2, \ldots, \mathbf{a}_n]$. The determinant of a square $n \times n$ matrix A with entries a_{ij} is defined as

$$\det(A) = \sum_P (-1)^P a_{1P_1} a_{2P_2} \cdots a_{nP_n} \tag{5.22}$$

Where the sum is over all $n!$ permutations P of the numbers $1, 2, \ldots n$, $(-1)^P$ is 1 for even and -1 for odd permutations, and i is mapped onto P_i by the permutation P.

---

3. These results generalize to higher dimensions; the appropriate mathematical objects are called "forms" and will not be discussed here in detail. The important point to note here is that the generalized volumes of the k-dimensional parallelepipeds, or "volume elements," with edges given by a set of k vectors in n-dimensional space may be expressed analytically in a simple form in terms of the coordinates of the vectors. Forms and related concepts are fundamental to thinking about the geometry of high-dimensional spaces.

5.2.3 Linear Independence and Basis Sets

An important concept for a collection of vectors is that of linear independence. Linear dependence is a generalization of the geometrical notion of collinear or coplanar sets of points. For example, in two dimensions, two vectors picked at random will not in general point in the same direction (i.e., will not be collinear). Two vectors that are not collinear are said to be linearly independent. On the other hand, three vectors in two dimensions will of course lie on the same plane. This means that in two dimensional space, three vectors must be linearly dependent. This generalizes, so that in n-dimensional space, at most n vectors can form a linearly independent set. Formally, a vector $\mathbf{x}$ is said to be linearly dependent on a set of other vectors $(\mathbf{x_1}, \mathbf{x_2}, \ldots, \mathbf{x_n})$ if it can be expressed as a linear combination of those vectors, that is, if one can find scalars $c_1, c_2, \ldots, c_n$ such that

$$\mathbf{x} = c_1\mathbf{x_1} + c_2\mathbf{x_2} + \cdots + c_n\mathbf{x_n} \tag{5.23}$$

The scalars may be either real or complex numbers; the latter is distinguished by talking about a complex vector space. If such a linear combination cannot be found, then the vector $\mathbf{x}$ is said to be independent of the vectors $(\mathbf{x_1}, \mathbf{x_2}, \ldots, \mathbf{x_n})$. A set of vectors is defined to be independent if each vector in the set is linearly independent of the remaining set of vectors.

In n-dimensional space, there can be at most n linearly independent vectors in a given set (although the choice of a set of n linearly independent vectors is not unique). Such a maximal set of independent vectors is called a *basis set*. Basis sets play an important role, because any vector in the vector space may be written as a linear combination of vectors from the basis set. Of particular importance are basis sets where all pairs of basis vectors are orthonormal; such a basis set is termed an orthonormal basis.[4]

The reader unfamiliar with basis sets and linear independence is invited to explore these concepts in two- or three-dimensional spaces, using geometric constructions, in the following exercises:

- In a two-dimensional real Euclidean vector space (the two-dimensional plane with a Cartesian coordinate system set up for purposes of the exercise), a vector (x_1, x_2) can be visualized as an arrow joining the origin to the point with coordinates (x_1, x_2). Find formulae for the length of the vector, and angles made by the vector with coordinate axes, in terms of (x_1, x_2).
- Using Euclidean geometry, demonstrate that vector addition satisfies the parallelogram law. Consider the vectors $\mathbf{x_1} = (x_1, 0)$ and $\mathbf{x_2} = (x_2, y_2)$. Construct the parallelogram with adjacent sides given by the vectors $\mathbf{x_1}$ and $\mathbf{x_2}$. Show using a geometrical construction that the vector joining the

---

4. Sets of n-dimensional vectors with more than n members are also of interest and are called frames or overcomplete bases.

coordinate origin to the fourth vertex of the parallelogram thus constructed has coordinates given by $(x_1 + x_2, y_2)$.

- Demonstrate geometrically in two dimensions that any three vectors must
  be linearly dependent. Using the parallelogram construction, show that by
  adding suitable multiples of two of the vectors, one can always obtain the
  third vector.
- Repeat this exercise in three dimensions. Find a geometrical criterion in
  three dimensions to guarantee that a given set of three vectors are linearly
  independent.
- In two dimensions, consider two sets of orthogonal coordinate axes, with the
  same origin, but with the second set of axes rotated by an angle of θ from the
  first set. In each coordinate system, choose basis vectors of unit length along
  the coordinate axes. Using a geometrical construction, express the vectors of
  the second coordinate system in terms of the vectors of the first basis set.

5.2.4   Subspaces and Projections

Given a set of vectors, the set of all linear combinations of these vectors (the
"linear span" of the given set of vectors) forms a *vector space*. Two vector spaces
that will be of most use to us are R^n and C^n, consisting of n-tuples of real or
complex numbers, which can be thought of geometrically as position vectors in
n-dimensional space. R^1, R^2, and R^3 correspond to straight lines, planes, and
ordinary three-dimensional space.

Consider a line or a plane passing through the coordinate origin. These are
examples of lower dimensional subspaces (a line being a one-dimensional
subspace and a plane being a two-dimensional subspace) of the larger three-
dimensional space. More generally, a subspace is a lower dimensional vector
space embedded in the original space. In three dimensions, given any plane
(or two-dimensional subspace), a vector can be decomposed uniquely into
a component that lies in the plane, and a perpendicular component. This is an
important notion that generalizes to higher dimensions. Formally, a subspace
consists of a set of vectors that is closed under addition and multiplication by a
scalar number. In other words, adding two vectors belonging to a subspace
gives a third vector that must also lie in the subspace. Similarly, multiplying a
vector in the subspace should give a vector lying in the subspace as well.

- Given a set of vectors $(\mathbf{u_1}, \mathbf{u_2}, \ldots, \mathbf{u_k})$, consider the set U of all possible linear
  combinations of these vectors. Show that U is a subspace as defined above.

Given a vector space V and a subspace P, any vector $\mathbf{x}$ belonging to V can
be written uniquely as a sum of two vectors, $\mathbf{x} = \mathbf{x}_P + \mathbf{x}_{P\perp}$ where $\mathbf{x}_P$ lies in
the subspace P, and $\mathbf{x}_{P\perp}$ has no component in P (i.e., is orthogonal to P).[5] $\mathbf{x}_P$ is

---

5. The fact that any vector in V can be decomposed in this way is also expressed by saying that the
vector space itself can be decomposed into a direct sum of the subspace P and its orthogonal complement
$P^\perp$ (i.e., $V = P \oplus P^\perp$).

the vector lying in the subspace P that best approximates the vector $\mathbf{x}$, in the sense that $|\mathbf{x} - \mathbf{x}_P| \leq |\mathbf{x} - \mathbf{x}_1|$ for all $\mathbf{x}_1$ in subspace P. One refers to $\mathbf{x}_P$ as the projection of $\mathbf{x}$ into the subspace P. The notion of projection into a subspace plays an important role in making approximations, and in linear regression. In both cases, the geometrical picture is of intuitive value.

5.2.5   Matrices: Linear Transformations of Vectors

Vectors written in component form are given by lists of numbers. One can also make lists of vectors, and if the vectors are of the same dimensions, then this gives a matrix, which is a table or two-dimensional array of numbers, real or complex. In geometrical terms, a matrix can be thought of as a linear transformation that takes one vector to another. Given a matrix with entries M_{ij}, $i = 1, \ldots, m$, $j = 1, \ldots, n$ and a vector $\mathbf{v} = (v_1, v_2, \ldots, v_n)$ one can get a second vector $\mathbf{u} = (u_1, u_2, \ldots, u_m)$ with elements given by $u_i = \sum_j M_{ij} v_j$. One also writes this without explicit reference to the components as $\mathbf{u} = M\mathbf{v}$. The fact that the transformation is linear is the same as saying that the following two conditions hold ($\mathbf{u_1}$ and $\mathbf{u_2}$ are vectors and c is a scalar constant):

$$M(\mathbf{u_1} + \mathbf{u_2}) = M\mathbf{u_1} + M\mathbf{u_2} \tag{5.24}$$
$$M(c\mathbf{u}) = cM\mathbf{u} \tag{5.25}$$

If M is a square matrix with $m = n$, then the vectors $\mathbf{v}$ and $\mathbf{u}$ live in the same dimensional space. A vector in n-dimensional real space can be thought of geometrically as an arrow pointing away from the coordinate origin, and a square $n \times n$ matrix operating on this vector produces a second vector. In general, this second vector is different from the first vector. A special case of particular importance is when the vector produced after the action of a matrix is parallel to the original vector, so that its direction is left unchanged. Such a vector $\mathbf{u}$ is called an *eigenvector* or *special* vector of the matrix M and satisfies the *eigenvalue equation*:

$$M\mathbf{u} = \lambda\mathbf{u} \tag{5.26}$$

λ is called the eigenvalue of the matrix M corresponding to the vector $\mathbf{u}$. The null vector $\mathbf{u}$ with all entries zero is a *trivial* eigenvector of a matrix with eigenvalue 0. A matrix does not necessarily have nontrivial eigenvectors (namely eigenvectors which are not identically zero).

- Show that the set of all eigenvectors of a matrix with eigenvalue equal to zero form a subspace. This is called the null space of the matrix (or kernel of the matrix).
- Show that given a set of eigenvectors, the subspace obtained by taking all possible linear combinations of these eigenvectors is left invariant by the matrix M. Namely, show that M acting on a vector from this subspace

produces a second vector that also lies in the subspace. Such a subspace is also called an invariant subspace or *eigenspace* of the matrix M.

- Is there a matrix for which every vector is an eigenvector?
- Construct a 2×2 matrix that has no nonzero eigenvector.

To recapitulate, matrices are linear transformations of vectors. If a vector is left unchanged in direction by the matrix, it is called an eigenvector. It should be kept in mind that for a rectangular matrix which is not square, the transformed vector lives in a space of different dimensions than the original vector.

Matrices may be added, multiplied by scalars, and multiplied by each other as long as their corresponding dimensions match. The product MP of two matrices M and P with entries M_{ik} and P_{kj} is well defined as long as the second dimension of M matches the first dimension of P. If M is an $n \times q$ matrix and P is a $q \times r$ matrix, then the product matrix MP has dimensions $n \times r$ with the $(i, j)^{th}$ entry given by $\sum_{k=1}^{q} M_{ik} P_{kj}$. Square matrices may possess an inverse. For a square matrix M_{ij}, if the inverse matrix M^{-1} exists, then the products MM^{-1} and $M^{-1}M$ are both equal to the identity matrix.

If a matrix is picked at random, then its row vectors and column vectors will in general form independent sets of vectors (an independent set of vectors is such that no vector from the set can be expressed as a linear combination of the remaining vectors). However, this is not always the case. The number of independent row vectors is called the row rank, and the number of independent column vectors is called the column rank. If the matrix is square, then it can be shown that the row rank is equal to the column rank and is simply called the rank of the matrix. This number can be shown to be equal to the number of nonzero eigenvalues of the square matrix. If an $N \times N$ matrix has rank less than N, then it is said to be rank deficient.

Eigenvalues and eigenvectors of a matrix play central roles in the theory of ordinary differential equations, and the importance of gaining a firm grasp of these concepts for understanding dynamical systems can hardly be overemphasized. It should be noted, however, that eigenvalues and eigenvectors do have limitations in their utility. In particular, we will discuss in later sections the singular values and the pseudospectrum of a matrix; these are of more general utility.

5.2.6 Some Classes of Matrices

For square matrices, several special classes are of particular note. Diagonal matrices have only nonzero elements on the diagonal. An upper triangular matrix has zeros below the diagonal, and a lower triangular matrix has zeros above the diagonal. A tridiagonal matrix has nonzero entries only on the main diagonal, and the entries adjacent to the main diagonal.

Toeplitz, circulant, and Hankel matrices play special roles in time series analysis. These matrices are best denoted in pictorial form.

In circulant matrices, all rows are circular permutations of one row:

$$\begin{pmatrix} a_1 & a_2 & \cdots & a_n \\ a_n & a_1 & \cdots & a_{n-1} \\ \cdots & \cdots & \cdots & \cdots \\ a_2 & a_3 & \cdots & a_1 \end{pmatrix}$$

Toeplitz matrices are similar, except that the rows do not wrap around but slide to the right:

$$\begin{pmatrix} a_1 & a_2 & \cdots & a_n \\ a_0 & a_1 & \cdots & a_{n-1} \\ \cdots & \cdots & \cdots & \cdots \\ a_{-(n-1)} & a_{-(n-2)} & \cdots & a_1 \end{pmatrix}$$

Hankel matrices are like Toeplitz matrices, except that the rows slide to the left instead of to the right.

Permutation matrices are obtained by shuffling either the rows or columns of an identity matrix, for example:

$$\begin{pmatrix} 0 & 1 & 0 & 0 \\ 0 & 0 & 0 & 1 \\ 1 & 0 & 0 & 0 \\ 0 & 0 & 1 & 0 \end{pmatrix}$$

For a matrix M and a permutation matrix P, the matrix PM corresponds to a shuffling of the rows of the matrix M, and similarly the matrix MP has its columns shuffled.

A symmetric matrix is unchanged under transposition, $M_{ij} = M_{ji}$. The trans-transpose of a matrix, obtained by interchanging the indices, is written as M^T; for a symmetric matrix, $M = M^T$. The complex conjugate of the transpose of a matrix is also called the Hermitian conjugate and is denoted with a dagger symbol:

$$(M^\dagger)_{ij} = M_{ji}^* \tag{5.27}$$

A Hermitian matrix is one that is equal to its Hermitian conjugate,

$$H^\dagger = H \tag{5.28}$$

A Hermitian matrix has the property that all its eigenvalues are real. If the matrix leaves the length of the vector unchanged, then it is called a unitary matrix. For such a matrix,

$$\|U\mathbf{x}\| = \|\mathbf{x}\| \tag{5.29}$$

Unitary matrices have the special property that their inverse is given by the hermitian conjugate. As a result, their determinant has unit magnitude.

$$U^\dagger = U^{-1} \tag{5.30}$$

$$|det(U)| = 1 \tag{5.31}$$

Unitary matrices have the property that all their eigenvalues are of the form $e^{i\theta}$ for some real number θ. Real unitary matrices are also called orthogonal matrices or rotation matrices, because they simply rotate vectors. Another simple class of matrices are the diagonal matrices, with the only nonzero elements on the diagonal.

5.2.7 Functions of Matrices: Determinants, Traces, and Exponentials

There are a number of important functions of square matrices, with outputs given by numbers or by other square matrices. One such matrix function, the determinant, has been defined earlier. Another function is the trace, given by the sum of the diagonal entries

$$Tr(M) = \sum_i M_{ii} \tag{5.32}$$

The determinant and the trace are left invariant if the matrix is "rotated" with a unitary matrix

$$det(U^\dagger MU) = det(M) \tag{5.33}$$

$$Tr(U^\dagger MU) = Tr(M) \tag{5.34}$$

In fact, these are special cases of a more general set of invariants, given by the eigenvalues of the matrix (note that rotating a matrix does not change its eigenvalues). It can be shown that the eigenvalues λ satisfy the characteristic equation

$$det(M - \lambda I) = 0 \tag{5.35}$$

The left-hand side of the equation is a polynomial in λ of degree n for an $n \times n$ matrix, termed the characteristic polynomial,

$$\lambda^n - p_1 \lambda^{n-1} + \cdots + (-1)^n p_n = 0 \tag{5.36}$$

The eigenvalues λ_i, $i = 1, \ldots, n$ are the roots of this equation. From the properties of polynomials, $p_1 = \lambda_1 + \lambda_2 + \ldots + \lambda_n$, and $p_n = \lambda_1 \lambda_2 \ldots \lambda_n$. From the definitions of trace and determinant it follows that $p_1 = Tr(M)$ and $p_n = det(M)$. The other polynomial coefficients give other invariants, which are not particularly useful: it is simpler to think in terms of the eigenvalues.

Some simple properties of the determinant and the trace are noteworthy: For $n \times n$ matrices A, B and numbers a, b:

$$det(AB) = det(A)det(B) \tag{5.37}$$
$$det(aA) = a^n det(A) \tag{5.38}$$
$$Tr(A+B) = Tr(A) + Tr(B) \tag{5.39}$$
$$Tr(aA) = aTr(A) \tag{5.40}$$
$$Tr(AB) = Tr(BA) \tag{5.41}$$

Following the series definition of the exponential function, one can define the exponential of a matrix as

$$\exp(M) = \sum_n \frac{1}{n!} M^n \tag{5.42}$$

An important property of the matrix exponential is given by the identity

$$\det(e^M) = e^{Tr(M)}, \tag{5.43}$$

which is also written as

$$\log(\det(M)) = Tr(\log(M)) \tag{5.44}$$

- Demonstrate these identities starting from the expressions for trace and determinant in terms of eigenvalues.

5.2.8 Classical Matrix Factorization Techniques

A matrix can be represented as a product of other matrices, a process referred to as a matrix factorization or a matrix decomposition. A number of classical matrix factorization algorithms play a central role in linear algebra and, for that matter, in much of the subject matter covered in this book. We list some of them here along with some of the contexts in which they arise.

LU Decomposition

Under certain circumstances, a matrix can written as a product of a lower triangular (entries above the diagonal are zero) and an upper triangular matrix,

$$M = LU \tag{5.45}$$

This factorization is associated with the Gauss-Jordan elimination method for solving linear systems of equations. The decomposition is not unique, because the right hand side has $N^2 + N$ nonzero entries, but this nonuniqueness can be removed by rescaling the diagonal entries of either L or U. More generally, any square matrix can be written in the form

$$M = PLUQ \tag{5.46}$$

where P and Q are permutation matrices.[6] If the matrix M is nonsingular (has a nonzero determinant), then one can always find the decomposition

$$M = PLU \tag{5.47}$$

The LU factorization is sensitive to numerical error and has to be treated carefully; this is in fact the case with many of the decomposition methods. Fortunately, the associated numerical analysis methods have been well studied, and robust algorithmic implementations are available as standard libraries and are incorporated into a number of open source and commercial software platforms.

If the original matrix M is hermitian, then $U = L^{\dagger}$, and an LU factorization can be written alternatively in the form $M = LL^{\dagger}$, which is referred to as a Cholesky factorization.

QR Factorization

Given a set of vectors that are not necessarily orthogonal, the Gram-Schmidt procedure iteratively constructs a set of orthogonal vectors, a process that leads to the factorization of a matrix M into a product of a unitary matrix Q and an upper triangular matrix R, with appropriate generalizations to the case where the matrix M is rectangular.

$$M = QR \tag{5.48}$$

- Consider the columns of an $N \times N$ matrix M as a set of vectors $x_1, x_2, \ldots, x_n$. Normalize the first vector by its length to obtain a unit vector e_1.
- Construct a second unit vector e_2 by taking the vector x_2, subtracting the projection of this vector onto e_1, and normalizing the results. Show that e_1 and e_2 are orthonormal (namely $e_1 \cdot e_2 = 0$, $|e_1| = 1$ and $|e_2| = 1$.).
- Use this procedure iteratively to construct a sequence of orthonormal vectors e_i. Rearrange the results to obtain the QR decomposition of the matrix.

6. Permutation matrices are obtained by taking the identity matrix and permuting either the rows or the columns. If P is a permutation matrix, then the product PM is a matrix with its rows shuffled, and MP is a matrix with its columns shuffled.

Eigenvalue Decomposition, Similarity Transformations, and Jordan Normal Form

A square matrix with all eigenvalues distinct has an eigenvalue decomposition

$$M = S\Lambda S^{-1} \tag{5.49}$$

$$S^{-1}MS = \Lambda \tag{5.50}$$

Here, Λ is a diagonal matrix with the eigenvalues of M along its diagonal. Another way of saying this is that a square matrix with distinct eigenvalues can always be diagonalized by a similarity transformation (defined by the second equation). If the original matrix M is hermitian, then the matrix S is unitary—this is the case most familiar to physicists. If all eigenvalues are not distinct, then in general the matrix cannot be "diagonalized." For such matrices, the analogous decomposition is given by the Jordan normal form

$$M = SJS^{-1} \tag{5.51}$$

$$S^{-1}MS = J \tag{5.52}$$

where the matrix J is bidiagonal and has the following properties: the diagonal entries consist of the eigenvalues arranged in blocks where repeats of the same eigenvalue are grouped together. For each of these blocks, the upper diagonal consists of ones. The form of the matrix is illustrated below, with the first eigenvalue being twofold degenerate:

$$\begin{pmatrix} \lambda_1 & 1 & 0 & \cdots & 0 \\ 0 & \lambda_1 & 0 & \cdots & 0 \\ 0 & 0 & \lambda_2 & \cdots & 0 \\ \cdots & \cdots & \cdots & \cdots & \cdots \\ 0 & 0 & \cdots & \cdots & \lambda_n \end{pmatrix}$$

For a pair of matrices A, B one can define generalized eigenvalues by means of the equations

$$A\mathbf{u} = \lambda B\mathbf{u} \tag{5.53}$$

$$\det(A - \lambda B) = 0 \tag{5.54}$$

Generalized eigenvalues and eigenvectors play an important role in solving linear inverse problems.

Singular Value Decomposition

Perhaps the most important of these decompositions is the singular value decomposition, which is defined for any matrix, and is given by

$$M = U\Sigma V^{\dagger} \tag{5.55}$$

where M is a $p \times q$ matrix (we assume $p \geq q$), U is a $p \times q$ matrix with orthonormal column vectors, Σ is a diagonal $q \times q$ matrix with non-negative entries on the diagonal, called singular values, and V is a $q \times q$ unitary matrix.

The singular values and singular vectors satisfy the equation

$$Mv = s\mathbf{u} \tag{5.56}$$

For physicists who are used to thinking about the eigenvalue decompositions of hermitian matrices, it is easier to think about the singular value decomposition in terms of the eigenvalue decompositions of the hermitian matrices $MM^\dagger$ and $M^\dagger M$

$$MM^\dagger = U\Sigma^2 U^\dagger \tag{5.57}$$
$$M^\dagger M = V\Sigma^2 V^\dagger \tag{5.58}$$

If the matrix M is Hermitian ($M = M^\dagger$), then the singular values of M are the squares of the eigenvalues; however, this is not in general true. In particular, note that the singular values are defined for an arbitrary (in general rectangular) matrix and are real non-negative, whereas eigenvalues are only defined for square matrices and are in general complex. The SVD plays a central role in the analysis techniques discussed later in this book and will be treated extensively in later chapters.

5.2.9 Pseudospectra

Linear algebra is an old subject, and it would be excusable to think that the subject is conceptually mature with no changes expected in the broad ideas. Nevertheless, this is precisely what has happened recently in the case of eigenvalue decompositions of matrices. It is not an exaggeration to say that in certain circumstances, eigenvalues have been demoted in status. For a class of matrices known as non-normal matrices, it is now understood that eigenvalues are of limited practical utility and may in realistic cases be impossible to estimate due to extreme sensitivity to numerical error. This is not mathematical esoterica; it has practical implications for circumstances where eigenvalues have traditionally been used as a tool in theoretical work, both in physics and biology. Instead of the set of eigenvalues of a matrix, the appropriate quantity is now understood to be the so called *pseudospectrum* of the matrix. Although the subject is too recent and complex for us to detail here, we briefly outline some of the basic ideas in this section.

A matrix is non-normal if it fails to commute with its hermitian conjugate, $AA^\dagger \neq A^\dagger A$. Equivalently, a normal matrix has a complete set of orthonormal eigenvectors. A normal matrix can be diagonalized by a unitary transformation, but a non-normal matrix cannot. A simple example of a non-normal matrix M is given by

$$\begin{pmatrix} 0.9 & A \\ 0 & 0.9 \end{pmatrix}$$

- What are the eigenvalues of M?
- Perturb M by a small amount, and calculate the eigenvalues for the perturbed matrix. Show that for A large, even small perturbations cause large changes in the eigenvalues.
- Consider the discrete dynamical system given by $\mathbf{x}_{n+1} = M\mathbf{x}_n$, with $\mathbf{x}_n$ being a 2×1 column vector. Show that $\mathbf{x}_n = M^n \mathbf{x}_0$.
- Study the behavior of $\mathbf{x}_n$ as a function of n for $\mathbf{x}_0 = (0,1)$ using analytical or numerical means. Show that the Euclidean norm $\|\mathbf{x}_n\|$ shows an initial growth followed by an eventual exponential decline.

The exercise above points to one of the problems with characterizing non-normal matrices using eigenvalues. The matrix M above has eigenvalues less than 1, and the corresponding discrete dynamical system given above is therefore asymptotically stable. However, this is misleading in two ways. First, the size of M^n initially grows before eventually declining. Depending on the size of A, this growth can be substantial. Because linear dynamical systems such as this one are usually approximations, the growth can take the system into a nonlinear regime, causing a qualitative change in the behavior and invalidating the asymptotic stability analysis using eigenvalues. Similarly, small perturbations to the matrix entries can make the matrix unstable.

Pseudospectra are defined in terms of the so-called resolvent. For a matrix M, the resolvent $G(z)$ is a matrix that is a function of a complex parameter z, defined by

$$G(z) = (z - M)^{-1} \tag{5.59}$$

The resolvent is well defined unless $(z - M)$ is singular and is not invertible. This is precisely what happens when $z = \lambda$, one of the eigenvalues of the matrix M. Therefore, the resolvent is not defined at the eigenvalues of the matrix M and the norm of the resolvent diverges near these values of z. Note that different definitions of matrix norm is possible, one of the most useful one being the Euclidean norm, given by $\|G\|^2 = Tr(GG^\dagger)$, the sum of the absolute squared values of all matrix entries.

The norm of the resolvent diverges when z belongs to the eigenvalue spectrum. The pseudospectrum is given by the region in the complex plane where $\|G(z)\|$ is large; in general the pseudospectrum covers a two-dimensional region of the complex plane and contains the eigenvalue spectrum. The definition of pseudospectrum depends on what is considered "large." This may seem ad hoc, but for large matrices, appropriate limiting procedures exist that make the pseudospectrum a well-defined region of the complex plane, which can in general be quite different from the spectrum. The significance of the pseudospectrum is that if the original matrix is perturbed by a small amount, then the perturbed eigenvalues are scattered in the region described by the pseudospectrum. The initial growth phenomenon described above can also be related to the pseudospectrum. For more details, the interested reader is referred to the definitive text on pseudospectra by Trefethen and Embree.[7]

5.3 Fourier Analysis

Fourier (fig. 5.2) analysis plays a central role in signal processing. The reasons for this are many: some are mathematical, but other reasons arise from the nature of signals that one observes in the world. Fourier representations are ubiquitous in physics; this may be epitomized by the fact that even the unit of time is defined via frequency, based on a narrow spectral peak corresponding to an atomic resonance. The invariance of physical laws under translational invariance in space and time directly lead to the use of Fourier representations in terms of spatial and temporal frequencies.

Fourier analysis has also played an important role in neuroscience, particularly in vision and audition. The responses of neurons in early visual and auditory areas are formulated in terms of functions which have various degrees of localization in the Fourier domain. Nevertheless, it is often believed that Fourier analysis is useful only for analyzing "linear" systems, and that bio-

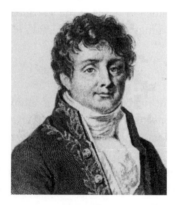

Figure 5.2: French mathematician and physicist Jean Baptiste Joseph Fourier (1767–1830) developed the theory of Fourier expansions in his studies of heat conduction. Fourier actively participated in the French Revolution and held a variety of military and administrative positions.

7. L. N. Trefethen, M. Embree. *Spectra & Pseudospectra: The Behavior of Nonnormal Matrices.* Princeton, NJ: Princeton University Press, 2005.

logical systems, being "nonlinear," need other methods of analysis. This criticism is misplaced. In fact, Fourier methods are of much broader utility than analyzing the input-output behavior of linear systems. This is true in physics—the vast majority of physical systems for which temporal and spatial frequencies are used either in an experimental or theoretical setting are in general interacting systems with strong nonlinearities in the interactions. Similarly, Fourier methods have proven valuable in analyzing biological signals, even in the presence of substantial nonlinearities. Fourier representations provide useful transformations of time series by separating slowly varying signals from rapidly varying ones. We list here a couple of the critiques and corresponding responses for the utilization of Fourier techniques in analyzing biological time series.

- *Critique:* Fourier analysis expands data into infinitely long sinusoids, which are inappropriate for biological data. *Response:* Most uses of Fourier analysis in signal processing involve simultaneous localization in time and frequency. Even in physical applications, one never deals with infinitely long sinusoidal trains, but rather with wave packets of defined duration. The Fourier decomposition is informative even if the function is not a narrowband oscillation.
- *Critique:* Fourier analysis presupposes that the data come from a linear system. *Response:* Fourier representations are demonstrably useful in investigating nonlinear dynamical systems in biology. For example, period doubling and transitions between periodic and chaotic states in animal vocalizations have been studied using time-frequency representations.

There are several natural questions one may ask about a function of time: How smooth is the function? Given part of the function, can one deduce or draw inferences about the rest of the function (e.g., predict the future from the past)? Can one approximate the function by taking combinations of a set of known functions? More generally, can one compress the information present in the function into a few parameters? How similar are two given functions? All these questions may be treated within the framework of Fourier analysis. The area in mathematics that deals with these sorts of questions is referred to as functional analysis, a subject area that is quite rich and complicated; for the purposes of simplicity we will mostly stick to the simpler machinery associated with finite dimensional vector spaces. In this setting, functions of time will be regarded as vectors in a finite dimensional space. The simplest case is when time is discrete and the length of the time interval is finite. If the duration of the experiment is T and samples are gathered at intervals of Δt so that $T = N\Delta t$, then measurements of a function $f(t)$ gives a vector $\mathbf{x} = [f(0), f(\Delta t), f(2\Delta t), \ldots, f(n\Delta t), \ldots, f(N\Delta t)]$.

It should be kept in mind that there are many subtleties that arise for infinite dimensional function spaces that are not apparent when dealing with finite dimensional vector spaces. We will occasionally comment on these subtleties; however, if the subtleties have real-life implications they can usually be examined through appropriate limiting procedures employing progressively larger spaces of finite dimensionality. Such discretizations are certainly necessary when working with real data on a digital computer.

5.3.1 Function Spaces and Basis Expansions

Informally, a function space is a set of functions along with some restrictions or properties. Such properties may include the domain over which the functions are defined, for example the real line $[-\infty,\infty]$, an interval $[a, b]$, the complex plane, or other more general sets. Because we are interested in time series, we will be dealing with functions defined on the real line or some subset of the line, or, in more practical terms, on a discrete time grid. Another set of properties have to do with how smooth the functions are; for example, we may want the functions to be continuous, or have various degrees of smoothness, which can be characterized by asking that derivatives of the function up to some order are well defined. A third set of properties deals with the "size" of the function: is $|f(t)|$ bounded? Does $|f(t)|$ have a finite integral? Does $|f(t)|^2$ have a finite integral? In real-life experiments we are dealing with functions that live on a finite interval of time, have a finite "size," and are sufficiently smooth. Different function spaces formalize these notions (table 5.1).

Moreover, there are more subtle concepts that nevertheless appear in practical settings: metrics or distances between functions, convergence of sequences of functions, approximations of a function by functions chosen from a class, and so on. Although limits, continuity, and convergence are familiar from elementary calculus, when dealing with function spaces, procedures to deal with these concepts become complex and cumbersome unless abstractions are introduced. Examples of such abstractions are constructs such as topologies (to deal with continuity and convergence), measures (to generalize the notion of Riemann integration), Hilbert and Banach spaces (infinite dimensional vector spaces with desirable properties), and so on. This is beyond of the scope of this text, so having briefly hinted at some of the topics studied in functional analysis we will proceed informally, assuming that the reader has some intuitive grasp of the relevant

Table 5.1: Some Function Spaces

Symbol	Description	Conditions
l_1	Sequences with bounded 1-norm	$\sum_i |f_i| < \infty$
l_2	Sequences with bounded 2-norm	$\sum_i |f_i|^2 < \infty$
l_p	Sequences with bounded p-norm	$[\sum_i (|f_i|^p)]^{\frac{1}{p}} < \infty$
$\mathcal{L}_1(R)$	Real functions with bounded 1-norm	$\int dx |f(x)| < \infty$
$\mathcal{L}_2(R)$	Real functions with bounded 2-norm	$\int dx |f(x)|^2 < \infty$
$C^n(R)$	Real functions with nth order derivatives	$\forall x f^{(n)}(x)$ exists
$S(R)$	Schwartz space: rapidly decreasing functions	$\forall n, m \max_x x^n \frac{d^m}{dx^m} f(x) < \infty$

ideas from elementary calculus. The reason we mention these subtleties has to do with the theory of Fourier transforms; although widely used in practice, the theoretical foundations of Fourier analysis are by no means elementary and have a number of complications that cannot be satisfactorily treated without the introduction of these abstractions. Although we will not enter into the abstractions, we will treat some important examples of the complications.

Given an observed time series (such as a voltage as a function of time), we will frequently expand the time series in terms of a set of basis functions, each being a function of time. We will also consider basis expansions of multichannel or image time series where basis functions across channels or in space will play a role. Some of the relevant concepts will hold whether we are dealing with functions of time or functions of space. Given some time series $x(t)$, consider the expansion in terms of a set of basis functions $x_k(t)$

$$x(t) = \sum_k a_k x_k(t) \tag{5.60}$$

The first question to consider for an expansion of this sort is the number of terms in the series. If for some set of functions, only a finite number of terms up to some maximum number are required for the basis expansion, then the situation is particularly simple. This is the situation for the discrete time case, with a finite time interval discussed in the last section. However, discretizing time is not necessary; one can simply construct a finite dimensional vector space by choosing a finite basis set. In general, this is not possible, and most interesting function spaces do not have a finite basis set. One may, however, demand that even if the basis set is not finite, only a finite number of basis functions are needed to expand any given function. It can be shown[8] that such bases, called Hamel bases, always exist for any vector space; however, they are not of much practical use. Unfortunately, unless more conditions are put on the vector space, these are the only types of bases that are guaranteed to exist.

If instead, one deals with basis expansions with an infinite number of terms, this immediately introduces the complexities associated with the convergence of infinite sums. At the very least, we need to define the notion of convergence; this can be done in so-called *topological* vector spaces. The function spaces of practical-interest to us in fact have even more structure; for example, in so-called Hilbert spaces one can define angles and orthonormality between vectors, thus allowing the geometrical notions developed for finite dimensional vector spaces to carry over.

It cannot be overemphasized that in practice, function spaces may be made finite dimensional through the usage of discrete time and a finite interval; however, this does not entirely get rid of the theoretical difficulties associated

---

8. This is a consequence of the set theoretical Axiom of Choice.

with infinite dimensional spaces, which could re-emerge, for example, in the form of numerical bad behavior.

Although the equality sign is used in equation (5.60), it should be understood that in many cases of practical interest the equality may not hold at every time point. For example, it may hold at all but a set of points "of measure zero" (a concept that we will not define but is adequately picturesque for the reader to form a rough idea of what is involved). Consider the partial sum $S_N(t)$ obtained by truncating the expansion at N terms. For the basis expansion to be sensible, it is desirable that the partial sums, obtained by keeping N terms, converge to the function $x(t)$ for large N.

Two distinct notions of convergence are applicable:

1. The series is said to converge pointwise at time t if $\lim_{N \to \infty} S_N(t) = x(t)$.
2. One may also define convergence more globally through the notion of uniform convergence. For any given ε, no matter how small, if there exists an integer M such that for all t, $|S_N(t) - x(t)| < \varepsilon$ when $N > M$, then the expansion is said to converge uniformly.

In words, if the absolute difference between the function and the partial sum can be made arbitrarily small for *all* times for sufficiently large N, then the series converges uniformly. Uniform convergence is a stronger condition than pointwise convergence: the latter does not imply the former.

Before entering into a discussion of Fourier series, it is useful to consider polynomial approximations, or expansions where the basis functions are polynomials. This is familiar to students of elementary calculus in the form of Taylor expansions, and indeed Fourier series may be understood in terms of polynomials on the unit circle in the complex plane.

Consider real functions that are defined on a finite time interval. Without loss of generality, consider a function $f(t)$ defined on [0 1]. One way to approximate this function with a polynomial would be to choose a discrete grid of distinct points t_i and find an interpolating polynomial that is equal to the function on that grid. Using the Lagrange interpolation formula, such a polynomial is given by

$$
\begin{aligned}
f_{Lagrange}(t) = f(t_1) &\frac{(t-t_2)(t-t_3)\cdots(t-t_n)}{(t_1-t_2)(t_1-t_3)\cdots(t_1-t_n)} \\
+ f(t_2) &\frac{(t-t_1)(t-t_3)\cdots(t-t_n)}{(t_2-t_1)(t_2-t_3)\cdots(t_2-t_n)} + \cdots
\end{aligned}
\tag{5.61}
$$

The reader can verify that $f_{Lagrange}(t)$ is a polynomial of degree $n-1$, $f_{Lagrange}(t) = \sum_{j=0}^{j=n-1} c_j t^j$ and it satisfies $f_{Lagrange}(t_i) = f(t_i)$. Therefore, given any function on the interval, one can explicitly construct a polynomial that agrees with the function on any fixed finite grid. By making this grid finer, one can expect that the approximation will improve and that one will end up with a series expansion of the original function in terms of integer powers of t. As it turns out, this is precisely the case for an appropriate class of functions. A famous theorem due to Wierstrass ensures that any continuous function $f(t)$ on the interval can be approximated arbitrarily well by a polynomial, both in the local sense of pointwise convergence, as well in the global sense of uniform convergence described above.

There is a subtlety, however, that underlines the difficulties lurking around the corner if one is not careful with the approximating functions. In the polynomial interpolation example above this shows up, for example, as Runge's phenomenon (similar to Gibbs' phenomenon for Fourier expansions to be studied next). Runge was able to find a simple, smooth function $f(x)$ for which the Lagrange interpolating polynomial oscillates wildly if the interpolation is made on a uniform grid $(t_i = i/n)$. For this example, it turns out that $\lim_{N \to \infty} \max_t |f(t) - f_N(t)| = \infty$.

One solution to this problem is to use a nonuniform grid (so much for the apparent simplicity of a uniform grid in this context!) in the form of the zeros of Tchebycheff polynomials. This gets rid of the nonuniformity of the convergence and is known as Tchebycheff interpolation. In practical interpolation problems, however, one does not use polynomials over the whole interval: rather, one uses piecewise polynomials or splines. This will take us too far afield, and we will postpone discussion of splines until later. However, this discussion should give the reader some flavor of the issues involved in expanding functions in terms of basis sets.

5.3.2 Fourier Series

A Fourier series is a sum of complex exponentials (or equivalently, sums over sines and cosines) of the form

$$\sum_{n=-\infty}^{n=\infty} c_n e^{if_n t} \tag{5.62}$$

Here c_n is a sequence of complex numbers and f_n are real numbers. We will be interested in series where $f_n = an$. It is of substantial interest to study series where f_n are not uniformly spaced, but we will not enter into this discussion here. Because $e^{2n\pi i} = 1$ for integer n, all terms in the sum above are periodic with a common period of $T = 2\pi/a$. For our initial discussion, we will choose $a = 1$, so that the series repeats itself with a time period of $T = 2\pi$.

We will explore three illustrative examples; intermediate steps in the derivation are elementary but the unfamiliar reader should work through them as exercises. We will require the formula that sums a geometric series

$$1 + r + r^2 \cdots + r^N = \frac{1 - r^{N+1}}{1 - r} \tag{5.63}$$

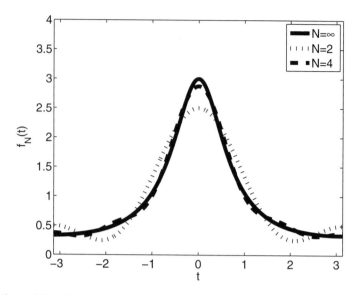

Figure 5.3: Convergence of Fourier series: first example, equation 5.65.

Consider the case where $c_n = A^{-|n|}$ with A a real number greater than 1, so that the coefficients decay exponentially. The sum can be then written as

$$f(t) = -1 + 2Re \sum_{n=0}^{\infty} A^{-n} e^{-int} \qquad (5.64)$$

Using the summation formula for geometric series, we obtain

$$f(t) = \frac{A^2 - 1}{A^2 - 2A \cos(t) + 1} \qquad (5.65)$$

This is a smooth periodic function ranging from $\frac{A-1}{A+1}$ to $\frac{A+1}{A-1}$, illustrated in figure 5.3 for $A = 2$. The figure also shows partial sums (ranging from $-N$ to N) for $N = 2$ and $N = 4$, illustrating the rapid convergence of the series.

- Study the behavior of the function 5.65 numerically for values of A close to 1.
- Try to take a continuous limit by setting $A = 1 + \varepsilon$ and rescaling time by setting $t = \varepsilon \tau$. Convert the sum to an integral, and evaluate it to obtain a function of τ.

As a second example, consider the case where $c_n = 1$. The partial sum $f_N(t)$ can be evaluated by applying the formula for the geometric series (the reader should work this out as an exercise),

$$f_N(t) = \sum_{n=-N}^{n=N} e^{int} = \frac{\sin\left(N + \frac{1}{2}\right)t}{\sin\left(\frac{t}{2}\right)} \qquad (5.66)$$

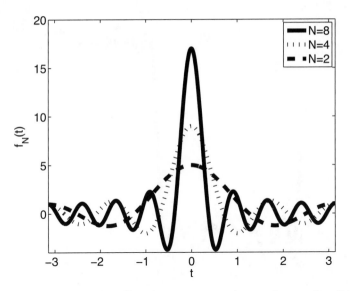

Figure 5.4: Convergence of Fourier series: second example, equation 5.66.

This is the so-called Dirichlet kernel or function that we will encounter repeatedly and which is plotted in figure (5.4). It can be seen from the figure that the partial sums have a sharp central peak. The height of this peak is obtained by setting $t = 0$ in the sum to obtain $f_N(0) = 2N + 1$. As N increases, this peak becomes sharper and narrower; however, its integral over time remains constant at 2π (the reader should show this by integrating the series for the partial sum, term by term). In the large N limit, this sum becomes a "delta function"; however, the oscillations around the central lobe also grow in height so that the area of each lobe goes to a constant value. This is not a very nice delta function; in fact, this oscillatory behavior is the source of the trouble when dealing with the convergence properties of Fourier series (and the source of bias in spectral estimation). We will discuss this in greater detail in later sections.

As a final example, consider the case

$$c_n = i((-1)^n - 1)/n \tag{5.67}$$

Here $i = \sqrt{-1}$. Note that in the two previous examples, the Fourier coefficients c_n are real, whereas in this example they are imaginary. The partial sums constructed by summing from $n = -N$ to $n = N$ are real, however. The partial sums for increasing N are shown in figure 5.5. As $N \to \infty$, the series converges to a step function. However, there are oscillatory overshoots on both sides of the step. The important point is that as N becomes large, these overshoots move

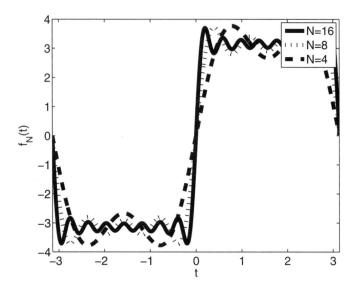

Figure 5.5: Convergence of Fourier series: third example, equation 5.67.

closer to the step, but *tend to a fixed limiting height.* It can be shown that the limiting size of the overshoot is about 10% of the height of the jump on either side (the precise factor is $\frac{1}{2\pi}\int_{-\pi}^{\pi} sinc(x)dx$, where $sinc(x) = \frac{sin(x)}{x}$). Clearly, this is not uniform convergence; $\lim_{N \to \infty} \max_t |f(t) - f_N(t)|$ is finite. This is the well known Gibbs's phenomenon (the oscillatory overshoots are sometimes referred to as Gibbs's ripples or Gibbs's oscillations).

How can this be fixed? There is a classical procedure for series such as these known as Cesaro summation, which has a direct analog in spectral estimation to be studied later. Consider the partial sums $f_N(t)$ defined above. The idea is that convergence can be improved by taking the average of the first N partial sums, defined as

$$S_N(t) = \frac{1}{N+1}\sum_{n=0}^{N} f_n(t) \qquad (5.68)$$

The corresponding partial sums $S_N(t)$ are shown in figure 5.6. It can be seen that the Gibbs's ripples have been diminished and the partial sums now converge more gracefully to a step. Note that if the limit exists, then $f_N(t)$ and $S_N(t)$ converge to the same limit at any given t; what the procedure above achieves is that the nonuniformity of the convergence is now removed. By rearranging the terms in the sum, it can be shown that the Cesaro partial sum is in fact a partial sum of the Fourier series obtained by taking the original series and multiplying by a "taper" before computing the partial sum. It is important to note that this is

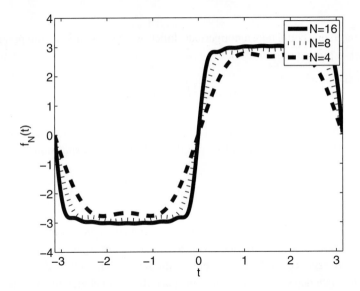

Figure 5.6: Convergence of Fourier series: Cesaro summation, equation 5.68.

not a new Fourier series; the taper depends on N and changes with the order of the partial summation.

$$S_N(t) = \sum_{n=-N}^{n=N} \left(1 - \frac{|n|}{N+1}\right) c_n e^{int} \qquad (5.69)$$

This is an indication of what is to come. The Cesaro summation procedure replaces the abrupt truncation of a partial sum, with the gradual truncation provided by a triangular "taper."

5.3.3 Convergence of Fourier Expansions on the Interval

So far we have discussed the convergence properties for specific Fourier series for some choices of c_n. If the partial sum does converge, how are the coefficients related to the function it converges to? First, note that for $n \leq N$, the partial sums satisfy the equation

$$c_n = \frac{1}{2\pi} \int_{-\pi}^{\pi} f_N(t) e^{-int} dt \qquad (5.70)$$

The usual procedure in defining Fourier expansions of functions is to start with the definition of the Fourier coefficients of the function $f(t)$, assumed to be integrable over the interval of choice. Note that by default we are considering the time interval $[-\pi \ \pi]$, and we assume that the function $f(t)$ is periodic (although one could take a nonperiodic function over an interval and periodize it with a jump discontinuity).

$$c_n = \frac{1}{2\pi} \int_{-\pi}^{\pi} f(t) e^{-int} dt \qquad (5.71)$$

One then asks if the partial sum $f_N(t)$ of the Fourier series converges to $f(t)$. If it does, then it is meaningful to write the corresponding expansion

$$f(t) = \sum_{n=-\infty}^{n=\infty} c_n e^{int} \qquad (5.72)$$

The conditions for convergence of the partial sums are complex. One may define convergence in a number of different ways: convergence at a point, uniform convergence, and convergence in the norm. For each of these notions, convergence depends on the function space that $f(t)$ belongs to. Here we will only state a few convergence theorems relevant to Fourier series; for more details the interested reader should consult a book on functional analysis. The subject has a rich history, some of which is recent.

1. If $f(t)$ has a continuous derivative on the (periodic) interval, then the partial sums of the Fourier series converge uniformly.

2. If $f(t)$ is continuous but does not have a derivative, then the partial sums of the Fourier series need not in general converge. However, it can be shown that the Cesaro sums are in fact uniformly convergent. This reiterates the importance of "tapers."

3. If $f(t)$ belongs to $L_2([-\pi\ \pi])$, the space of square integrable functions on the interval, then the partial sums converge in the L_2 norm.

$$\lim_{N \to \infty} \int_{-\pi}^{\pi} |f(t) - f_N(t)|^2 dt = 0 \qquad (5.73)$$

Note that this does not mean pointwise convergence; there could be a "set of measure zero" where the convergence does not occur.

4. If $f(t)$ belongs to $L_1([-\pi\ \pi])$, so that the function is absolutely integrable but not necessarily square integrable, then the Fourier series does not in general converge. It can in fact *diverge*, illustrating the subtleties involved in the convergence of Fourier expansions.

For the case of square integrable functions, the total power is the same, whether calculated in the time or Fourier domain (Parseval relation).

$$\frac{1}{2\pi} \int_{-\pi}^{\pi} |f(t)|^2 dt = \sum_{n=-\infty}^{n=\infty} |c_n|^2 \qquad (5.74)$$

5.3.4   Fourier Transforms

As in the case of Fourier series, for Fourier integrals one has to be cautious about convergence properties, domains of definition, and so on. Because we have more to do with Fourier series than with Fourier integrals, our discussion of these issues will be much more brief. The Fourier transform is well defined and has nice properties for the space of rapidly decreasing, smooth functions (Schwartz spaces) defined above. There is some latitude in defining the transform and its inverse, in terms of normalization, as well as whether to use circular frequencies ω or conventional frequency f, related by $\omega = 2\pi f$. In this section, we will continue using circular frequencies (as in the last section), whereas we will switch to using conventional frequencies in the next section. This can be a bit confusing. However, because both conventions are in use in the literature, it seems best to give the reader exposure to both conventions.

For functions belonging to Schwarz space, the Fourier transforms also live in Schwarz space, and the forward and inverse transforms are defined as

$$\hat{F}(\omega) = \int_{-\infty}^{\infty} dt F(t) e^{-i\omega t} \tag{5.75}$$

$$F(t) = \int_{-\infty}^{\infty} \frac{d\omega}{2\pi} \hat{F}(\omega) e^{i\omega t} \tag{5.76}$$

Note the asymmetrically placed factor of 2π; this can be placed more symmetrically but the convention given above is typical in the physics literature. One way to avoid the annoying factors of 2π is to use conventional frequency; in this case the factor of 2π appears in the exponential:

$$\hat{F}(f) = \int_{-\infty}^{\infty} dt F(t) e^{-2\pi i f t} \tag{5.77}$$

$$F(t) = \int_{-\infty}^{\infty} df \hat{F}(f) e^{2\pi i f t} \tag{5.78}$$

This is the convention we follow in the rest of the book. For this section, however, we will retain circular frequencies. Table 5.2 gives some examples of Fourier transform pairs, including examples of distributions, and illustrates some basic facts about Fourier transformations.

Table 5.2:   Some Fourier Transform Pairs

Time Domain	Frequency Domain
$\frac{1}{\sqrt{2\pi\sigma^2}} e^{-\frac{t^2}{2\sigma^2}}$	$e^{-\frac{1}{2}\omega^2\sigma^2}$
$\frac{d}{dt}$	$i\omega$
1	$2\pi\delta(\omega)$
$\int_{-\infty}^{\infty} F(t')G(t-t')dt'$	$\hat{F}(\omega)\hat{G}(\omega)$

1. The Fourier transform of a Gaussian is a rescaled Gaussian.
2. Derivatives in the time domain become multiplication by frequency after transformation; this makes Fourier transforms a basic tool in solving differential equations.
3. The Fourier transform of a constant is a delta function.
4. The Fourier transform of a convolution is the product of the Fourier transforms.

One has a continuous version of Parseval's theorem (conservation of total power)

$$\int_{-\infty}^{\infty} |f(t)|^2 dt = \int_{-\infty}^{\infty} \frac{d\omega}{2\pi} |\hat{F}(\omega)|^2 \qquad (5.79)$$

5.3.5 Bandlimited Functions, the Sampling Theorem, and Aliasing

Fourier transforms appear ubiquitously in physics, but in doing actual time series analysis one has to deal with time on a finite grid. This has become the only meaningful way in which we can deal with real-life time series, because modern measurements are based on computerized digital acquisition, which gives us samples of the series at discrete time points. Under what conditions does this still allow us to deal with underlying functions that are defined over continuous time?

Fortunately, there is a simple and practically meaningful criterion that when satisfied justifies the usage of a discrete time grid. If a function is bandlimited, so that its Fourier transform vanishes for large enough frequencies, then the function is fully characterized by its samples on a discrete time grid, provided the grid spacing is fine enough. Consider a real or complex valued function $F(t)$ defined on the real line, and let the Fourier transform $\hat{F}(f)$ vanish outside the interval $[-B\ B]$ so that $\hat{F}(f) = 0$ for $|f| > f_N$. Then the sampling theorem allows us to reconstruct the function $F(t)$ at arbitrary time t from the samples of this function $F(n\Delta t)$ on a uniform grid of spacing Δt as long as $\Delta t \leq 1/(2B)$. Let us assume that the bandwidth B is the smallest such bandwidth outside which the Fourier transform vanishes. Then B is called the Nyquist frequency, and the condition on the sampling frequency $1/\Delta t$ is that it has to be greater than twice the Nyquist frequency. Under these conditions, the relation between the discrete samples $F_n = F(n\Delta t)$ and the continuous time function $F(t)$ is given by (recall that $sinc(x) = \sin(x)/x$)

$$F(t) = \sum_n sinc[2\pi B(t - n\Delta t)]) F_n \qquad (5.80)$$

This interpolation is illustrated in figure 5.7. However, do bandlimited processes actually exist? If not, then this would not be a very useful formula in de-

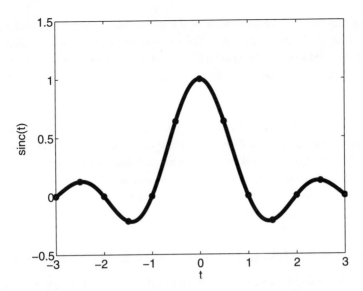

Figure 5.7: Interpolation of the samples of a bandlimited function (equation 5.82). In this case, the function is itself the sinc function, and the samples are at twice the Nyquist rate.

scribing digital signals. Also, what happens when the function is not bandlimited? These are questions of practical importance to real-life experiments, and they have practical answers. Even if natural processes are not bandlimited, they do tend to have power spectra that decay at large frequencies. This could be regarded as a deep fact about nature, that there is structure and predictability in the signals we observe; practically, this can make life simpler for the time series analyst. Thus, approximately bandlimited functions appear due to different reasons:

1. The foremost reason is that processes observed in nature are often smooth beyond some microscopic scale and have a natural frequency cutoff. A neurobiological example is the falloff of the EEG power spectrum at high frequencies.
2. Even if the natural process has high frequencies in it, the measurement may be made through an instrument that is sluggish at high frequencies and therefore has its own cutoff bandwidth.
3. The experimenter chooses to apply a low-pass filtering process explicitly into the measurement hardware. This is known as an anti-aliasing filter, because it prevents aliasing. In circumstances (such as in fMRI) where the measurement device does not permit the inclusion of an anti-aliasing filter, one has to be particularly careful in interpreting the spectrum of the digitized signal.

If a function is not bandlimited, or if it is bandlimited but sampled at a rate lower than the Nyquist rate (i.e., if Δt is larger than $1/(2f_N)$), then the spectrum of the digitized signal is distorted with respect to the original spectrum. In fact, this distortion has a fairly simple form; frequencies higher than the sampling rate are "reflected back" to lower frequencies. If the sampling rate is R, and if a frequency is present in the signal at $f_0 > R/2$, then it will appear at $R - f_0$ instead of R^9. As a practical example, say the cardiac rate is 1 Hz, corresponding to a period of one second. If this signal is sampled at less than 2 Hz sampling rate, then the fundamental frequency peak will appear at a lower value. For example, if the sampling time in the experiment is $0.75s$, corresponding to a sampling frequency of $1/0.75 = 1.33\,\text{Hz}$, then the heartbeat frequency will appear to have a peak at 0.66 Hz.

5.3.6 Discrete Fourier Transforms and Fast Fourier Transforms

In discussing Fourier series, we have effectively discussed the properties of the discrete Fourier transform (DFT). The DFT of a discrete time series x_t is defined as

$$X(f) = \sum_t e^{-2\pi i f t} x_t \qquad (5.81)$$

In this sum, t ranges over a discrete time grid. Note that $X(f)$ is a function of a continuous frequency variable. Now just as we had to discretize time in order to think of implementation on a digital computer, we have to discretize frequency in order to have a practical implementation.[10] By choosing the frequency grid to be sufficiently fine, one can approximate the DFT as closely as one likes. Once time and frequency have both been discretized, the computation of the Fourier transform reduces to a matrix multiplication. For N_f frequency grid points and N_t time grid points, computation of the DFT requires $N_f N_t$ steps. This is already too large for reasonable values of N_f and N_t. Fortunately, the matrix has special structure, which can be exploited to speed the computation up considerably. We are referring here to the fast Fourier transform (FFT), one of the most widely used algorithms: listening to music, talking on a cell phone, and almost any application using embedded signal processing uses the FFT. It should be noted that the DFT is a function of frequency, and the FFT is an *algorithm* to compute the DFT on a finite grid. Confusingly, the result of applying the FFT algorithm is also referred to as an FFT; more precisely, applying the FFT algorithm produces an estimate of the DFT on a finite frequency grid.

---

9. Here we are only considering positive frequencies and $R < f_0 < 3R/2$. Note that real signals will have a power spectrum that is symmetric around $f = 0$. More generally, the peak at f_0 will appear at $f_0 \bmod R/2$, and one has to take into account both positive and negative frequency peaks.

10. In the same vein, it is of course also true that numbers on a digital computer are also discretized; one cannot deal directly with a real number.

Let the unit of time be $\Delta t = 1$ and consider a series of length N. By default, the FFT algorithm evaluates the DFT on a grid with N frequency points given by $f_j = j/N$. A discrete time series may be viewed in two ways: as a sampled version of a bandlimited, continuous time series, or as a series that exists only for discrete time values. If one adopts the latter (unphysical) perspective,[11] then instead of being bandlimited, the frequency domain can be thought of as living on a circle, in this case $f \in [0\ 1]$. Because in this perspective the frequency domain is periodic, one can equally well think of the frequency domain as $[-1/2\ 1/2]$. The frequencies given by f_j with $j \leq N/2$ are usually designated positive, and for $j > N/2$, f_j are designated *negative* frequencies. This can be made clearer by considering the complex exponential in the DFT:

$$e^{-2\pi i f_j t} = e^{-2\pi i \frac{jt}{N}} \tag{5.82}$$

The reader should show that the above expression is unaltered if f_j is replaced by $-f_{N-j}$. It is convenient to write the above expressions in terms of the Nth root of unity, $\omega = e^{2\pi i/N}$. Note that $\omega^N = 1$. The FFT algorithm is used to evaluate

$$X_j = \sum_{t=1}^{N} \omega^{-jt} x_t \tag{5.83}$$

The speedup provided by the algorithm occurs when N is composite, with the maximum speedup obtained when $N = 2^k$ (i.e., the length of the series is a power of 2). To understand the basic idea, it is useful to consider the toy example for $N = 4$. In this case, the DFT consists of computing the four quantities

$$X_1 = x_1 + ix_2 - x_3 - ix_4 \tag{5.84}$$
$$X_2 = x_1 - x_2 + x_3 - x_4 \tag{5.85}$$
$$X_3 = x_1 - ix_2 - x_3 + ix_4 \tag{5.86}$$
$$X_4 = x_1 + x_2 + x_3 + x_4 \tag{5.87}$$

If each sum is computed separately, this requires 3 complex additions or subtractions for each term, for a total of 12 operations. However, examination of the equations show that one can reduce the number of operations by pre-computing certain sums. If one defines

$$A = x_1 + x_3 \tag{5.88}$$
$$B = x_1 - x_3 \tag{5.89}$$
$$C = x_2 + x_4 \tag{5.90}$$
$$D = x_2 - x_4, \tag{5.91}$$

---

11. Note that this is actually a physically relevant perspective in solid state physics when dealing with crystals; in that case, the atoms or molecules constituting the crystal are closer to being point like objects.

then the results can be obtained by fewer operations in terms of these intermediate quantities

$$X_1 = B + iD \tag{5.92}$$
$$X_2 = A - C \tag{5.93}$$
$$X_3 = B - iD \tag{5.94}$$
$$X_4 = A + C \tag{5.95}$$

In this second procedure, only 8 complex additions and subtractions are involved, compared with 12. The more general case can be illustrated by considering N to be even, so that $N = 2M$, and breaking the sum (equation 5.83) into odd and even terms. For $j \leq M$, one then has

$$X_j = \sum_{l=1}^{M} \omega^{-j(2l)} x_{2l} + \sum_{l=1}^{M} \omega^{-j(2l+1)} x_{2l+1} \tag{5.96}$$

Relabeling the even and odd parts of the series for clarity, $x_l^e = x_{2l}$ and $x_l^o = x_{2l+1}$, and noting that $\omega^2 = e^{4\pi i/(2M)} = e^{2\pi i/M}$ is an Mth root of unity, we have

$$X_j = \sum_{l=1}^{M} \theta^{-jl} x_l^e + \omega^j \sum_{l=1}^{M} \theta^{-jl} x_l^o \tag{5.97}$$

where $\theta = e^{2\pi i/M}$ is an Mth root of unity. Similarly, one can obtain the values of X_j for $j > M$ in terms of the sums over the odd and even terms (this is left to the reader as an exercise). The important thing to note about the above equation, is that the odd and the even sums are themselves DFTs, computed over $M = N/2$ terms in each case. Thus, the DFT over $2M$ terms can be written in terms of two DFTs each over M terms. If M is even, this procedure can be repeated; if $N = 2^k$ is a power of two, this procedure can be repeated k times. Suppose that $T(k)$ are the number of complex additions and multiplications needed for $N = 2^k$. Then applying the recursive procedure above, we see that

$$T(k) = 2T(k-1) + 2 \cdot 2^k \tag{5.98}$$

The second term in the equation is needed because there are $N = 2^k$ values of j, and for each j, given the transforms of the odd and the even series, one needs to do a multiplication and an addition. This is a recursive equation for the time complexity of the algorithm, and it can be solved by substituting $T(k) = R(k)2^k$. This yields a simpler recursion for $R(k)$, which is seen to satisfy $R(k) = R(k-1) + 2$, which has the solution $R(k) = 2k$. Therefore the number of complex multiplies and adds are $T(k) = 2k2^k = 2N\log_2(N)$. This is the well-known $O(N\log(N))$ result for the time-complexity of the FFT algorithm, for $N = 2^k$. If a number is not a power of two but is a power of three, then it is easy to see that the procedure generalizes, this time with three DFTs needed for one step of the recursion. More generally, some speedup is obtained as long as N is composite, by breaking N up into its prime factors. Thankfully, we do not have to worry about the implementations of these complex algorithms; they are available in prepackaged form for most computational platforms.

So far, we have assumed that the number of frequency grid points is equal to the number of time grid points in the series under consideration. Using the FFT in this default mode evaluates the DFT on a fairly coarse grid. How does one get the DFT on a finer grid? The answer is very simple: one "zero pads" the series (appends a string of zeros at the end of the series) before application of the FFT algorithm. For example, consider voltage data sampled at 1 kHz for one second. This gives us 1000 samples. A direct application of the FFT algorithm will return the DFT computed on a frequency grid with spacing given by 1 Hz. This may not be adequate to show the smooth shape of the spectrum, which may have peaks with widths close to 1 Hz. The usual procedure is to zero pad by some amount; say in this case we pad by 7192 zeros to obtain a total length of 8192 before application of the FFT. This has two benefits: first, the frequency grid is now refined to a spacing of about a tenth of a Hz; second, the number of grid points is now a power of 2 ($8192 = 2^{13}$). It is sometimes erroneously argued that padding is unnecessary because no extra information is being added to the series by adding zeros. Although it is true that the frequency grid points or the unpadded FFT carry a full complement of the information present in the data and the intermediate points are simply (sinc) interpolates, we are incapable of doing such interpolation visually and may easily draw the wrong inferences by looking at an inadequately smooth DFT. Moreover, if there were a frequency peak in the spectrum, it may well lie in between grid points, and choosing the DFT bin with maximal magnitude of the Fourier transform will lead to an inaccurate determination of peak location.

5.4 Time Frequency Analysis

Fourier transforms over infinite time intervals and Fourier series with an infinite number of terms is convenient mathematical fiction. In real life, the time interval is always finite; consequently one is interested in the properties of Fourier transforms over finite intervals. Finiteness of the data segment is, however, not the only consideration that forces finite time windows on us: the spectral content of the function we are interested in may change over time in a practically meaningful sense. Therefore, it is very often the case that signals are examined with small, moving time windows. This brings us to the important topic of simultaneous localization in the time and frequency plane. A variety of theorems assert that signals cannot be simultaneously localized in both time and frequency beyond a certain limiting resolution; the precise statement depends on the definition of localization. Signals that are strictly time localized (i.e., vanish outside a finite time interval) cannot also be strictly frequency localized (i.e., vanish outside a finite frequency interval). It is therefore important to understand the properties of the Fourier transform of a finite data segment.

5.4.1 Broadband Bias and Narrowband Bias

We consider a discrete time series x_t, where t takes integral values and ranges over the entire discrete time range $-\infty < t < \infty$. The Fourier transform of the infinite series is given in terms of a Fourier series

$$X(f) = \sum_{t=-\infty}^{\infty} x_t e^{-2\pi i f t} \tag{5.99}$$

Taking note of the discussion about convergence in an earlier section, under appropriate circumstances one has for the Fourier coefficients

$$x_t = \int_{-1/2}^{1/2} X(f) e^{2\pi i f t} df \tag{5.100}$$

Now suppose we are only given a finite segment of the time series of (even) length T given by x_t, $-T/2 \le t \le T/2$. From this, we can only compute the truncated Fourier series

$$\tilde{X}(f) = \sum_{t=-T/2}^{T/2} x_t e^{-2\pi i f t} \tag{5.101}$$

We might be interested in the function $X(f)$, the Fourier transform of the signal over all time. However, we only have access to $\tilde{X}(f)$. What is the relation between these two quantities? We can answer this question by substituting the form of x_t given in equation 5.100 in the equation for the truncated Fourier series equation 5.101. This yields the equation

$$\tilde{X}(f) = \sum_{t=-T/2}^{T/2} \int_{-1/2}^{1/2} X(f') e^{2\pi i (f'-f) t} df' \tag{5.102}$$

Rearranging terms, one obtains

$$\tilde{X}(f) = \int_{-\frac{1}{2}}^{\frac{1}{2}} D_T(f-f') X(f') df' \tag{5.103}$$

Where the kernel $D_T(f)$, also known as the Dirichlet kernel, is given by

$$D_T(f) = \sum_{t=-T/2}^{T/2} e^{-2\pi i f t} \tag{5.104}$$

Examination shows that this is precisely the second example of Fourier series discussed in a previous section (equation 5.66) and we can use the previously calculated partial sum to obtain a closed form for the kernel

$$D_T(f) = \frac{\sin(\pi f(T+1))}{\sin(\pi f)} \tag{5.105}$$

The cautious reader will have noted that in going from the previous example to the current one, the roles of time and frequency have been interchanged; in the example in the previous section, the Fourier series when summed gave a periodic function of time. In the present instance, $D_T(f)$, $X(f)$, and $\tilde{X}(f)$ are periodic functions of frequency with period 1. As discussed previously, $D_T(f)$ is approximately a delta function. If it were precisely a delta function (which happens when $T \to \infty$), then we would have $\tilde{X}(f) = X(f)$. For finite time windows, however, $\tilde{X}(f)$, the DFT of the data, is related to the underlying Fourier transform through an integral equation with kernel $D_T(f)$. This kernel is not a delta function for two reasons: the central peak has a finite width, given by $2/T$ if measured from node to node, and the first sidelobe has a finite height, which can be computed as follows. For large T, the numerator $\sin(\pi f(T+1))$ shows rapid oscillations, whereas the denominator is smooth, as long as f is much smaller than π but comparable to $1/(T+1)$. Therefore, defining a rescaled frequency $f = x/(T+1)$, we obtain for the Dirichlet kernel

$$D_T(f) \approx (T+1)\frac{\sin(\pi x)}{\pi x} \tag{5.106}$$

The Dirichlet kernel (fig. 5.8) is therefore approximately a rescaled sinc function near the origin. The location of the first sidelobe peak is given by the first extremum of the sinc function. This occurs when $\pi x = 1.43\ldots$, and the absolute value of the sinc function at this (minimum) is given by $0.2172\ldots$ Thus, the first sidelobe is 22% of the central lobe; importantly, it does not reduce in size if T becomes large. The sidelobes come closer to the central lobe as T becomes larger, but they decay slowly: the nth is of size $\sim 1/n$. In statistical parlance, $\tilde{X}(f)$ is a biased estimator of $X(f)$. Because one is talking about a function rather than a number, the bias cannot be characterized by a single number. It is customary to divide the bias into two contributions. The first comes from a finite width to the central lobe of the Dirichlet kernel and is called the *narrowband* bias. The second comes from the slowly decaying sidelobes, and this is called *broadband* bias. As we will see later, these two forms of bias are in some sense complementary: one can trade the one off against the other.

How to mitigate the slowly decaying sidelobes? The previous discussion of Cesaro summation gives a hint: one should multiply the data series by a *taper*,[12] a

---

12. In the signal processing literature the data taper is often referred to as the data window. We reserve the word window for the data segment under consideration and use the word taper to denote the function multiplying the data segment to suppress sidelobes.

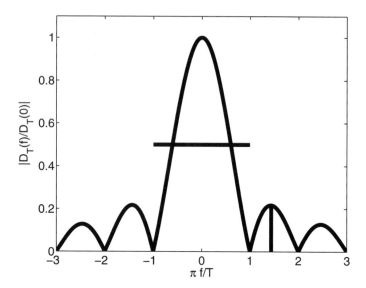

Figure 5.8: The normalized Dirichlet kernel. The central lobe width (narrow-band bias) and the first sidelobe magnitude (broadband bias) are indicated by bars on the figure.

function w_t with which the data time series is multiplied before performing the Fourier transformation. It is easy to verify that this leads to the Dirichlet kernel being replaced by a kernel that is the Fourier transform of the taper

$$D_T^w(f) = \sum_{t=-T/2}^{T/2} w_t e^{-2\pi i f t} \tag{5.107}$$

The bias properties of the taper is denoted by the function $D_T^w(f)$. A large number of data tapers have been used in the literature; these have different properties and reduce bias according to some criterion. Some examples are the "Hamming" taper and the "Hanning" taper (both of which are constructed out of cosines) as well as the triangular tapering function reminiscent of Cesaro summation. Using one of these tapers (a process also known as apodization) reduces the sidelobes at the expense of the width of the central lobe, as illustrated in figure 5.9 for the triangular taper

$$w_t = 1 - \frac{|t|}{T/2 + 1} \tag{5.108}$$

The kernel corresponding to the triangular taper (and to Cesaro summation) is known as the Fejer kernel and is given by

$$F_T(f) = \frac{1}{\frac{T}{2} + 1} \left(\frac{\sin\left(\left(\frac{T}{2} + 1\right)\pi f\right)}{\sin(\pi f)} \right)^2 \tag{5.109}$$

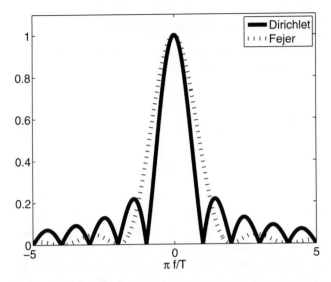

Figure 5.9: The Fejer kernel, corresponding to the triangular taper, compared with the Dirichlet kernel, corresponding to the rectangular taper. Note the broadening of the central lobe and the reduction of the side lobes. Both kernels are normalized to unity at zero frequency.

This kernel also integrates to unity and becomes more sharply peaked, like the Dirichlet kernel, and therefore behaves like a delta function for large T. In contrast with the Dirichlet kernel, however, the Fejer kernel is non-negative, and is a nicer way to approach delta function. The Dirichlet kernel is not absolutely integrable in the large T limit, namely $|D_T(f)|$ when integrated over frequency gives a value that diverges as $\log(T)$, whereas $|F_T(f)|$ when integrated over frequency is a constant.

The usage of taper functions leads naturally to the question: are there tapers which are in some sense optimal? The answer to this question will of course depend on how one defines optimality. In addition, however, there is another question: tapering a finite data segment downweights the two edges of the data window compared to the center of the window. This leads to loss of data, which seems artificial. Is there a way to rectify this and gain back the lost edges of the window? There is an elegant answer to this problem, which also provides an optimal set of tapers in a precise sense. This leads us to the spectral concentration problem, studied in a fundamental series of papers by Slepian, Landau, and Pollack[13-17].

13. D. Slepian and H. O. Pollack. Prolate spheroidal wave functions, Fourier analysis and uncertainty—I. *Bell Sys. Tech. J.* 40, 43–64, 1961.

14. H. J. Landau and H. O. Pollak. Prolate spheroidal wave functions, Fourier analysis and uncertainty—II. *Bell Sys. Tech. J.* 40, 65–84, 1961.

5.4.2 The Spectral Concentration Problem

Consider the DFT of a finite series w_t, $t = 1 \ldots T$. Note that in the previous section we have considered time series ranging from $-T/2 \cdots T/2$, which for T even have a length of $T + 1$. This is a minor modification in notation; it is simpler to use one or the other convention depending on the circumstance. The DFT $U(f)$ is given by

$$U(f) = \sum_{t=1}^{T} w_t e^{-2\pi i f t} \tag{5.110}$$

Because $\Delta t = 1$, the elementary frequency interval will be taken as $f \in [-1/2, 1/2]$. Note that $U(f)$ is periodic with period 1. It is easy to demonstrate that $U(f)$ can vanish only at isolated points and cannot vanish over an entire interval. To see this, let us define the variable $z = e^{-2\pi i f}$. Then $U(f) = P(z)$, where $P(z) = \sum_{t=1}^{T} w_t z^t$ is a polynomial in the complex variable z of order T. Because $P(z)$ is a polynomial, it only has T isolated zeros (which could be degenerate, namely the zeros can coincide). This implies $U(f)$ also has only isolated zeros, which in turn implies that the integral of $|U(f)|^2$ over any finite interval is nonzero. In particular, for any $W \neq -1/2$,

$$\int_{-1/2}^{-W} \|U(f)\|^2 df > 0 \tag{5.111}$$

This implies that the so-called spectral concentration $\lambda(W, T)$ of $U(f)$ on the interval $[-W, W]$, defined as ratio of the power of $U(f)$ contained in the interval $[-W, W]$ to the whole interval $[-1/2, 1/2]$, is strictly less than one.

$$\lambda(T, W) = \frac{\int_{-W}^{W} \|U(f)\|^2 df}{\int_{-1/2}^{1/2} \|U(f)\|^2 df} \tag{5.112}$$

In other words, for $0 < W < 1/2$, the fact that $U(f)$ has only isolated zeros implies that $0 < \lambda(T, W) < 1$. Thus, the spectral concentration is strictly less than one, and there is no finite sequence w_t for which the DFT can be confined to a band $[-W, W]$ and made to vanish outside this band. Note that in the above equation we have noted the explicit dependence of λ on W and T. In the following text, we will sometimes note this dependence explicitly and sometimes not, depending on notational convenience.

---

15. H. J. Landau and H. O. Pollack. Prolate spheroidal wave functions, Fourier analysis and uncertainty. III—*The dimension of the space of essentially time- and band-limited signals. Bell Sys. Tech. J.* 41, 1295–1336, 1962.

16. D. Slepian. Prolate spheroidal wave functions, Fourier analysis and uncertainty—IV: Extensions to many dimensions; Generalized prolate spheroidal functions. *Bell Sys. Tech. J.*, 43 3009–3058, 1964.

17. D. Slepian. Prolate spheroidal wave functions, Fourier analysis, and uncertainty. V—The discrete case. *Bell Sys. Tech. J.* 57, 1371–1430, 1978.

This leads naturally to the question: for given time window T and half bandwidth W, is there a sequence for which the spectral concentration is maximized? In other words, is there a sequence for which the sidelobe energy outside a frequency range $[-W, W]$ is minimal? The answer to this question is: yes, such a sequence exists, and it can be found by a simple procedure. Minimizing $\lambda(T, W)$ defined above is the same as minimizing the power $\int_{-W}^{W} \|U(f)\|^2 df$, with the constraint that the total power is held fixed, $\int_{-1/2}^{1/2} \|U(f)\|^2 df = 1$. This is a constrained optimization problem that can be solved using the method of Lagrange multipliers. The interested reader is urged to work this out as an exercise, to derive the following equation satisfied by the optimal sequence w_t:

$$\sum_{t'=1}^{T} \frac{\sin 2\pi W(t-t')}{\pi(t-t')} w_{t'} = \lambda w_t \qquad (5.113)$$

This is an eigenvalue equation, for a symmetric matrix given by $M_{t,t'} = \sin(2\pi W(t-t'))/(\pi(t-t'))$. The largest eigenvalue of this equation corresponds to the largest possible spectral concentration λ, and the corresponding eigenvector is the sought after optimal sequence w_t. We have already proven that the spectral concentration is between 0 and 1. It is also easy to show that the matrix above is positive definite, so that the eigenvalues λ are between 0 and 1. The eigenvectors are known as Slepian sequences and are illustrated in figure 5.10. The Slepian sequence corresponding to the largest value of λ gives the unique taper that has maximally suppressed sidelobes.

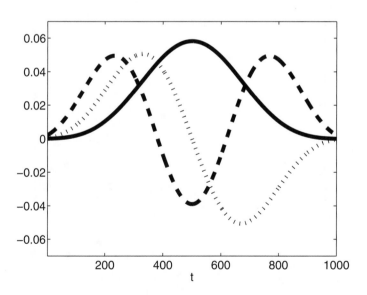

Figure 5.10: The three leading Slepian sequences for $T = 1000$ and $2WT = 6$. Note that each higher order sequence has an extra zero-crossing.

Some of the subleading eigenfunctions also have good spectral concentration properties. If one arranged the eigenfunctions in the order of decreasing λ, then the second Slepian sequence provides the best sidelobe suppression (in the sense of maximizing λ), among all functions that are orthogonal to the first Slepian sequence. This procedure may be continued recursively; the $(n+1)^{th}$ Slepian sequence provides best sidelobe suppression in the space of sequences orthogonal to the first n sequences. One then asks: until what value of n is the amount of sidelobe suppression good; namely how many Slepian sequences have λ close to one? The answer to this question is both elegant and a fundamental result in signal processing (and led to the utility of this theoretical framework in communication engineering).

It turns out that the subspace of well-concentrated functions has a dimensionality given by the product of the time interval and the frequency interval, $N \approx 2WT$. About $2WT$ of the functions have $\lambda \approx 1$, and the rest have $\lambda \approx 0$, as illustrated in figure 5.11. The transition zone is in fact quite narrow; it can be shown that it is only logarithmically dependent on the time bandwidth product. Let λ_n be the nth eigenvalue, in decreasing order. As $T \to \infty$, it can be shown that for any small ε, $\lim_{T \to \infty} \lambda_n(T, W) = 1$ if $n < 2WT(1 - \varepsilon)$, and on the other hand $\lim_{T \to \infty} \lambda_n(T, W) = 0$ if $n > 2WT(1 + \varepsilon)$.

This implies that the width of the transition zone can be made arbitrarily small compared to $2WT$, for T large enough. In a quite precise sense, therefore, the space of strictly time-limited functions that are also optimally bandlimited

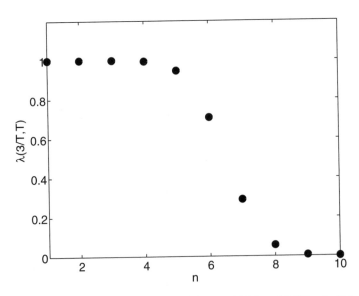

Figure 5.11: The ten leading values of λ for $T = 1000$ and $2WT = 6$. Note the sharp falloff around $n = 6$.

within a bandwidth $[-W, W]$ has a dimensionality of $2WT$. This space is spanned by the first $n \approx 2WT$ Slepian sequences. In practise, it is customary in spectral analysis to take n to be the integer closest to $2WT - 1$, although somewhat smaller values of n may be chosen if better spectral concentration is desired.

This may seem abstract, so consider a practical example of a sequence of EEG data 10 seconds long, sampled at 1 kHz. This gives us 10,000 data samples. Now suppose we are performing spectral analysis, and wish to allow for a spectral resolution of 2 Hz. Because the alpha rhythm is a few hertz wide, this may be a reasonable thing to do. What is the dimensionality of the space of functions that are 10 seconds long and 2 Hz in bandwidth? To answer this question, we take the product of the time and the frequency intervals, to obtain the dimensionless number $10 \times 2 = 20$. This is the number of *degrees of freedom* we have in that time-frequency window. Note that in the above example we computed the product using time and frequency measured in real units of seconds and hertz. What is the relation between this calculation and the considerations in the sections, where we considered dimensionless units where $\Delta t = 1$? The answer is that one may work with dimensional or dimensionless units, as convenient, as long as the units are consistent. One could work in dimensionless units where $T = 10000$, and $2W = 2\,\mathrm{Hz}/1\,\mathrm{kHz} = 0.002$: if time is measured in units of $\Delta t = 1$, then frequency should be measured in units where the total frequency range is also 1, so that a bandwidth of 2 Hz would then be normalized by the sampling frequency, 1 kHz. In either case, the time-bandwidth product is a dimensionless quantity and remains the same.

The reader might ask for the relationship between the leading Slepian function and the Gaussian, which also has a rapidly decaying Fourier transform and in the physics literature is used as a function that minimizes time-frequency uncertainty. Under appropriate circumstances, the leading Slepian function does indeed resemble a Gaussian but is not identical to it. The reason for the difference is that the Slepian function is defined through a criterion that maximally suppresses sidelobes for a finite sequence; the Slepian sequence is defined on a finite window.[18] The Gaussian also optimizes spectral concentration in the following sense: let $g(t)$ be a function defined over all time and $G(f)$ be its Fourier transform. If the time spread is defined as $\int_{-\infty}^{\infty} t^2 |g(t)|^2 dt$, and frequency spread is defined symmetrically as $\int_{-\infty}^{\infty} f^2 |G(f)|^2 dt$, then the function that minimizes frequency spread for a fixed time spread (with the size constraint $\int_{-\infty}^{\infty} |g(t)|^2 dt = 1$) is a Gaussian.

In analogy with the procedure we followed for the Slepian sequences, the minimization condition for the Gaussian leads to a eigenvalue problem, whose

---

18. The Slepian sequence can be extrapolated outside the window $t = 1 \cdots T$ by using equation 5.113 as the definition of the sequence outside of this window. This procedure in fact yields a sequence which is now extended over all time, but in turn strictly bandlimited.

solutions are given by the Hermite functions well known in physics. In a certain sense, therefore, the Slepian sequences are analogous to Hermite functions. Why not just use Hermite functions instead of the lesser known Slepian sequences? This might be useful in some circumstances; note, however, that the optimality properties of the Hermite functions no longer hold on a finite interval. Infinite ranges of time and frequency are mathematical fictions that are useful when doing analytical calculations, but must be treated with caution when dealing with finite time series data. The Slepian functions explicitly take into account the finiteness of the data window, and with modern day computers these are numerically no more difficult to compute than the Hermite functions.

5.5 Probability Theory

Probability theory is a branch of mathematics that formalizes the treatment of randomness or chance. It is important to note that a probabilistic formalism is not the only way to deal with uncertainty. There is an equivalent formulation in terms of game theory, where chance experiments may be regarded as "games with nature" in an appropriate formal sense. Another example is the use of set-based methods where the only structure imposed on uncertain parameters, which may vary in time, is that they belong to a given set, and performance guarantees are desired without imposing any further structure. Although these formulations will not appear in this book, the reader should be alerted that such alternative treatments do exist and have their domains of usage.

Probability theory has had a colorful history, including consultations between gamblers and mathematicians, analysis of the behavior of the stock market, and the building of instruments of war. It has also been intimately associated with twentieth century physics and biology. As a fully developed formal mathematical theory, it is relatively recent and dates to the middle of the twentieth century. There are different philosophical approaches that may be adopted when thinking about probability theory, and these can lead to heated debates that are not easy to resolve. The main fault line lies between what might be called the objective and subjective views: whether probabilities are objective properties of the external world that are at some level empirically accessible, or whether they reflect the subjective state of belief of a human observer. In this book we adopt an objective perspective following that of Kolmogorov, the famous Russian mathematician who formalized probability theory through an elegant set of axioms that remove philosophical uncertainties from the realms of probabilistic reasoning. Fortunately, however one conceptualizes what probabilities truly mean, Kolmogorov's formalism has been more or less universally adopted for mathematical manipulations involving probabilities.

The objective perspective overlaps with, but is not the same as, the so-called frequentist viewpoint in which probabilities are regarded as the limiting values of empirical frequencies of event occurrences. This view is articulated informally by Kolmogorov as follows (italics added):

> The assertion that the event A occurs under conditions S with a definite probability
>
> $$P(A|S) = p \qquad (5.114)$$
>
> amounts to saying that in a sufficiently long series of tests (i.e., realizations of the complex of conditions S) the frequencies
>
> $$v_r = \frac{\mu_r}{n_r} \qquad (5.115)$$
>
> of the occurrence of the event A (where n_r is the number of tests in the rth series, and μ^r is the number of tests of this series for which event A occurs) will be *approximately identical with one another* and will be *close to p.*
>
> The existence of constant $p = P(A | S)$ (objectively determined by the connection between the complex of conditions S and the event A) such that the frequencies v get closer "generally speaking" to p as the number of tests increase is well borne out in practice for a wide class of events.

The explicit emphasis placed on the "complex of conditions" S is worth noting: it is the relation between the event A and the background conditions S that determine the corresponding probabilities. Also, it is not necessary that all probabilities of interest be conceptualized this way; Kolmogorov is quick to point out in the same essay that once some basic probabilities have been established empirically, other probabilities may be deduced using the formal apparatus of probability theory. This does not resolve all the difficulties; although the above procedure is empirically pleasing, it is cumbersome as a formal means of defining probabilities. A more abstract but less cumbersome framework is provided by the set theoretic and measure theoretic setting for defining probabilities. We will outline the basic notions involved below without being formal.

However, before doing this we would like to note the other component of the objective view of probabilities that makes it more than just the frequentist view, which is the role of the laws of physics. Probabilistic laws are the bread and butter of much of modern physics, whether one thinks of quantum mechanics, where outcomes of experiments are fundamentally regarded as probabilistic, and the theoretical apparatus is used to compute these probabilities— or classical statistical mechanics, where probability theory is the natural mathematical framework, and which provides a bridge between deterministic microscopic dynamics and macroscopic thermodynamic behavior. Most physicists would agree that the laws of physics deal with objective reality,[19] subject

---

19. Including quantum mechanics, notwithstanding ongoing but unnecessary confusion about the role of a conscious observer.

to empirical falsification. In this sense, probabilities in physical law are objective quantities; nevertheless, they are part of a predictive, a priori theoretical framework and not necessarily regarded as the limiting values of empirical frequencies. This is not to say that the empirical procedure to determine probabilities in terms of frequencies will fail; on the contrary, it provides a route to verifying a particular physical law (for example, wave function amplitudes may be empirically measured from empirical frequencies of particle counts). Nevertheless, limiting frequencies and physical probabilities are both objective in nature and do not have to involve questions about states of belief.

We should note that probability theory certainly provides a consistent framework for reasoning; quantifying a set of subjective beliefs in probabilistic terms and deducing the consequences of these quantified beliefs using the machinery of probability theory is a coherent exercise, as long as one does not lose track of the self evident truth that what will come out of such an exercise will only be as good as what goes in. Consistent reasoning based on false premises will still lead to false conclusions, no matter how elegant and seductive the reasoning apparatus is in its mathematical precision.

5.5.1   Sample Space, Events, and Probability Axioms

In defining probabilities, one starts with some elementary concepts: sample spaces and events. The sample space is a set of "elementary events." The usual examples given in textbooks to illustrate sample spaces include the two element set (heads, tails) as the sample space for outcomes of a coin toss, the six-element set consisting of the numbers one through six, for outcomes of the throw of a die, and so on. In an idealized experimental measurement where the outcome is a real number, the sample space is the real line. In an experiment where the measurements are voltages, measured at discrete times in a finite interval with n time points, the sample space could be taken to be the n-dimensional space R^n.

Events, sometimes called compound events (to distinguish them from elementary events, which are the members of the sample space) are defined as subsets of the sample space. The idea is that even though what happens at any given time is an elementary event, we may not be interested in the precise identity of the event, but whether the event belongs to a particular well-defined class. For example, if the experiment consists of N tosses of a coin, the sample space is the set of binary sequences of length N (consider heads to be represented by 1 and tails to be represented by 0). We may be interested in the event that the number of heads is bigger than the number of tails, which is the subset of binary sequences of length N where the number of ones exceeds the number of zeros.

A probability "measure" is a function defined on the set of events, taking values in the interval [0 1], with certain properties to be outlined below. In the axiomatic framework devised by Kolmogorov, these axioms are quite simple and intuitive. Things are straightforward if the sample space Ω is finite dimensional. In such cases, the set of events is almost always taken to be the power set F of the sample space Ω. In words, all possible subsets of samples are allowed as events. Things become substantially more complicated if the sample space is infinite dimensional. Even for the elementary case where the sample space is the real line, constructing a set of events and a probability measure that satisfies our intuitions about probability is not in general trivial. In particular, in order to avoid paradoxical outcomes, it becomes necessary to restrict the events to which probabilities will be ascribed to some specific subsets of the sample space and not to allow other subsets. Matters are even more complicated formally when the elementary events themselves are stochastic processes or functions defined on the line, because one now has to consider sets of functions as events and ascribe probabilities to sets of functions. We simply point to these difficulties but will not enter into the details because the material is outside of the scope of this book. Fortunately, these more subtle considerations do not prevent us from proceeding in an elementary manner and obtaining the results of practical interest that concern us.

It is worthwhile to note that the theory of probability measures goes hand in hand with the theory of integration. Even though probabilities were first conceived in the context of chance experiments or occurrences, it is easiest to formalize them in terms that relate to integration. The difficulties in defining probabilities for infinite dimensional sample spaces and those of integrating functions defined on the same sets go hand in hand and have a common set of solutions. From this perspective, although probability theory originates in an attempt to mathematically formalize the notion of uncertainty, in the axiomatic framework for probability theory one can dispense with philosophical discussions about what uncertainty really means either in objective or subjective terms and still capture the formal essence of such discussions.

If one dispenses of the subtleties of defining the set of events, then Kolmogorov's axioms are very simple. The only requirements are that probabilities are real non-negative numbers not greater than one, that the whole sample space has probability one, and that probabilities for mutually exclusive events add.

- For all events $0 \leq P(E) \leq 1$
- For the whole sample space Ω, $P(\Omega) = 1$
- For the union of disjoint events $E_1 \cap E_2 = \phi$ the probabilities add, $P(E_1 \cup E_2) = P(E_1) + P(E_2)$

For infinite sample spaces, the last condition has to be extended over a countable infinity of events, $P(\cup_{i=1}^{\infty} E_i) = \sum_{i=1}^{\infty} P(E_i)$ if the events are mutually exclusive, $E_i \cap E_j = 0$ for any pair of events.

If $P(E_2) > 0$, then the conditional probability of event E_1 given E_2 is defined as

$$P(E_1 | E_2) = \frac{P(E_1 \cap E_2)}{P(E_2)} \tag{5.116}$$

From this definition, one immediately obtains Bayes' theorem,

$$P(E_1|E_2) = \frac{P(E_2|E_1)P(E_1)}{P(E_2)} \qquad (5.117)$$

The notion of independence is central to probability theory. Two events are said to be independent if the probability of joint occurrence of the events is the product of the corresponding event probabilities

$$P(E_1 \cap E_2) = P(E_1)P(E_2) \qquad (5.118)$$

If two events are independent, then $P(E_1|E_2) = P(E_1)$ and $P(E_2|E_1) = P(E_2)$.

5.5.2 Random Variables and Characteristic Function

After sample spaces and events, we come next to random variables. The phrase "random variable" is used in different contexts in the statistics literature, but we will adopt the standard definition that a random variable is a (typically real or complex valued) function defined on the sample space. This means that for each point in sample space, there is a unique value of the random variable. For example, for the sample space H, T, we could define the function σ such that $\sigma(H) = 1$ and $\sigma(T) = -1$. Here σ is a random variable. If the sample space is the real line, and the random variable is defined as the identity function $\sigma(x) = x$, then it seems pedantic to emphasize the distinction between the sample point or elementary event x, and the random variable $\sigma(x)$ that has the value x. Usually, such a formal distinction is not maintained.

If the sample space is finite, then a probability measure can be simply specified by listing the probabilities associated with each sample point (considered as elementary events). If the probabilities p_i of all sample points are added up the sum must be one, $\sum_i p_i = 1$. If the sample space is the real line, then one has to consider the subtleties indicated earlier when constructing probability measures. Without going into formal details, two types of probability measures will be sufficient for our discussions. The first type corresponds to cases where a *probability density function $p(x)$* can be defined, so that the probability of an event corresponding to the interval [a b] is given by $\int_a^b p(x)dx$. The second type corresponds to cases where isolated points have nonzero probability (which can also be thought of as having a set of delta functions for the probability density function). More generally, the probability density function can contain both a delta function part and a continuous part.[20]

---

20. Other kinds of densities are also possible; for example, one could define a probability measure that lives on a fractal set with nonintegral dimension, such as the Cantor set in one dimension. This does not correspond to either of the cases noted in the text. Such probability measures are relevant more as mathematical curiosities than models of natural phenomena, although some phenomena may indeed be concisely modeled using such measures.

Given a random variable, one defines the mean or expectation value $E[X]$ of the random variable with respect to a probability measure by taking the integral of the random variable over the sample space with respect to the probability measure. For a finite sample space, the expectation of a random variable X_i is given by

$$E[X] = \sum_{i=1}^{N} p_i X_i \qquad (5.119)$$

The expectation is a linear functional, and because it involves multiplication by non-negative numbers and integration, it preserves inequalities, so that

$$E[aX + bY] = aE[X] + bE[Y] \qquad (5.120)$$
$$X \leq Y \rightarrow E[X] \leq E[Y] \qquad (5.121)$$

The moments of a random variable X are defined as the expectations of powers of the random variable, $\mu_n = E[X^n]$. The variance is defined as $E[|X - E(X)|^2]$, and is a measure of departure from the mean. The covariance between two random variables X and Y is defined as $cov(X, Y) = E[(X - E[X])(Y - E[Y])]$.[21] Two random variables are said to be uncorrelated if their covariance is zero.

In analogy with independent events, two random variables X, Y are said to be independent if the distribution of X conditional on Y does not depend on Y, and vice versa: $P(X | Y) = P(X)$ and $P(Y | X) = P(Y)$. Independence is a much stronger condition than decorrelation and therefore harder to satisfy.

The moments of a random variable X can all be computed from the *moment-generating* function or the *characteristic function* $F(k)$ corresponding to the random variable, defined as

$$F(k) = E[e^{-ikX}] \qquad (5.122)$$

Note that the characteristic function is precisely the Fourier transform of the probability distribution corresponding to the random variable. The reader can easily verify that

$$i^n \frac{d^n F(k)}{dk^n}\Big|_{k=0} = \mu_n = E[X^n] \qquad (5.123)$$

Assuming a moment exists, it can be obtained by taking the appropriate derivative of the characteristic function and setting the argument to zero. The characteristic function is also used to define the cumulants of the distribution κ_n,

$$\kappa_n = i^n \frac{d^n \log (F(k))}{dk^n}\Big|_{k=0} \qquad (5.124)$$

---

21. For simplicity we have implicitly assumed that the variables are real; if they are complex, then one typically defines $cov(X, Y) = E[(X - E[X])^*(Y - E[Y])]$.

The relation between the moments and the cumulants may be computed by using the above expressions. Note that the second cumulant is the variance. The first few cumulants are given by

$$\kappa_1 = \mu_1 \tag{5.125}$$

$$\kappa_2 = \mu_2 - \mu_1^2 \tag{5.126}$$

$$\kappa_3 = \mu_3 - 3\mu_1\mu_2 + 2\mu_1^3 \tag{5.127}$$

$$\kappa_4 = \mu_4 - 4\mu_3\mu_1 - 3\mu_2^2 + 12\mu_1^2\mu_2 - 6\mu_1^4 \tag{5.128}$$

The lower order cumulants can be used to summarize the overall shape of the probability distribution. The variance $\kappa_2 = \sigma^2$ measures the width of the distribution. The third cumulant can be normalized to obtain a measure of "skewness," κ_3/σ^3. Similarly, the fourth cumulant is used to define the "kurtosis," κ_4/σ^4. This is a measure of the "flatness" or "peakiness" of the distribution.

Given two random variables X and Y one can define a third random variable $E[Y|X]$, the *conditional expectation* of Y given X. Note that this is a random variable that depends on the value of X. Conditional expectations generalize the notion of conditional probabilities to random variables.

Two random variables are said to be independent if the joint probability distribution of the two is equal to the product of the individual probability distributions, $P(X, Y) = P_1(X)P_2(Y)$. The characteristic function of the sum of two independent random variables, is therefore the product of the individual characteristic functions:

$$E[e^{-it(X+Y)}] = E[e^{-itX}]E[e^{-itY}] \tag{5.129}$$

From this it is easy to show that the characteristic function of the sum of n independent random variables with the same distribution is the nth power of the individual characteristic function, a result that will be used later to prove the central limit theorem: if X_i are independent random variables with the characteristic function $F(t)$, then the sum $\sum_{i=1}^{n} X_i$ has the characteristic function

$$F_{sum}(t) = F(t)^n \tag{5.130}$$

Finally, for a discrete probability measure specified by the probabilities $p_1, p_2, \ldots, p_n$, one defines the entropy $H(p)$ as

$$H(p) = -\sum_i p_i \log(p_i) \tag{5.131}$$

Note that the base of the logarithm is a matter of convention, if it is taken in base 2 then the entropy is in "bits," where if it is the natural logarithm, then the entropy is in "nats." The entropy is a theoretical quantity of fundamental importance and measures the uniformity or "randomness" of the probability measure. If all points in the sample space of size n are equally likely, then

$H(p) = \log(n)$. On the other extreme, of the probability measure is concentrated on only one point, then $H(p) = 0$. All other probability measures on the same sample space have their entropies between 0 and $\log(n)$.

Another quantity of theoretical importance, defined for a pair of probability measures p and q, is the Kullback-Leiber (KL) divergence $D(p\|q)$. This is an asymmetrically defined quantity given for discrete probability distributions by

$$D(p\|q) = \sum_i p_i \log (p_i/q_i) \tag{5.132}$$

It can be shown that $D(p\|q) \geq 0$, equality being achieved only when $p = q$. The KL divergence is like a distance but lacks an important defining property of distances or norms, namely it does not satisfy the triangle inequality. Therefore, although of theoretical importance, it should not be interpreted as a distance between probability distributions. One can also define a symmetrized quantity, $D(p\|q) + D(q\|p)$.

5.5.3 Some Common Probability Measures

In this subsection we discuss three of the most commonly encountered probability measures. Rather than talk about the underlying probability measures, it is customary to talk about the probability distributions of random variables. Recall that the random variables are functions, with the sample space being the domain of the function. The probability measures in the sample space "induce" corresponding measures in the space in which the random variables take their values. These are called the probability distributions of the corresponding random variable.

Bernoulli and Binomial Distributions

The Bernoulli distribution corresponds to the simplest nontrivial sample space, with two elements, which could be the two sides of a coin, the two responses in a two-alternative forced choice task, success or failure in some binary trial, and so on. The probabilities corresponding to the two outcomes are p and $1 - p$, where p is the single parameter characterizing the distribution. Define the random variable X with value 1 for the first outcome (e.g., success, heads). Then $E[X] = p$, the variance $V[X] = p(1 - p)$, and the entropy of the distribution is given by $H(p) = -p\log(p) - (1 - p) \log(1 - p)$. The variance and the entropy are both maximum when $p = 1/2$.

The binomial distribution corresponds to a repeated sequence of independent Bernoulli trials, which could be used to model a sequence of coin tosses, a series of choices in a psychophysical experiment offering two alternatives, and so on. Let the random variable X denote the number of trials in which the first alternative occurs (we will label these trials as successful trials). Assuming that the individual Bernoulli probabilities are all p and there are n trials, the probability distribution of the total number of successful trials X, which takes integer values ranging from 0 and n, is given by

$$P(X = m) = \binom{n}{m} p^m (1-p)^{n-m} \tag{5.133}$$

This distribution is illustrated for $p = 0.3$ and $n = 10$ in figure 5.12. The mean and variance of X can be worked out to be $E(X) = np$ and $V(X) = np(1-p)$. Consider the random variable X/n, the fraction of successful trials, $E(X/n) = p$, and $V(X/n) = p(1-p)/n$. It should be noted that as n becomes large with p fixed, the fraction of successful trials goes to a fixed value given by p, and the variance of this fraction goes to zero. For a large number of trials, therefore, the *fraction of successful trials* converges to the *probability of a successful trial*. This is a preliminary example of the law of large numbers which will be treated in some more detail in the next section.

The characteristic function of the binomial distribution is easy to compute. By definition, the characteristic function is given by

$$F(t) = \sum_{m=0}^{m=n} \binom{n}{m} p^m (1-p)^{n-m} e^{-itm} \tag{5.134}$$

The reader should show (using the binomial expansion formula) that

$$F(t) = ((1-p) + pe^{-it})^n \tag{5.135}$$

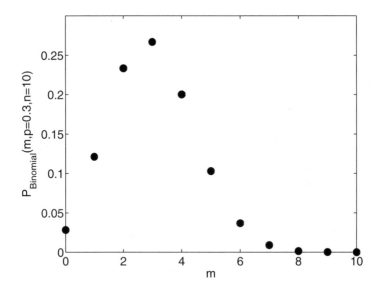

Figure 5.12: The binomial distribution illustrated for $p = 0.3$ and $n = 10$.

- By taking derivatives of the characteristic function, compute the first three moments of the binomial distribution.
- Compute the skewness of the binomial distribution, and plot it as a function of p for fixed n as well as a function of n for fixed p.
- Show that the characteristic function of the sum of two binomial random variables with parameters (n_1, p) and (n_2, p) is the characteristic function of another binomial distribution with parameter $(n_1 + n_2, p)$.

The Poisson and the Gaussian distributions may both be regarded as limiting cases of the binomial distribution. This is interesting because it shows how all three widely used distributions may be built up, starting from the elementary Bernoulli distribution with only two alternatives. This observation is useful to keep in mind when dealing with stochastic processes, where one can start with discrete time bins, each containing zero or one points, and can build up a Poisson or a Gaussian process through appropriate coarse-graining procedures.

Poisson Distributions

We first consider the Poisson limit. This corresponds to taking $n \to \infty$ and $p \to 0$ while keeping np fixed at some value, $np = \Lambda$. In words, this is the limit of a large number of Bernoulli trials where the probability of success in each individual trial becomes vanishingly small. Because $E(X) = np$ and $V(X) = np(1 - p)$ for the binomial distribution, we can read off that $E(X) = \Lambda$ and $V(X) = \Lambda$ for the Poisson distribution. The characteristic function of the Poisson distribution, defined through this limiting procedure, can be worked out as follows (set $p = \Lambda/n$ in the above formula for the characteristic function of the binomial distribution):

$$F_{Poisson}(t) = \lim_{n \to \infty} \left(1 + (e^{-it} - 1)\frac{\Lambda}{n}\right)^n = \exp\left(\Lambda(e^{-it} - 1)\right) \qquad (5.136)$$

Expanding the exponential, we can get the characteristic function of the Poisson distribution:

$$F_{Poisson}(t) = e^{-\Lambda} \sum_{n=0}^{\infty} \frac{\Lambda^n}{n!} e^{-itn} \qquad (5.137)$$

So that the distribution is given by

$$P_{Poisson}(X = n) = e^{-\Lambda} \frac{\Lambda^n}{n!} \qquad (5.138)$$

Note that the Poisson distribution is characterized by a single parameter, and the mean and variance are equal. In fact, as the reader can show, all cumulants are equal; this fact also uniquely characterizes the distribution. Also, by multiplying the characteristic functions together, it can be seen that the sum of two independent Poisson variables with parameters Λ_1 and Λ_2 is also a Poisson distribution with parameter $\Lambda_1 + \Lambda_2$.

Gaussian Distributions

A second limiting case can be obtained from the binomial distribution by letting $n \to \infty$ while keeping p finite. In this case, both the mean and the variance diverges, so a normalization procedure has to be adopted to keep them finite. How should this normalization work? This is dictated by the form of the variance; it is straightforward to verify that for a binomial random variable X with parameters (n, p), if we define a rescaled random variable Y as

$$Y = \sigma \frac{X - np}{\sqrt{np(1-p)}} \qquad (5.139)$$

Then $E(Y) = 0$ and $V(Y) = \sigma$. What is the limiting probability distribution of Y as $n \to \infty$? To answer this question, we start with the characteristic function of Y. The reader should show, starting from the characteristic function of the binomial distribution, that this is given by

$$E[e^{-itY}] = \left(1 - p + p \exp\left(-i \frac{\sigma t}{\sqrt{np(1-p)}} \right) \right)^n \exp\left(it\sigma\sqrt{np/(1-p)} \right) \quad (5.140)$$

In order to take the limit corresponding to large n, it is convenient to take the logarithm of the above expression and to expand the argument of the logarithm. This yields

$$\log\left(E[e^{-itY}] \right) = it\sigma\sqrt{np/(1-p)}$$
$$+ n \log\left[1 - p + p\left(1 - i \frac{\sigma t}{\sqrt{np(1-p)}} - \frac{(\sigma t)^2}{2np(1-p)} + O\left(\frac{1}{n^{3/2}} \right) \right) \right]$$
$$(5.141)$$

The logarithm can be expanded, and it is left as an exercise to the reader to show that for large n,

$$\log\left(E[e^{-itY}] \right) = -\frac{1}{2}t^2\sigma^2 + O\left(\frac{1}{\sqrt{n}} \right) \qquad (5.142)$$

Thus, the limiting characteristic function of the normalized and mean-subtracted success rate Y is given by

$$E[e^{-itY}]) = e^{-\frac{1}{2}t^2\sigma^2} \qquad (5.143)$$

Fourier transforming the characteristic function, we obtain the Gaussian probability density function

$$p(Y) = \frac{1}{\sqrt{2\pi\sigma^2}} e^{-\frac{y^2}{2\sigma^2}} \qquad (5.144)$$

We have therefore shown that for fixed p and large n, after appropriate scaling the distribution of a binomial random variable tends to the Gaussian distribution. This is a special case of the Central Limit Theorem, which underlies that widespread appearance of the Gaussian distribution in a number of natural phenomena. This theorem will be further discussed in a later section; we now continue our discussion of random variables with a Gaussian distribution.

As can be seen from the characteristic function, all cumulants of the Gaussian distribution with order higher than two vanish, and the distribution is fully specified by its first two cumulants (or equivalently, the first two moments. This will be useful when defining stochastic processes; the Gaussian stochastic process is completely specified by its first and second moments, which in turn can be estimated from observations. To make the connection, it is useful to study the properties of a multivariate Gaussian distribution, where the random variable $\mathbf{X}$ is now a real or complex vector. The probability distribution function of a real multivariate Gaussian distribution with mean μ and covariance matrix C is given by

$$p(\mathbf{X}) = K \exp -\frac{1}{2}(\mathbf{X}-\mu)^{\dagger} C^{-1}(\mathbf{X}-\mu) \qquad (5.145)$$

The random variable X is a real n dimensional vector. For the probability distribution to be well defined, it is required that C be a positive definite Hermitian matrix. This means that $C^{\dagger} = C$, and that $\mathbf{X}^{\dagger} C \mathbf{X} > 0$ for all non-zero $\mathbf{X}$. The normalization constant K is given by $K = \det(2\pi C)^{-1/2} = (2\pi)^{-n/2}\det(C)^{-1/2}$. The matrix C is the so-called covariance matrix of the Gaussian distribution and is equal to the covariance defined in analogy with the one-dimensional case,

$$C_{ij} = cov(X_i, X_j) = E[(X_i - \mu_i)(X_j - \mu_j)] \qquad (5.146)$$

For notational simplicity, let us assume that the distribution has zero mean, $\mu = 0$. The characteristic function of the multivariate Gaussian distribution is defined analogous to the one-dimensional case and is given by

$$E[e^{-i\mathbf{J}^{\dagger}\mathbf{X}}] = \exp\left(-\frac{1}{2}\mathbf{J}^{\dagger}C\mathbf{J}\right) \qquad (5.147)$$

In analogy with the one-dimensional case, note that all moments of the multivariate Gaussian distribution are given by the covariance matrix (we have assumed that the mean is zero). A particularly simple case is when the covariance matrix is diagonal; in this case, the multivariate Gaussian distribution becomes the product of univariate distributions. Since the covariance matrix is Hermitian, it can be diagonalized by a suitable choice of basis for the vectors $\mathbf{X}$. In a statistical context, the eigenvectors of the matrix C are called principal components; clearly, the eigenbasis of the covariance matrix is a useful basis to work in, because one can then work simply with univariate distributions. However, sometimes it is easier to work with a nondiagonal covariance matrix.

So far, we have dealt with real random variables. It is also very useful to work with complex random variables and define probability distributions on the complex plane, or more generally, work with complex vectors. The reader can think of a complex random variable as a pair of real random variables. Usage of complex notation can simplify calculations, although care must be exercised in interpreting integrals over complex random variables. In the present context, all such integrals should be interpreted as separate integrals over the real and imaginary parts of the variable. For example, consider the Gaussian distribution of a single complex random variable $z = x + iy$

$$p(z) = \frac{1}{\pi S} e^{-\frac{|z|^2}{S}} \tag{5.148}$$

This can be thought of as a short-hand notation for the bivariate real Gaussian distribution

$$p(x, y) = \frac{1}{\pi S} e^{-\frac{x^2 + y^2}{S}} \tag{5.149}$$

The reader should verify as an exercise that $\int dz p(z) = 1$ with the convention $dz \equiv dx dy$ noted above, with the integral extending over the entire complex plane. Note also that $E[|z|^2] = S$, so the distribution is parameterized with respect to the variance of the complex variable z. Note the slight difference in the form of the distribution compared to the univariate real Gaussian: some factors of 2 are missing. More generally, a complex multivariate Gaussian distribution may be defined, for the complex vector $\mathbf{Z}$, mean μ, and covariance matrix S

$$p(\mathbf{Z}) = K \exp -(\mathbf{Z} - \mu)^\dagger S^{-1} (\mathbf{Z} - \mu) \tag{5.150}$$

Where the normalization constant $K = [\pi^n \det(S)]^{-1}$. Note that $p(\mathbf{Z})$ is real and nonnegative, even though $\mathbf{Z}$ is a complex vector; this is of course necessary for the probability distribution to be well defined.[22] The correlation structure of the Gaussian variable $\mathbf{Z}$ is captured by the covariance matrix S, and one way to examine this correlation structure is to diagonalize S and examine the ei- genvalues s_j, which are real and nonnegative by construction. The set of these eigenvalues constitutes the *spectrum* of the covariance matrix. Consider two extreme cases: if only one eigenvalue is nonzero, and the rest zero, then the variables are maximally correlated. On the other hand, if all eigenvalues are equal, the spectrum is "white," and the variables are maximally uncorrelated. These concepts will go over directly to the treatment of stochastic processes.

One can define a measure of how close the spectrum is to a white spectrum by taking the ratio W of the geometric mean (GM) to the arithmetic mean (AM) of the eigenvalues.

---

22. It should be noted that although probabilities cannot be complex, measures *can*; this is a reminder that probability measures are special kinds of measures or that the notion of measure is a nontrivial generalization of the notion of probability.

$$W = \frac{(\prod_{i=1}^{n} \lambda_i)^{\frac{1}{n}}}{\frac{1}{n}\sum_{i=1}^{n} \lambda_i} \qquad (5.151)$$

$$\log(W) = \frac{1}{n}\sum_{i=1}^{n} \log(\lambda_i) - \log\left(\frac{1}{n}\sum_{i=1}^{n} \lambda_I\right) \qquad (5.152)$$

Because $GM \leq AM$, this ratio W is a number between zero and one, and in the context of spectral analysis is known as the "Wiener entropy."[23] The logarithm of W may be more convenient to deal with, and can be interpreted as the KL divergence between the Gaussian distribution, and a white Gaussian distribution with the same "total power" (i.e., $E[|\mathbf{Z}|^2]$. We will use this to measure the "whiteness" of Gaussian stochastic processes.

5.5.4   Law of Large Numbers

The law of large numbers or the law of averages provides a precise way to relate probabilities to empirical frequencies. In its weak form, the law states that the arithmetic average of a sequence of uncorrelated random variables X_i with identical mean μ and variance σ^2 (assumed finite) tends to μ with probability one. In more precise terms, for any small ε,

$$\lim_{n\to\infty} P(|\bar{X}_n - \mu| < \varepsilon) = 1 \qquad (5.153)$$

This confirms the intuitively plausible idea that averaging over many independent trials reduces stochastic fluctuations, and the average tends to the underlying mean value of the random variable in question. The proof is quite simple and employs an important inequality due to Tchebychev, so we will present it here, starting with the proof of the Tchebychev inequality ($\theta(x)$ is the step function, $\theta(x) = 0$ for $x < 0$ and $\theta(x) = 1$ for $x \geq 1$):

$$\theta(|Y| - 1) \leq |Y|^2$$
$$\Rightarrow E(\theta(|Y| - 1)) \leq E(|Y|^2)$$
$$\Rightarrow P(|Y| \geq 1) \leq E(|Y|^2)$$

Substituting $Y = (X - E(X))/c$, where c is an arbitrary positive constant, and noting that the variance $V(X) = E(|X - E(X)|^2) = E(|Y|^2)$, we obtain

$$P(|X - E(X)| \geq c) \leq \frac{1}{c^2} V(X) \qquad (5.154)$$

Now substitute $\bar{X}_n = \frac{1}{n}\sum_{i=1}^{n} X_i$ for X. Note that the assumption that X_i are uncorrelated, with mean μ and variance σ^2, implies that $E(X) = \mu$ and $V(X) =$

---

23. The logarithm of the ratio of arithmetic to geometric means also appears in the Bartlett M-ratio statistic for testing the homogeneity of variance.

σ^2/n. Substituting the corresponding quantities in the inequality above and replacing c by ε, we obtain

$$P(|\hat{X}_n - \mu| \geq \varepsilon) \leq \frac{\sigma^2}{n\varepsilon^2} \qquad (5.155)$$

Noting that $P(|\hat{X}_n - \mu| \leq \varepsilon) = 1 - P(|\hat{X}_n - \mu| \geq \varepsilon)$, we obtain

$$P(|\hat{X}_n - \mu| \leq \varepsilon) \geq 1 - \frac{\sigma^2}{n\varepsilon^2} \qquad (5.156)$$

Letting n go to infinity, we get the weak law of large numbers stated above. Now consider a repeated sequence of identical experiments (trials) performed independently from each other, where the probability of a given event occurring in any of the trials is p. For the ith trial, define the random variable $X_i = 1$ if the event occurs, and $X_i = 0$ otherwise. This is a Bernoulli random variable, as discussed earlier, and $E(X_i) = p$, $V(X_i) = p(1 - p)$ and $cov(X_i, X_j) = 0$. Therefore, the random variables X_i satisfy the conditions of the weak law of large numbers. Further, the average of X_i over all trials is nothing but the empirical frequency $f_n = r/n$ where r is the number of times the desired event occurred in n trials. We therefore obtain

$$\lim_{n \to \infty} P(|f_n - p| < \varepsilon) = 1 \qquad (5.157)$$

Therefore, as the number of trials goes to infinity, the difference between the empirical frequency f_n and the event probability p goes to zero with probability one.

5.5.5 Central Limit Theorems

We saw earlier how the Gaussian distribution may arise as a limiting case of the Binomial distribution: the average value of a large number of Bernoulli distributed variables eventually becomes Gaussian distributed. This is a special case of the central limit theorem: under appropriate conditions, the rescaled mean of a large number of random variables becomes Gaussian distributed. Here we will consider the simplest case of N independent variables X_i that have identical distributions $p(X)$. Instead of dealing with the probability distributions, it is simpler to work with the characteristic functions $F(t) = E[e^{-itX}]$. The characteristic distribution of the rescaled sum of two variables is given by

$$F_{sum}(t) = E[e^{-it(X_1 + X_2)/h}] = E[e^{-itX/h}]^2 = F(t/h)^2 \qquad (5.158)$$

A natural question is, what are the *stable* distributions, such that characteristic function of the rescaled sum of variables is the same as that of the variables themselves (mathematically, $F_{sum}(t) = F(t)$)? For this to happen, one requires that $\log(F(t)) = 2\log(F(t/h))$, which means that after rescaling, $\log(F(t))$ should retain its form. It can be seen by inspection that this will happen if

$\log(F(t)) = c|t|^\alpha$, for constants c and α that do not depend on t. In fact, it can be shown that this exhausts all the possibilities for obtaining stable distributions. The Gaussian distribution corresponds to the case $\alpha = 2$, because $\log(F(t)) \propto t^2$. If the distribution has finite variance, then the second derivative of the characteristic function with respect to t is well defined at the origin; this constrains α to be two. Therefore, the only stable distribution with finite variance is precisely the Gaussian distribution!

The distributions that correspond to more general values of α are the so-called Levy distributions. The case $\alpha = 1$ is particularly simple because it corresponds to a Lorentzian distribution, $p(x) \sim (1 + ax^2)^{-1}$. Note that it does not have a finite variance. Distributions without finite variance are pathological, because physical causes will always provide an appropriate cutoff for the value of the random variable; however, such distributions may occasionally be useful to model "heavy tailed" distributions, where large values of the random variable are rare, but occur more frequently than a Gaussian distribution would imply. It can be shown that the Levy laws are defined for $0 < \alpha < 2$, and for these values of α the distribution falls off as $X^{-(1+\alpha)}$ for large values of X.

So far, we have considered stable distributions that maintain their form when the corresponding random variables are added together. What happens to more general random variables on addition? It turns out that the resulting sum, when rescaled appropriately, tends to one of the stable distributions. As long as the variance is finite, this limiting distribution is the Gaussian; the reader is invited to prove this following the lines of the argument for the binomial case discussed earlier. This captures most cases of practical interest. If the variables in question do not have a finite variance, then the limiting distribution will be one of the Levy laws, depending on how rapidly the original distribution decays at large values of X.

5.6 Stochastic Processes

Stochastic processes are fundamental to the analysis of neural signals, because in many applications the signals are theoretically modeled as stochastic processes. Canonical examples include extracellular and intracellular voltage time series, spike trains, sequences of images, or behavioral time series. There are two broad classes of stochastic processes that are relevant for our discussion—continuous processes such as voltage time courses, where the observed quantity varies continuously with time, or point processes, such as a sequence of spike times. Needless to say, our observations are collected and analyzed using digital computers, time is always on a discrete grid, and variables can only take discrete values. The mathematical fictions of real valued functions of continuous time and point processes where time points are chosen from the real line rather than from a discrete grid, are of course conceptually convenient. However, a discrete treatment of time has more to it than just being an artifact imposed on us by the limitations of our computational devices. In fact, it allows us to avoid difficulties in treating stochastic processes that are functions of continuous time.

5.6.1 Defining Stochastic Processes

The definition of a stochastic process in a formal setting such as an advanced text on probability theory is quite formidable. The formal treatment of even elementary facts about well-known stochastic processes can be impenetrably abstruse to the uninitiated reader. In keeping with the tone of this book, our discussion will be informal and elementary. The formal difficulties can be entirely avoided by keeping everything discrete and finite and taking appropriate limits; this is the attitude usually adopted in statistical physics, where stochastic processes are basic to much of the subject matter. In fact, such discretization and limiting procedures are the easiest ways of understanding the formal difficulties and of circumventing them.

There are two ways of thinking about a stochastic process $x(t)$. One way is to think of the process as a random variable that takes values in some function space; the whole process $x(t)$ is a single random variable. A second way is to think of the process as a collection, or family, of random variables $x(t)$, one for each time; it is to be understood that there is an underlying sample space, such that for each choice of the underlying elementary event in the sample space, the whole collection of random variables $x(t)$ is simultaneously determined. The first view is usually adopted in the statistical physics literature, whereas the second view is more frequently encountered in the statistics literature. We will illustrate the difference in the two perspectives with an example.

Stochastic Processes as High-Dimensional Random Variables

In keeping with our discussion about discretizing time, let us think about a voltage measurement, carried out for a finite time interval. This gives us a vector of numbers, $V_j = V(j\Delta t)$, where Δt is the discrete time grid, and $j = 1 \dots N$, where $N\Delta t = T$, the observation interval. Therefore, a voltage time series in this discrete, finite setting can be thought of as a vector valued random variable, with values in R^n. Recall that a random variable is a function defined on a sample space; however, it is convenient to dispense with the sample space in most discussions and deal only with the probability distributions of the random variables in question. Therefore, in specifying a stochastic process to model the voltage waveform, we need to specify a probability distribution $p_N(V_1, V_2, \dots, V_N)$ in an N-dimensional space.

This is the first view described above. This view makes it clear why doing statistical analysis with stochastic processes presents inherent difficulties: there is no hope of estimating such high-dimensional distributions from experimental observations without making strong assumptions. Note that given the N-dimensional distribution of the vector $(V_1, V_2, \ldots, V_N)$, one can obtain the marginal distributions[24] of a subset of the vector indices; in particular one can obtain the distributions of the marginals $p(V_1), p(V_2), \ldots, p(V_j)$. Note however that this procedure cannot be reversed in general: information is lost in going from the full N dimensional distribution to the one dimensional marginals $p(V_j)$. This is a very important point that is not always well appreciated, and conflation of the full distribution with the marginals can lead to serious conceptual error. For example, if one were interested in evaluating the entropy of the original distribution, this cannot in general be done by obtaining the entropies of the marginal distributions. The one dimensional marginals can be estimated from a reasonable amount of data, but the high dimensional distribution is pretty much hopeless to estimate.

Subtleties in Taking the Continuum Limit

The discussion so far has been elementary, in the sense that the probability distribution associated with a discretized, finite length stochastic process can be regarded simply as a multivariate probability distribution. If we now let the time spacing shrink to zero, we get a hint of the kind of formal difficulty that may arise in the continuous time limit. For example, let us consider the probability distribution $p(V_1, V_2, \ldots, V_N)$, where each V_i is uniformly and independently distributed over the interval $[0 \ V_{max}]$. For finite N, the distribution is given simply by the normalization constant, $p(V_1, V_2, \ldots, V_N) = 1/V_{max}^N$. However, if we now let N go to infinity, then the normalization constant is well defined only if $V_{max} = 1$; otherwise it is zero, or infinity. This is a hint that there are constraints in what kind of probability distributions may be well defined in the large N limit. Moreover, there are constraints on what kind of events can be ascribed nonzero probability. For example, consider the event that some of the V_is are constrained to the interval $[0 \ 1/2]$ and the rest range over the entire interval $[0 \ 1]$. Clearly, only a finite number of V_i's may be so constrained; otherwise, we would end up with driving the probability of the event to zero. These are only indications of the complexities that may arise in the $\Delta t \to 0$ limit, and further discussion is beyond the scope of this text. Fortunately, for a very important class of processes (namely Gaussian stochastic processes) to be discussed in further detail below, the formalism can be satisfactorily worked out in the continuous time limit, and most practical questions relating to such processes can be answered without having to resort to technical subtleties.

---

24. The marginal distributions are those obtained from the original distribution by integrating out some of the variables.

Stochastic Processes as Indexed Families of Random Variables

To discuss the second perspective where a stochastic process is regarded as a family of random variables, it is necessary to keep explicit track of the underlying sample space Ω. Recall that a random variable is defined as a function defined on Ω; a real valued random variable is real function $x(\omega)$, where $\omega \in \Omega$. A stochastic process can be defined as a collection or family of random variables $x_t(\omega)$, where t belongs to a continuous time interval $[0\ T]$ or to a discrete index set $t = 0, 1, 2, \ldots$. So in distinction with the first approach, where the process is a single random variable, taking its value in a space of functions, here we have a whole set of random variables. Note, however, that the random variables are not necessarily independent; once we have picked the sample point ω, the entire collection of variables $x_t(\omega)$ now have well defined values. Superficially, this perspective seems to simplify things a lot, because we now have to apparently deal with random variables that are individual real numbers rather than whole functions. Unfortunately, this simplicity is deceptive: we have hidden the complexity of defining the sample space Ω. For example, in analogy with the previously discussed example, a suitable sample space would be R^n, and each sample or elementary event would be a vector in R^n. The collection of random variables would be given by the coordinates of this vector. So we are back to the problems with high-dimensional spaces. However, this second approach does have its advantages; for example, we could choose the sample space Ω to be finite and still allow $x_t(\omega)$ to be continuous functions of time chosen from some appropriate function space.

How to specify the probability distribution of a stochastic process x_t with a continuous time parameter? It would be nice if this could be done by specifying the set of finite dimensional distributions $p(x(t_1), x(t_2), \ldots, x(t_n))$, for all finite, ordered sets of points $t_i | t_1 \leq t_2 \leq t_3 \ldots$ It turns out that this can indeed be done, as long as an intuitive consistency condition (due to Kolmogorov) is satisfied: clearly, the distribution for n points should equal the appropriate marginal of the distribution for $n + m$ points. Therefore, these finite dimensional distributions cannot be chosen arbitrarily. In the simple case of the finite dimensional example given above, this simply means that the marginal distributions have all to be consistent with the full distribution for N points. The infinite dimensional case is more subtle, but nevertheless comes along with the same consistency requirements.

5.6.2   Time Translational Invariance

If we do an experiment repeatedly, and there is some stochastic element to the outcome, we do not in general expect the results to be exactly the same every time. However, we would hardly be in the business of doing science if *something* about the outcome were not repeatable. This is the idea behind time translation invariance of a stochastic process. Supposing we are given a realization of a stochastic process $x(t)$. Consider the process $x(t+T)$ given by a shift in the time origin. As long as the experimental conditions remained relatively constant, one would expect that shifting the time origin would not make a difference. This cannot of course be interpreted to mean that the function itself remains the same; this would be only possible if $x(t+T) = x(t)$, which would imply (assuming the relation holds for all T) that $x(t)$ is a constant independent of time. Such a process possesses time translational invariance but is not a particularly interesting process. A more useful criterion is that whereas a particular $x(t)$ has a time dependence, its statistical properties are time independent. For example, one would ask that $E[x(t+T)] = E[x(t)]$, which would mean that the average value of the process is time invariant. Similarly, one would expect the second moment of the process to satisfy $E[x(t'+T)x(t'+T)] = E[x(t)x(t')]$. This condition implies that the second moment depends only on the time difference, $E[x(t)x(t')] = E[x(t-t')x(0)]$.

The above discussion motivates the definition of a stationary process. A stationary stochastic process is one with a probability distribution that is left invariant by a time shift. This can be specified by requiring that all moments are time shift invariant (which also implies that the nth order correlation function depends on $n-1$ time differences):

$$E[x(t+T)] = E[x(t)] \tag{5.159}$$

$$E[x(t+T)x(t'+T)] = E[x(t)x(t')] \tag{5.160}$$

$$E[x(t_1+T)x(t_2+T)\ldots x(t_n+T)] = E[x(t_1)x(t_2)\ldots x(t_n)] \tag{5.161}$$

5.6.3   Ergodicity

A more demanding condition than time translational invariance is that of ergodicity. A process is said to be ergodic if averages over the probability distribution of the process, or ensemble averages, are equivalent to time averages. Again, this condition can be given in terms of the moments of the process:

$$\lim_{T \to \infty} \frac{1}{T} \int_0^T x(t+T) = E[x(t)] \tag{5.162}$$

$$\lim_{T \to \infty} \frac{1}{T} \int_0^T x(t+T)x(t'+T) = E[x(t)x(t')] \tag{5.163}$$

$$\lim_{T \to \infty} \frac{1}{T} \int_0^T x(t_1+T)x(t_2+T)\cdots x(t_n+T) = E[x(t_1)x(t_2)\cdots x(t_n)] \tag{5.164}$$

Because one only has experimental access to time averages, ergodicity is a condition that is often assumed in the statistical analysis of stochastic processes.

However, one can easily imagine realistic processes which are not ergodic; one simple example of a time translational invariant process which is not ergodic, is given simply by $x(t) = constant$, with a different choice of the constant for different samples of the process (for example, consider the stochastic process obtained by observing the height of an individual over time). Clearly, the time average is not equal to the ensemble average unless the ensemble has only one constant in it.

5.6.4 Time Translation Invariance and Spectral Analysis

Time translational invariance of a stochastic process directly leads us to spectral analysis. The reason behind this is that the exponential function is an eigenfunction of the time translation operator. What does this statement mean? Let us define the operator $\mathcal{T}x(t) = x(t+T)$. Then it is easy to verify that e^{at} satisfies $\mathcal{T}e^{at} = e^{a(t+T)} = e^{aT}e^{at}$. Therefore, the function $x(t) = e^{at}$ satisfies the eigenvalue equation $\mathcal{T}x(t) = \lambda x(t)$, where $\lambda = e^{aT}$. This means in particular that the Fourier basis is an eigenbasis of the time translation operator. Now consider the second moment of the stochastic process—in the Fourier basis, $E[X(f)^*X(f')]$ instead of the time basis. If the process is time translation invariant, then the second moment should be left unchanged under a time translation; this means that $E[\mathcal{T}X(f)^*\mathcal{T}X(f')] = E[X(f)^*X(f')]$. However, we have $\mathcal{T}X(f) = e^{-2\pi i f T}X(f)$. These two equations together imply that

$$e^{2\pi i(f-f')T}E[X(f)^*X(f')] = E[X(f)^*X(f')] \qquad (5.165)$$

For $f \neq f'$, in general $e^{2\pi i(f-f')T} \neq 1$, so that this equation can be satisfied only if $E[X(f)^*X(f')] = 0$. Therefore, we conclude that for a time translation invariant stochastic process, $E[X(f)^*X(f')] = 0$ for $f \neq f'$. Thus the second moment of the process is diagonalized in the frequency basis; this is in contrast with the time basis, where in general $E[x(t)x(t')] \neq 0$ for arbitrary t, t'.

5.6.5 Gaussian Processes

Gaussian processes are fundamental to the study of stochastic process theory and are also the most tractable. A Gaussian stochastic process is fully characterized by the mean $\mu(t) = E[x(t)]$ and covariance function $C(t, t')$, a real or complex function of two times. To simplify the discussion we assume $\mu(t) = 0$, since this is a simple shift of the variables and can be easily reincorporated.

For any collection of times t_i, the random variable $x(t_1), x(t_2), \ldots, x(t_n)$ has a multivariate Gaussian distribution with covariance function $E[x(t_i)x(t_j)] = C(t_i, t_j)$. The function $C(t, t')$ cannot be arbitrary: it has to be positive definite, in the sense that $\sum_{ij} a_i^* C(t_i, t_j) a_j > 0$ for any collection of time points t_i and a corresponding list of numbers a_i not all of which are zero. We can write out the probability distribution of the vector $x_i = x(t_i)$ explicitly in terms of the covariance matrix $C_{ij} = C(t_i, t_j)$ as[25]

$$p(x_1, x_2, \ldots, x_n) = \frac{1}{(2\pi)^{n/2} \det(C)} e^{-\frac{1}{2} \sum_{ij} x_i (C^{-1})_{ij} x_j} \tag{5.166}$$

Stationary Gaussian Processes

If the process is stationary, then the covariance function depends only on the difference between the times, $C(t, t') = C(t - t')$. The Fourier transform of the covariance function is the spectrum

$$S(f) = \int_{-\infty}^{\infty} dt\, C(t) e^{-2\pi i f t} \tag{5.167}$$

For a stationary Gaussian process, the Fourier transform of the process $X(f)$[26] is uncorrelated for different frequencies. Therefore, prescribing the joint distribution of $X(f_1), X(f_2), \ldots, X(f_n)$ is even simpler than prescribing the joint distribution in the time domain. In the Fourier domain, the joint distribution becomes the product of independent univariate distributions (each being a complex Gaussian). If the normalization is chosen such that $X_T(f) = \frac{1}{\sqrt{T}} \int_{-T/2}^{T/2} x(t) e^{-2\pi i f t}$, then in the large T limit, one obtains $\lim_{t \to \infty} E[|X_T(f)|^2] = S(f)$.[27] Loosely speaking, we can write $E[|X(f)|^2] = S(f)$, and similarly $E[X^*(f)X(f')] = 0$ if $f \neq f'$. With this normalization, the joint distribution in the frequency domain (for a translation invariant process) is given in the product form

$$p(X_1, X_2, \ldots, X_n) = \prod_i \frac{1}{\pi S_i} e^{-\frac{|X_i|^2}{S_i}} \tag{5.168}$$

Clearly, it is easier to work with uncorrelated variables and not to have to worry about the correlations between different elements of a vector random variable. This explains why spectral estimation plays a basic role in analyzing time series data.

25. We give the expression for a real valued process. The distribution for a complex process can be read off from the earlier discussion about complex Gaussian distributions.

26. For a stochastic process of infinite length, one has to exercise caution in defining the Fourier transform, which is only defined if appropriately normalized and a proper limiting procedure applied.

27. With a different normalization, $X(f) = \int_{-T/2}^{T/2} x(t) e^{-2\pi i f t}$, one has instead $E[X^*(f)X(f')] = S(f)\delta(f-f')$.

Nonstationary Processes and Dynamic Spectrum

If there is no time translational invariance, one can define a *dynamic* spectrum, by Fourier transforming the correlation[28] matrix $C(t, t')$ along its diagonal:

$$S(f, t) = \int_{-\infty}^{\infty} dt' C(t + t'/2, t - t'/2) e^{-2\pi i f t'} \tag{5.169}$$

Because in most neurobiological experiments there are explicit external sources of nonstationarity (such as input stimuli), the dynamic spectrum is in general the quantity we use in our analysis.

Ornstein Uhlenbeck Process

We will now consider some examples of a Gaussian stochastic process. Our first example will be that of a stationary stochastic process with an exponentially decaying correlation function, $C(t, t') = \sigma^2 e^{-|t - t'|/\tau}$. Such a process is also called an Ornstein Uhlenbeck process and has a Lorentzian power spectrum:

$$S(f) = \frac{\sigma^2 \tau}{1 + (2\pi f \tau)^2} \tag{5.170}$$

The Ornstein Uhlenbeck process $x(t)$ can be obtained from a white noise process $\eta(t)$ (with delta-function correlations, $E[\eta(t)\eta(t')] = \sigma^2 \tau \delta(t - t')$, by passing it through a "leaky integrator":

$$\tau \frac{d}{dt} x(t) + x(t) = \eta(t) \tag{5.171}$$

The correlation function for the process decays at long times; if we look at time scales long compared to τ (or equivalently frequency scales much less than $1/\tau$) the process should look like white noise. This is indeed true: if we let $f\tau \ll 1$, then the power spectrum is a constant given by $\sigma^2 \tau$. On the other hand, if we let the time constant of the integrator become long, then $x(t)$ is simply the integral of a white noise process, or Brownian motion. In this limit the spectrum becomes proportional to $1/f^2$.

Apart from being a Gaussian process, the Ornstein Uhlenbeck process is also a Markovian process. Let us denote the joint probability density for n time points $x_1 = x(t_1)$, $x_2 = x(t_2), \ldots, x_n = x(t_n)$ of the stochastic process be given by $p(x_1, x_2, \ldots, x_n; t_1, t_2, \ldots, t_n)$. We assume that the time points are in increasing order. We have emphasized the explicit dependence on time and not made assumptions about time translational invariance. A stochastic process

---

28. The words correlation and covariance are being used in an interchangeable manner.

is said to have the Markovian property if the dependence on the past at a given time point can be fully captured by specifying the value of the process at the last time point. In equations, the conditional probability satisfies if $p(x_n; t_n | x_1, x_2, \ldots, x_{n-1}; t_1, t_2, \ldots, t_{n-1}) = p(x_n; t_n | x_{n-1}, t_{n-1})$. For a Markovian process, the joint probability distribution can be written in factorized form as

$$p(x_1, x_2, \ldots, x_n; t_1, t_2, \ldots, t_n) = p(x_1; t_1)p(x_2; t_2 | x_1, t_1) \ldots p(x_n; t_n | x_{n-1}, t_{n-1}) \tag{5.172}$$

Therefore, a Markovian stochastic process is specified by the initial probability $p(x; 0)$ and the transition probability function $p(x; t | x'; t')$.

Stochastic processes have to satisfy the Kolmogorov consistency condition: any marginal obtained by integrating out a variable should lead to the probability distribution of the remaining variables. For a Markovian process, this leads to the Chapman-Kolmogorov equation for the transition probability function $p(x; t | x'; t')$

$$p(x; t | x'; t') = \int dx'' p(x; t | x''; t'') p(x''; t'' | x'; t') \tag{5.173}$$

If the process in question is time translation invariant, then the transition probability depends only on a the time difference.

- We have asserted that the Ornstein Uhlenbeck process is Markovian and has a correlation function given by $C(t, t') = \sigma^2 e^{-|t-t'|/\tau}$. Show that the transition probability for this process $(t > 0)$ is given by

$$p(x; t | x', 0) = \frac{1}{\sqrt{2\pi\sigma^2(t)}} \exp\left(-\frac{(x - x'e^{-t/\tau})^2}{2\sigma^2(t)}\right) \tag{5.174}$$

  where $\sigma^2(t) = \sigma^2(1 - e^{-t/\tau})$.
- Therefore show that for this process, $E[x(t) | x(0) = x'] = x'e^{-|t|/\tau}$. This means that if we initially observe the process at some nonzero value, it is subsequently expected to decay back to the origin.
- Take the limit $\tau \to \infty$ and $\sigma \to \infty$ with $D = \sigma^2/(2\tau)$ being held constant. Show that this in this limit, the transition probability becomes the diffusion propagator

$$p(x; t | x', 0) = \frac{1}{\sqrt{4\pi Dt}} \exp\left(-\frac{(x - x')^2}{4Dt}\right) \tag{5.175}$$

Wiener Process or Brownian Motion

The last exercise leads us to perhaps the most widely known stochastic process, namely Brownian motion, or the Wiener process. This is a Markovian stochastic process, and although in the above exercise it was obtained as a limiting case of a stationary stochastic process, it is not in itself stationary! The correlation function for Brownian motion is given by $C(t, t') = E[x(t)x(t')] = 2D \min(t, t')$, where we assume $t, t' > 0$ and that $x(0) = 0$. The Brownian motion starting at the origin has a mean square displacement that grows linearly with time. Although not stationary, the Brownian motion or Wiener process is Markovian, with the transition probability given by the Gaussian function as above. For this process, $x(t) - x(t')$ is distributed as a Gaussian with zero mean and variance given by $2D|t - t'|$. Now suppose we were interested in the time derivative of the process $x(t)$, and we started with the slope for a finite time increment $\Delta x(t)/h = (x(t+h) - x(t))/h$. This slope has zero mean; however, the variance of this slope is $E[(x(t+h) - x(t))^2]/h^2 = 2D/h$, and diverges as $h \to 0$. Therefore, the magnitude of the slope diverges with probability one at any time point.[29]

The Wiener process or Brownian motion is therefore a continuous but *rough* function of time; almost none of the sample paths of the process possess a well defined derivative at any given time point. This may seem unphysical, and indeed for a real Brownian particle, the Wiener process is not a good model at microscopic time scales corresponding to ballistic motion of the particle in between collisions. This sort of caveat should be kept in mind when we apply stochastic process theory to real neurobiological processes; the mathematical singularities that may appear in a theoretical setting are going to be smoothed out or regularized by some physical cutoff. Real voltages in real neurons will look smooth if one looks at sufficiently small timescales; however, measured voltages may indeed appear somewhat rough in an appropriate frequency range, and then they could be modeled as a Wiener process in that frequency range. Such power law spectral shapes for neuronal time series often excite attention due to (at least superficial) similarity to analogous power laws in statistical physics. However, one should not get too carried away by f^{-2} behavior in estimated power spectra; this can sometimes happen due to bad estimation techniques (e.g., leakage from a finite data window without appropriate tapering), or due to some conceptually less interesting frequency filtering imposed by the instrumentation or the underlying biophysics.

Although we have confined our discussion to one dimensional Gaussian processes, the above discussion goes over with little change to vector valued Gaussian processes. We will not clutter this chapter with the laborious but straightforward corresponding mathematical formulae, but one has to simply keep track of the covariance both as a function of the vector indices, as well as of time. The interested reader should write out the formulae corresponding to the discussions above, but for vector valued Gaussian stochastic processes.

---

29. Because $\Delta x(t)/h$ has a Gaussian distribution with variance $2D/h$, we have $P(|\Delta x(t)/h| > (2D/h)^\alpha) = 2(1 - Erf((h/2D)^{1/2 - \alpha}))$. Taking $0 < \alpha < 1/2$ and letting $h \to 0$, we obtain $P[\lim_{h \to 0}|\Delta x(t)/h| = \infty] = 1$

5.6.6 Non-Gaussian Processes

Except for some very special classes of stochastic processes, once the process becomes non-Gaussian it also reaches the realms of computational intractability. This can be understood by thinking about arbitrary multivariate distributions; computing anything for such distributions involves doing high-dimensional integrals, and this is in general not possible. There are indeed a number of exactly soluble models in statistical field theory, but these are exceptions to the rule; one either has to resort to perturbative methods or to numerical methods. There is a large literature on both topics in physics, because non-Gaussian stochastic process models are the basic tools in condensed matter physics and field theory.

Markovian Non-Gaussian Processes

Here we only indicate the one broad class of tractable stochastic processes, given by Markovian processes, which are formally related to quantum mechanics (but note that nothing quantum mechanical is implied about the domain of application of such process models).[30] We have already encountered one such process, namely the Ornstein Uhlenbeck process; the quantum mechanical analog is the staple of theoretical physics, the simple harmonic oscillator. More generally, consider the stochastic differential equation or Langevin equation describing a Brownian particle moving in a potential V (equivalently, in a force field proportional to dV/dx),

$$\frac{dx}{dt} = -D\frac{dV(x)}{dx} + \eta(t) \qquad (5.176)$$

where $\eta(t)$ is white noise and the diffusion constant of the corresponding Brownian motion is D. We will state without proof the following results that allow a full characterization of the corresponding Markovian stochastic process. The finite distributions of the process $p(x_1, t_1; x_2, t_2; \ldots; x_n, t_n)$ are given by

$$p(x_1, t_1; x_2, t_2; \ldots; x_n, t_n) = \prod_{k=2}^{k=n} p(x_k, t_k | x_{k-1}, t_{k-1}) p(x_1, t_1) \qquad (5.177)$$

Therefore, one only need specify the marginal distribution $p(x, t)$ and the transition probability $p(x, t | x', t')$. If we further assume time translational invariance, the process simplifies further, $p(x, t)$ does not depend on time and is given by the equilibrium distribution $p_0(x)$, and the transition probability depends on a

---

30. The formulation presented here also requires going to an imaginary time variable $t \to it$, so the relationship is only a formal one. There is, however, a bona fide formulation of quantum mechanics in terms of stochastic processes with *complex* measures, namely the Feynman path integral formulation.

single time $p(x, t|x')$. It is not too difficult to show that the transition probability satisfies the *Fokker Planck* equation

$$\frac{\partial}{\partial t} p(x, t|x') = D \frac{\partial}{\partial x} \left(\frac{\partial}{\partial x} + \frac{dV(x)}{dx} \right) p(x, t|x') \qquad (5.178)$$

The steady state distribution is given by setting the right-hand side to zero,

$$\frac{\partial}{\partial x} \left(\frac{\partial}{\partial x} + \frac{dV(x)}{dx} \right) p_0(x) = 0 \qquad (5.179)$$

This leads to $p_0(x) = \frac{1}{Z} e^{-V(x)}$, where Z is a normalization constant. Defining the quantity $G(x, t|x') = e^{V(x)/2} p(x, t|x') e^{-V(x')/2}$, it can be shown that G is given by the eigenfunction expansion

$$G(x, t|x') = \sum_{n=0}^{\infty} \psi_n(x) \psi_n(x') e^{-E_n t}, \qquad (5.180)$$

where $\psi_n(x)$ and E_n are the eigenfunctions and eigenvalues of the single particle Schrodinger equation in one dimension (with the identification of the diffusion constant D with $\hbar^2/(2m)$) and an effective potential $V_{eff}(x) = D ((V'(x))^2/4 - V''(x)/2)$

$$-D \frac{d^2}{dx^2} \psi(x) + V_{eff}(x)\psi(x) = E\psi_n(x) \qquad (5.181)$$

The potential $V_{eff}(x)$ has the important property that the lowest energy eigenfunction has eigenvalue zero. The analytical forms of the eigenfunctions and eigenvalues of the Schrodinger equation are available for a variety of potentials; by choosing potentials that have zero ground state energy and for which the solutions are available in analytical form, one can obtain analytical expressions for the finite distributions, moments, and so on. Non-Gaussian Markovian models of this sort have not yet seen much use in theoretical neuroscience, but their analytical tractability may make them interesting for future use.

5.6.7 Point Processes

The general theory of point processes is quite involved. On the other hand, some point processes such as the Poisson process or renewal processes can be understood without invoking heavy machinery. Unfortunately, this has also biased thinking about point processes in applications to neural spike trains; there is a tendency to straightjacket all spike trains into these well understood categories. To some extent, endless debates about the "neural code" originate in confusion about the mathematical structure of point processes. Given the importance of this subject to understanding neural time series, our treatment of point process theory is relatively advanced. It is meant for the reader with some experience in point process theory and may not be accessible to the general reader.

Our coverage of the material in this section borrows in part from the books by Snyder [208] and Daley and Vere-Jones [54] to which the mathematically sophisticated reader is directed for fuller coverage. However, we have tried to emphasize and clarify concepts that can get buried in the mathematical formalism. Further, the formalism developed for point processes in the statistics literature has a different emphasis than that developed in the physics literature, where there also exists a vast body of work involving point processes, especially in the statistical mechanics of fluids. Our coverage tries to strike a balance between these two sets of approaches.

Point Processes as Delta Function Trains

There are a number of ways of thinking about point processes. Recall that we defined continuous stochastic processes as random variables that take their values in a function space (which in our discussion consisted of functions of time $x(t)$). Now consider the formal expression

$$x(t) = \sum_i \delta(t - t_i) \tag{5.182}$$

so that a sample path of the process consists of a sum over delta functions. This is one way to think of a point process. Point processes may be defined in higher dimensions, but we will stick to the one-dimensional case, relevant for treating neural spike train data.

Apart from being described as a sum over delta functions, the sample path of a point process can be alternatively specified in two other ways: as a set of points on the line, or a specific number of points in arbitrary intervals. These specifications are equivalent; a sum over delta functions can be specified by giving the locations of the delta functions, the number of points in an interval can be obtained by integrating the delta functions over that interval, and so on.

Point Processes as Counting Measures

The intuitive picture of the sample path of a point process as a series of delta functions can be formalized by thinking of a *counting measure*. Recall our discussion of a probability measure as a countably additive set function, so that for "measurable" sets $A_1, A_2, A_3, \ldots$

$$p(A_1 \cup A_2 \cup A_3 \cdots) = p(A_1) + p(A_2) + p(A_3) + \cdots \tag{5.183}$$

Namely, probabilities add when the sets A_i are disjoint. Along the same vein, a counting measure takes integer values, so that $N(A_i)$ is a non-negative integer, and for a countable collection of disjoint measurable sets A_i

$$N(A_1 \cup A_2 \cup A_3 \cdots) = N(A_1) + N(A_2) + N(A_3) + \cdots \qquad (5.184)$$

Although N is a non-negative measure defined on the line, it is not in general possible to define a corresponding probability measure by appropriate normalization, since the total number of points may be infinite. In terms of such counting measures, a point process may simply be defined as a random counting measure, in the same way a continuous valued stochastic process is a random function of time. Although one does not explicitly keep track of it for most applications, one assumes that there is an underlying sample space Ω, with elements being sample points ω. Recall that a random variable is a *function* defined on the sample space, so that for each sample point, the random variable has a unique value associated with it. In the present instance, for an elementary event ω, the corresponding value is itself a complicated object, namely a counting measure on R, as described above. Moreover, to define the point process, one assumes there is a probability measure on the sample space Ω. These two measures are completely different constructs and have nothing to do with each other.

Considerations of the Underlying Sample Space

Because this discussion is quite abstract, consider a trivial example, where the sample space Ω has only two elements, $\Omega = \omega_1, \omega_2$. The point process is a random variable defined on this sample space; therefore for each elementary event ω_i, the point process specifies a unique counting measure $N_i(A)$. The probability space is of course elementary: it is the previously encountered Bernoulli distribution with two outcomes and one parameter p, say $p(\omega_1) = p$ and $p(\omega_2) = 1 - p$. The counting measures $N_1(A)$ and $N_2(A)$ could be complicated; this does not make this particular point process a complicated object from a probabilistic perspective.

More generally, it is unnecessary and quite difficult to keep track of the sample space Ω and the corresponding probability measure. Instead, one can work with the analogs of the finite dimensional distributions, by specifying the joint probability of $N(A_1)$, $N(A_2)$, ..., $N(A_n)$ of a finite number of nonintersecting sets A_i. This is similar to specifying $p(x(t_1), x(t_2), \ldots, x(t_n))$ as in the earlier discussion on stochastic processes. Further, for technical reasons we will not discuss, it is enough to keep track of these joint probabilities for sets of the form $A_i = (\tau_i, t_i]$. Thus, one needs to only specify joint probabilities of the form $p(N_1, N_2, \ldots, N_n)$, where N_n is the number of points in the interval $(\tau_i, t_i]$.[31]

---

31. The meaning of the notation is that the point t_i is included but the τ_i is not included; one could also choose the convention the other way around, including the initial point and excluding the final point.

Point Processes Starting at a Time of Origin

We have implicitly assumed that the number of points is countable; we cannot pick arbitrary sets of points on the line and think of them as sample paths of a point process. It is tempting to simply enumerate the points $t_1, t_2, \ldots$, starting from some initial time point. We will adopt this strategy in the following discussion. However, such a description is in fact limited and needs to be used with care, if we are really interested in point processes that live over the entire real line.

The reason for this is the following: suppose we arbitrarily choose our time origin at $t = 0$, such that all the points we are interested in occur after this point of time. The problem is that to deal with those points in the process that happen before $t = 0$, namely the "boundary conditions" we need to impose on the process. One could imagine averaging over what happened in the past, or conditioning over the past through some boundary variables or state variables that we have to keep track of, and so on; however, this introduces extra complications. It is also not very elegant, particularly for processes that were time translation invariant to begin with, because the boundary artificially breaks that translational invariance. Of course, it may be that we are dealing with phenomena where there is a privileged time of origin from which the process did start, in which case fixing the time of origin is not an issue; however, we are not able to deal with stationary processes in a straightforward way.

Boundary Effects

This is not just a theoretical quibble. It is true that when observing a neural spike train the experimental measurements have a well-defined time of origin, but that is an experimental artifact, because the measurements could have been started at any given time point. In fact, to deal with this precise issue, it is customary to gather data for a *baseline* period before the start of the experimental trial. However, the baseline period itself has a beginning, so the issue is not entirely eliminated, especially because experimental contingencies often dictate that the baseline period is short. We have encountered the impact of such boundary phenomena before, in our discussion of the spectral analysis of continuous processes based on a finite window of observation. It is therefore important to be explicitly aware of the boundary effects, rather than ignoring them because one is using a formalism that explicitly assumes a finite time of origin.

If we do specialize to point processes that start from a specific time of origin $t = 0$, the discussion simplifies substantially, because we can now keep track of a single function of time, the counting process $N(t)$, which counts the number of points in the interval from zero to t. Two conventions are possible: to allow a point at the origin but not include the point at t, and vice versa, to exclude the origin and allow at t. Both these conventions are in use, and as long as one maintains a consistency of notation, either can be used. It is unnecessary for our purposes to maintain a pedantic distinction between the two, but the reader should be aware of this subtlety when defining the counting process. Further, it is sometimes useful to consider the *Palm* process of a given stochastic process, where the process is made conditional on a point at the origin. In considering the Palm process, depending on the convention, $N(t)$ will have a minimum value of 0 or 1, the former being the more natural choice.

Specifying Point Processes Starting at a Time of Origin

We will now restrict ourselves to the case where we consider processes originating at $t = 0$, and we will return to the real line and the issues of stationarity in the section on general point processes. In discussing Poisson processes, this makes little difference, because Poisson processes do not have memory. However, it makes the discussion simpler, and it is the more familiar setting. In keeping with the earlier discussion, the point process can be specified by fixing the finite dimensional distributions for $N(t_1)$, $N(t_2)$, ... $N(t_n)$.

We can consider two cases: the times are bounded on the right so that $t_i \in [0\ T]$, or the times are unbounded. In the former case, one can specify the point process fairly arbitrarily by fixing the *sample function density* [208] or the configuration probability,[32] $p(t_1, t_2, \ldots, t_n | N(T) = n)$ for a fixed number of points, along with the probability of finding n points in the interval, $p(N(T)) = n$.

If T is not bounded, we can specify the joint distribution of the *first n time* points of the process starting at the time origin, $p(t_1, t_2, \ldots, t_n)$, for all n. This quantity is called the *joint occurrence density* and has to satisfy the consistency condition, that integrating out the last time point from the $(n+1)^{th}$ joint occurrence density gives back the one corresponding to n points.

Recall the earlier discussion about subtleties that can occur for general stochastic processes defined as a continuous function of time. Similar subtleties can also occur for point processes, and it is useful to have a finite and discretized description of the process and to employ appropriate limiting procedures. In our earlier discussion, we saw that continuous valued stochastic processes could be approximated by distributions in a finite dimensional vector space. Along similar lines, a point process on a finite time interval can be discretized and thought of as a finite binary sequence consisting of non-negative integers: if one takes a sufficiently fine time bin, and if the point process is well behaved, then this becomes a sequence of zeros and ones (analogous to one dimensional ising spin chains familiar to statistical physicists).[33]

---

32. These are also referred to as Janossy densities.
33. More generally, the integers in a given bin need not be constrained to zero or one even in the small time bin limit, but we will not discuss such cases.

Poisson Processes

Because this is all quite abstract, we illustrate the specification methods for the Poisson process, which plays the same central role in point process theory as does Brownian motion does for continuous stochastic processes. Recall that for Brownian motion, the increments of the process $x(t) - x(t')$ have a Gaussian distribution with zero mean and variance given by $2D|t - t'|$. Similarly, for the Poisson process, the increments $N(t) - N(t')$ have a Poisson distribution with Poisson parameter $\Lambda = \lambda(t - t')$, $(t > t')$. Moreover, successive increments are distributed independently. The joint distribution for $N(t_1) = N_1$, $N(t_2) = N_2, \ldots$, $N(t_n) = N_n$ $(N_1 \leq N_2 \leq N_3 \cdots)$ for the Poisson counting process is therefore given by

$$
\begin{aligned}
p(N_1, N_2, \ldots, N_n) \\
= f(N_1, \lambda t_1) f(N_2 - N_1, \lambda(t_2 - t_1)) \ldots f(N_n - N_{n-1}, \lambda(t_n - t_{n-1}))
\end{aligned}
\tag{5.185}
$$

where $f(n, \Lambda) = \Lambda^n e^{-\Lambda}/n!$ is the Poisson distribution discussed in an earlier section.

The joint occurrence density for the Poisson process, for the first n time points starting at $t = 0$, is given by

$$
p(t_1, t_2, \ldots, t_n) = \lambda^n e^{-\lambda t_n}
\tag{5.186}
$$

We have assumed that the points are ordered, namely $t_1 < t_2 < t_3 \ldots$ The sample function density, on the other hand, includes the extra information that only n points occur in the interval $[0\ T]$ and is given (for the Poisson process) by

$$
p(t_1, t_2, \ldots, t_n; N(T) = n) = \lambda^n e^{-\lambda T}
\tag{5.187}
$$

The relation between the two quantities is simply that the sample function density is the joint occurrence density multiplied by the probability that no point occurs in the interval $[t_n\ T]$. Although these relations look very similar, they have different domains of definition: for the joint occurrence density $t_1 < t_2 < \cdots < t_n < \infty$, whereas for the sample function density or configuration probability $t_1 < t_2 < \cdots < t_n < T$.

Note that $p(N(T) = n) = (\lambda T)^n e^{-\lambda T}/n!$. Therefore, for fixed $N(T) = n$, the conditional probability density for the ordered points $t_1, t_2, \ldots, t_n$ is given by

$$
p(t_1, t_2, \ldots, t_n | N(T) = n) = \frac{1}{n! T^n}
\tag{5.188}
$$

The factor of $n!$ comes from the fact that we have ordered the points; if we instead consider the probability density for finding the *unordered* points t_1, $t_2, \ldots, t_n$, then this is given by

$$
p(t_1, t_2, \ldots, t_n | N(T) = n)_{unordered} = \frac{1}{T^n}
\tag{5.189}
$$

This is just the uniform distribution over the hypercube T^n. If we fix n, then a sample of the Poisson process is easy to generate: we just pick the n points randomly in the interval $[0\ T]$. In fact, this is the way one simulates Poisson processes, including rate varying and doubly stochastic Poisson processes to be discussed next. However, it is crucial to note that the uniform distribution of the time points for fixed n *does not* mean that the process is Poisson. For example, if the distribution of the number of points is chosen to be a non-Poisson distribution, then the corresponding stochastic process is no longer Poisson, even if for *fixed N* the points are distributed uniformly over the interval. One example is

$$p(N(T) = n) = \frac{\mu^n}{(1+\mu)^{n+1}} \tag{5.190}$$

This process can also be obtained by considering a doubly stochastic Poisson process, where the rate λ is itself a random variable, chosen from an exponential distribution $p(\lambda) = (1/\mu)e^{-\lambda/\mu}$.

- Show that the joint occurrence probability and the sample function density for the Poisson process are appropriately normalized, and both integrate to one.
- Prove the assertion in the last paragraph.

Note that the Poisson process is time translation invariant, but the counting process is not; this is the analog of Brownian motion not being time translation invariant, because Brownian motion can also be obtained by integrating a stationary stochastic process, the white noise process. The Poisson distribution has the same mean and variance; therefore, one has $E[N(T)] = V[N(T)] = \lambda T$. Consider the process $\delta N(T) = N(T) - \lambda T$ obtained by subtracting the average growth of the number of counts from the counting process. Then we have $E[\delta N(T)] = 0$ and $E[\delta N(T)\delta N(T')] = \lambda \min(T, T')$, which is the same expression as for Brownian motion.

The process $\delta N(T)$ is not Gaussian distributed; however, due to the central limit theorem, one can indeed go over to Brownian motion by taking an appropriate limit: consider the process $x(t) = \delta N(t)/\sqrt{\lambda}$. Note from the earlier section on Poisson distributions that all cumulants of the Poisson distribution are identical; therefore, the kth cumulant of $\delta N(t)$ is λt. Now $x(t)$ is related by a simple rescaling; therefore, the kth cumulant of $x(t)$ is proportional to $\lambda^{1-k/2}$, so that as λ becomes large (corresponding to a large number of points per unit time), all cumulants higher than 2 tend to zero. In this limit, the rescaled process becomes Gaussian distributed. This is an important point, because in dealing with spike trains, neuroscientists have considered smoothed versions of spike trains, which could in turn be modeled as continuous stochastic processes.

Inhomogeneous Poisson Process

So far we have considered a constant rate Poisson process. This is not a very good model of a neuronal spike train, because spike rates vary with input stimuli and also exhibit spontaneous variations in rate due to intrinsic dynamics in the brain. Also, spike trains may exhibit complex correlation patterns in time. Therefore, more complicated point process models are needed to model observed point processes in the context of neural dynamics. We consider a series of such models in turn.

First consider the inhomogeneous or rate varying Poisson process, where the Poisson rate is no longer a constant but a function of time $\lambda(t)$. One way to obtain such a process is to take a Poisson process and rescale time. The number of points in an interval $[t\ t']$ is still Poisson distributed, but the Poisson parameter is given by $\int_t^{t'} \lambda(\tau)d\tau$. The sample function density for this process is given by

$$p(t_1, t_2, \ldots, t_n; N(T) = n) = \prod_{i=1}^{n} \lambda(t_i)e^{-\int_0^T \lambda(\tau)d\tau} \qquad (5.191)$$

This is no longer a stationary stochastic process. Inhomogeneous Poisson processes have been used to describe the response of neurons to external stimuli; in a prototypical experiment, the experimentalist provides the experimental subject with a set of stimuli (or perhaps a stimulus time course) and measures the corresponding spike trains. The most widely used characterization of spike trains is in the form of a time-dependent rate. This can be taken to correspond to $E[\rho(t)]$, the first moment of the process described as a sequence of delta functions, $\rho(t) = \sum_i \delta(t - t_i)$. If the process is an inhomogeneous Poisson process, then $E[\rho(t)] = \lambda(t)$, and this quantity captures all that is to be known about the process. On the other hand, if the process is not an inhomogeneous Poisson processes, then this rate function does not fully characterize the process.

There is a long-standing debate in the neuroscience literature about whether the rate function is sufficient to characterize a neuronal spike train. Even if the original process were not inhomogeneous Poisson, it is of course possible that the higher order correlations do not carry additional information about the stimulus. This is the so called *rate code* versus *temporal code* debate.[34] The answer to the question seems to be that inhomogeneous Poisson processes are sometimes suitable for describing spike trains, but not always; the higher order correlations, particularly the second-order correlations as quantified by spectra and cross coherences, can also be informative. It is certainly inadequate to stop at the inhomogeneous Poisson process in building models of neuronal spike trains.

---

34. At least this is a well-formulated version of that debate; often the debate originates in an imprecise formulation and is then a conceptual confusion about the problem to be studied as opposed to a well-posed question that can be answered in the affirmative or negative.

Doubly Stochastic Poisson Process

The next modification to consider starting from the inhomogeneous Poisson is that the rate function $\lambda(t)$ is itself a stochastic process; such a process is called a doubly stochastic Poisson process or Cox process. We have examined an example in the subsection on Poisson processes, where $\lambda(t)$ was stochastic (from sample to sample) but constant in time. Such processes may provide useful models for neurophysiological experiments where the stimulus response has a stereotypical shape as a function of time, but has a gain that varies from trial to trial (due to changes in neuronal excitability, for example).

To specify a doubly stochastic Poisson process, one has to do two things: specify the stochastic rate process $\lambda(t)$, then given $\lambda(t)$, specify the corresponding inhomogeneous Poisson process. Because one does not observe the rate process directly, one might be tempted to average or marginalize over the rate process in order to obtain the sample function density just in terms of the points of the process. Although this is possible to do in theory in formal terms, in practice one cannot obtain a closed form expression for the density except for the simplest cases, so that the doubly stochastic description is still the most parsimonious one.

General Point Process Models

To specify a general point process on the real line, one needs to specify the finite distribution of the counting measure $N(t, t+T)$ on collections of disjoint intervals $(t_1, t_1 + T_1), (t_2, t_2 + T_2), \ldots, (t_n, t_n + T_n)$. This is in general too difficult to do except for the simplest situations. Consider a Poisson process defined on the real line. Although we have discussed only processes starting at a time origin so far, because the Poisson process has no memory, it is easy to specify the finite distributions of the counting measure on collections of disjoint intervals. By definition, this distribution is a product of individual Poisson distributions

$$
\begin{aligned}
&p(N(t_1, t_1 + T_1), N(t_2, t_2 + T_2), \ldots, N(t_n, t_n + T_n)) \\
&= \prod_i p(N(t_i, t_i + T_i))
\end{aligned} \tag{5.192}
$$

Here $p(N(t_i, t_i + T_i))$ is the Poisson distribution with parameter given by λT_i, where λ is the rate of the process and T_i is the length of the ith interval. This distribution is also translationally invariant. In analogy with the continuous process case, the point process is said to be translationally invariant if the joint distribution function remains invariant under arbitrary time translations τ

$$
\begin{aligned}
&p(N(t_1 + \tau, t_1 + \tau + T_1), N(t_2 + \tau, t_2 + \tau + T_2), \ldots, N(t_n + \tau, t_n + \tau + T_n)) \\
&= p(N(t_1, t_1 + T_1), N(t_2, t_2 + T_2), \ldots, N(t_n, t_n + T_n))
\end{aligned} \tag{5.193}
$$

Note that the average number of time points in the interval is given by λT_i, so that the average number of points goes to infinity as the interval length goes to infinity. In fact, any stationary point process with a finite rate will have this property. This means that we cannot specify the process by specifying the configuration probability $p(t_1, t_2, \ldots, t_n \mid n)p(n)$ for a finite number of points n: for any finite n, $p(n) = 0$. The reader should verify this for the Poisson process by considering $p(n \mid T)$, the number distribution on a finite interval of length T, and letting T become large.

One way around this difficulty is to specify the process on a finite interval and then apply some appropriate limiting process in which the interval size become large. A variant on this is to keep the number of points finite (in the parlance of statistical physics, apply "soft walls" rather than "hard walls" to confine the particles). In both cases, the $p(n)$'s are nonzero, and the processes are referred to as finite point processes [54]. In this description, translational invariance is lost due to the presence of the walls; however, by receding the walls to infinity, translational invariance can be regained. The earlier discussion of point processes with a finite time of origin may be regarded as having a "hard wall" at the time origin.

A different alternative is to not specify n but give the joint density of some distinct points $t_1, t_2, \ldots, t_k$ of the process. Such quantities are called product densities or moment densities; the idea is that there are other points in the sample path, but we do not fix their locations. In this way of specifying the process, translational invariance can be retained. Moreover, these product densities are what come out of physical measurements and are also easier to estimate from samples of the process in a nonparametric manner. We will discuss these in a later section.

Gibbs Distributions

The most general finite point process is specified by an arbitrary set of joint occurrence densities or sample function densities. At this level of generality, there is little to be said; one needs to look at special model classes in order to make any progress. Moreover, it is desirable to have a specification that allows us to systematically push the confining walls to infinity in order to remove boundary effects.

Two somewhat different approaches have been adopted by physicists and by statisticians studying point processes. In the context of statistical physics, point processes appear as models describing the behavior of interacting point particles (for example, atoms or molecules in some state of matter), in the form of Gibbs-Boltzmann distributions. The Gibbs-Boltzmann distribution has the general form $p(X) = e^{-H(X)}/Z$, where X is the random variable in question, $H(X)$ is some real function of X (known as the energy function or Hamiltonian) and Z is a normalization constant (known as the partition coefficient). Consider the one-dimensional case, and let us confine our attention to a finite time interval $[0\ T]$. The sample function density can be written in the Gibbs-Boltzmann form (usually, the points are considered as unordered):

$$p(t_1, t_2, \ldots, t_n; n, T) = \frac{e^{\mu n}}{n! Z(\mu, T)} e^{-H(t_1, \ldots, t_n)} \qquad (5.194)$$

The parameter μ is called the *chemical potential* and controls the number of particles. The partition function $Z(\mu, T)$ (usually designated the grand canonical partition function, to differentiate from the canonical partition function for fixed n) is obtained by the normalization condition

$$Z(\mu, T) = \sum_{n=0}^{\infty} \int dt_1 \ldots dt_n \frac{e^{\mu n}}{n!} e^{-H(t_1, \ldots, t_n)} \qquad (5.195)$$

At this point, nothing seems to have been added to the discussion, because one can always define H as the logarithm of p in order to obtain this form. However, the utility of this description stems from specific forms of the energy function H that have simple physical interpretations as well as associated computational strategies.

The energy function is typically written as a sum over single particle terms, pair terms, and so on. The simplest energy function is given by $H = 0$, which the reader should verify corresponds to the Poisson process with rate $\lambda = e^{\mu}$. In fact, for more general stationary processes, the parameter μ has the significance that the average rate of the process is given by $\lim_{T \to \infty} E[N(T)]/T = e^{\mu}$, which is referred to in statistical physics as the *chemical potential*.

Gibbs Forms for Inhomogeneous Poisson Process and Renewal Process

The inhomogeneous Poisson process corresponds to a sum over one-particle energies,

$$H_1 = -\sum_i V_1(t_i) \qquad (5.196)$$

The identification with the Poisson parameter of the inhomogeneous process is that $\log(\lambda(t)) = \mu + V_1(t)$. A stationary process would necessarily have V_1 equal to a constant, which can be absorbed into μ; the next set of terms corresponds to pairwise interactions between points

$$H_2 = \sum_i \sum_j V_2(t_i - t_j) \qquad (5.197)$$

At this point, it is no longer possible to compute the partition coefficient analytically, except for rare exactly soluble instances of V_2, and one needs to resort to numerical, Monte Carlo methods. However, there is a special case, in which the particles are ordered in time, and the interaction energy is only between neighboring particles

$$H_2 = \sum_i V_2(t_i - t_{i-1}) \qquad (5.198)$$

This corresponds to a renewal process, and the partition function can again be computed analytically. For more general energy functions or Hamiltonians, there is a large array of approximation techniques, which are beyond the scope of this chapter. The reader is referred to standard textbooks in statistical physics [103, 122, 177].

Discretizing the point process into bins leads to another well-studied class of Hamiltonians, known as Ising models. In this case, the configuration space consists of binary sequences $(\sigma_1, \sigma_2, \ldots, \sigma_n)$, where $\sigma_i = 0$ or 1 according to whether there is a point in the ith time bin. Note that in this description, one no longer sums over the number of particles, but over the occupancy of time bins. The classical Ising model contains only nearest neighbor interactions J_i

$$H = -\sum_i h_i \sigma_i - \sum_i J_i \sigma_i \sigma_{i+1} \qquad (5.199)$$

The translational invariant case corresponds to $h_i = h$ and $J_i = J$. Without interactions and taking appropriate limits, the Ising model reduces to a Poisson process. The partition function of the Ising model can be calculated exactly using the transfer matrix method [122]. Again, there is a large literature on the Ising model, and it will not be discussed here further.

Conditional Intensity Process

An alternative approach for specifying point processes, which is popular in the engineering and statistics community, and better suited for likelihood based estimation and analysis, employs the *conditional intensity process*. Not every point process can be specified using conditional intensities (for example, see p. 212 [54]). Even if the conditional intensity process can be defined, it is not necessarily the most convenient description of all point processes. Analytical forms are not in general available for most quantities of interest for a general point process (such as the number distribution in a finite interval). Nevertheless, there are a number of merits to the conditional intensity approach, particularly the evolutionary nature of the description, which makes it similar to auto-regressive modeling for continuous stochastic processes.

The conditional intensity process can be explicitly constructed as follows for processes that begin at a given time origin and for which the joint occurrence density for the first n points $p(t_1, t_2, \ldots, t_n)$ is given for all n. We assume that the densities satisfy the Kolmogorov consistency conditions, so that integrating out t_n yields the density function for one fewer time point. Note first that a repeated conditioning on previous time points can be used to factorize this density

$$p(t_1, t_2, \ldots, t_n) = p(t_1)p(t_2|t_1) \ldots p(t_n|t_{n-1}, \ldots, t_1) \qquad (5.200)$$

For all k, define the *survival function*, which gives the probability that no point occurs in the specified interval after a given point

$$S(t|t_{k-1}, \ldots, t_1) = Prob(t_k \geq t|t_{k-1}, \ldots, t_1) = \int_t^\infty p(t_k|t_{k-1}, \ldots, t_1)dt_k \qquad (5.201)$$

For $k = 1$ there is no conditioning on previous points because t_1 is the first point of the process.

By taking a time derivative of this equation, we obtain

$$\frac{d}{dt}S(t|t_{k-1}, \ldots, t_1) = -p(t|t_{k-1}, \ldots, t_1) \qquad (5.202)$$

Now define the *hazard function* (also for each k) as the ratio

$$h(t|t_{k-1}, \ldots, t_1) = \frac{p(t|t_{k-1}, \ldots, t_1)}{S(t|t_{k-1}, \ldots, t_1)} \qquad (5.203)$$

The reader should verify that for a Poisson process, the hazard function is a constant and is equal to the Poisson rate. From the definition of the hazard function and the equation just prior to that it follows that

$$\frac{d}{dt}S(t|t_{k-1}, \ldots, t_1) = -h(t|t_{k-1}, \ldots, t_1)S(t|t_{k-1}, \ldots, t_1) \qquad (5.204)$$

This equation can be integrated to obtain

$$S(t|t_{k-1}, \ldots, t_1) = \exp\left(-\int_{t_{k-1}}^t h(\tau|t_{k-1}, \ldots, t_1)d\tau\right) \qquad (5.205)$$

From the definition of the hazard function, one then obtains the following expression for the conditional probability $p(t_k|t_{k-1}, \ldots, t_1)$

$$p(t_k|t_{k-1}, \ldots, t_1) = h(t_k|t_{k-1}, \ldots, t_1)\exp\left(-\int_{t_{k-1}}^{t_k} h(\tau|t_{k-1}, \ldots, t_1)d\tau\right) \qquad (5.206)$$

To simplify notation, we abbreviate the set of points $t_{k-1}, \ldots, t_1$ as H_k, with H_1 being the null set. The equation above can be rewritten as

$$p(t_k|H_k) = h(t_k|H_k)\exp\left(-\int_{t_{k-1}}^{t_k} h(\tau|H_k)d\tau\right) \qquad (5.207)$$

The joint occurrence density, or the likelihood of the first n points, can therefore be written as

$$p(t_1, t_2, \ldots, t_n) = \prod_{k=1}^{n} p(t_k|H_k) = \prod_k h(t_k|H_k) \exp\left(-\int_{t_{k-1}}^{t_k} h(\tau|H_k)d\tau\right) \quad (5.208)$$

Formal Resemblance to Inhomogeneous Poisson

Now *formally*, this resembles the likelihood of an inhomogeneous Poisson process. Let us define $H(t)$ to be the set H_k where t_{k-1} is the point just before t, or in other words, the history of the process up to, but not including t. The reason for this "left continuity" in defining t is to make sure the conditional intensity does not depend on what happens at t itself. As t increases, the set $H(t)$ changes discontinuously to a different set as t crosses one of the points in the process. With this convention, the hazard function can be written formally as a function of continuous time, $h(t|H(t))$. The joint occurrence density can therefore be expressed as

$$p(t_1, t_2, \ldots, t_n) = \prod_k h(t_k|H(t_k)) \exp\left(-\int_0^{t_n} h(\tau|H(\tau))d\tau\right) \quad (5.209)$$

This looks like the joint occurrence density of the first n points of an inhomogeneous Poisson process, with a time-dependent intensity given by the conditional intensity process

$$\lambda_{CI}(t) = h(t|H(t)) \quad (5.210)$$

It is very important to note that the conditional intensity process is a *random variable*; it is a function of the sample path, and should more explicitly be written as $\lambda_{CI}(t, \omega)$, where ω denotes the sample. In general, $\lambda_{CI}(t)$ is discontinuous with time, showing jumps at the points constituting a sample of the process. The conditional intensity process can generally only be computed once the sample of the process is given! This is in contrast with the inhomogeneous Poisson process, where the intensity function is first fixed, *then* a sample is drawn. This is no surprise, because the above manipulations have been formal and apply to arbitrarily complicated occurrence densities or likelihoods; the underlying problems have not been made any simpler through these formal manipulations.

It is also important to note that the process cannot be regarded as a Poisson process given the conditional intensity, because the conditional intensity depends in general on the realization of the process itself. One cannot first fix the conditional intensity, then sample the process (except, of course, for the trivial case when the conditional intensity is the same for all process samples, corresponding to the inhomogeneous Poisson process).

Closed Form Expressions for the Conditional Intensity

With the exceptions of processes that are otherwise tractable, such as renewal processes or some classes of doubly stochastic Poisson processes and so-called Poisson cluster processes, it is not in general possible to obtain a closed form expression for the conditional intensity process in terms of the sample path. This parallels the difficulty of computing the partition function for the Gibbs-Boltzmann distributions for most classes of interactions. To make things concrete, we consider a simple example, that of a doubly stochastic process where the rate function is constant in time but exponentially distributed for different sample paths, $p(\lambda) = e^{-\lambda/\lambda_0}/\lambda_0$. We have encountered this process in an earlier section, and it is a useful model to consider for treating rate fluctuations across trials in neurophysiological experiments. The joint occurrence density is given by

$$p(t_1, t_2, \ldots, t_n) = E_\lambda[\lambda^n e^{-\lambda t_n}] = \frac{n! \lambda_0^n}{(1 + \lambda_0 t_n)^{n+1}} \tag{5.211}$$

The conditional probability required to calculate the hazard function is therefore given by

$$p(t_n | t_{n-1}, \ldots, t_1) = n\lambda_0 \frac{(1 + \lambda_0 t_{n-1})^n}{(1 + \lambda_0 t_n)^{n+1}} \tag{5.212}$$

A simple integration as above shows that the survival function is given by

$$S(t | t_{n-1}, \ldots, t_1) = \frac{(1 + \lambda_0 t_{n-1})^n}{(1 + \lambda_0 t)^n} \tag{5.213}$$

Note in particular that $S(0) = 1$ and $S(\infty) = 0$. The hazard function is given by the ratio

$$h(t | t_{n-1}, \ldots, t_1) = \frac{\lambda_0 n}{1 + \lambda_0 t} \tag{5.214}$$

The history $H(t)$ for this process is captured by the number of time points up to but not including t, given by $n(t)$. We can therefore write the conditional intensity process as

$$\lambda_{CI}(t) = h(t | H(t) = \frac{\lambda_0 (n(t) + 1)}{1 + \lambda_0 t}. \tag{5.215}$$

This explicitly exhibits jumps at the sample points, because $n(t)$ is the counting process. This is illustrated in figure 5.13. It is important to note that we have been careful to refer to the conditional intensity *process* and not the conditional intensity *function*: $\lambda_{CI}(t)$ is not mathematically speaking a function of time, because it is not uniquely specified if the time point is given but is a stochastic process.

Another useful example is that of the renewal process, where both the Gibbs-Boltzmann distribution and the conditional intensity process have simple forms.

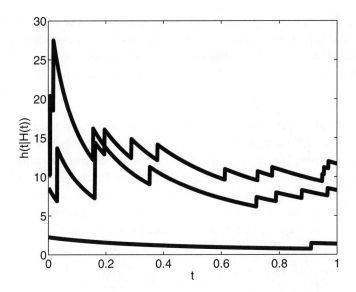

Figure 5.13: Hazard function. Three samples of the conditional intensity process for a doubly stochastic Poisson process, obtained by choosing a poisson rate from an exponential distribution with mean $\lambda_0 = 10$. Note the jump discontinuities in $\lambda_{CI}(t) = h(t|H(t))$.

A stationary renewal process is fully specified by the transition probability function $p(t_k | t_{k-1}) = q(t_k - t_{k-1})$. The likelihood for n points in an interval $[0\ T]$ has the Gibbs form, with an energy function corresponding to pairwise interactions between neighbors, $H = \sum_i V(t_i - t_{i-1})$, where

$$e^{-V(\tau)} = q(\tau) \tag{5.216}$$

On the other hand, the conditional intensity process is given by $\lambda_{CI}(t) = h(t - t_i)$, where t_i is the point in the process just preceding t, and the hazard function is given by

$$h(\tau) = \frac{q(\tau)}{1 - \int_0^\tau q(u)du} \tag{5.217}$$

Hawkes Process

A different example of a conditional intensity process is given by

$$\lambda_{CI}(t) = \sum_i \mu(t - t_i) \tag{5.218}$$

Here $\mu(t)$ is a positive function with an integral that is less than one. This conditional intensity corresponds to the so-called *Hawkes* process, which can be constructed recursively by starting from an initial generation of points, chosen according to a Poisson process. Successive generations are created from previous generations by constructing a set of daughter points that form a Poisson process with intensity $\mu(t - t_i)$ for each point t_i in the parent generation. The condition on the integral makes sure that the total number of points generated by a point from the first generation has remains finite (in probability).

As can be seen from the description of the process, the corresponding Gibbs distribution does not in general have a simple form. On the other hand, this process resembles autoregressive stochastic processes and has an evolutionary character that makes it suitable for prediction and filtering applications. Multivariate versions of this process have been used to model spike train likelihoods.

Compensator Process

The conditional intensity process can be used to construct the *compensator* process $\Lambda_C(t) = \int_0^t \lambda_{CI}(u)du$. Note as before, that the compensator process is a stochastic process and not a fixed function of time. Because the conditional intensity process has jump discontinuities, the compensator process is continuous and increasing but has discontinuities in slope. The importance of this process lies in the *time rescaling* theorem, which states that if the points of the original process are t_i, then the rescaled times $\tau_i = \Lambda_C(t_i)$ form a Poisson process with unit rate.

If a point process has a probability measure specified through a conditional intensity process with known form, then the time rescaling using the compensator function can be used to produce a second process, which should be Poisson with unit rate, under the null hypothesis that the sample path was generated according to the specified measure. Therefore, the hypothesis that a sample path of a process was generated by the specified likelihood can be tested by means of a simpler hypothesis test that the rescaled process is Poisson with unit rate. This latter hypothesis can be subjected to parametric or nonparametric tests.

Although this seems like an attractive procedure and is in current use, a note of caution should be taken into account in all instances where the probability measure has a high-dimensional parameter space. The space of all possible point process measures, if such a space can be meaningfully defined, is severely infinite dimensional, and data sets are of course quite finite. An infinite number of measures are therefore consistent with the finite sample of a point process. To reduce this to a unique measure one of course needs an infinite number of prior constraints; obviously, one cannot turn the procedure around to use the data set to justify the prior constraints. Therefore, it is not very clear what the meaning is of "testing" that a particular process model fits the data.

Of course, this is not a new problem; the same kind of arguments could be advanced against hypothesis testing of any sort about the probability distributions even for scalar random variables. However, the qualitative difference lies in the size of the space of models being considered. In the language of statistical inference, such tests have very little power in the sense that the number of alternative models that are consistent with the data for a given test is very large.

Specifying Stochastic Processes in Terms of Moments

One way to characterize the probability distribution of a random variable is in terms of its moments.[35] This can be done constructively by calculating the cumulants of the distribution from its moments, constructing the characteristic function (which is the Fourier transform of the probability distribution), and then taking a Fourier transform.

Note that the moments cannot be specified arbitrarily; for example, the variance cannot be negative. If only a finite number of the moments are specified instead of a full set, then in general an infinite number of distributions can be found consistent with these moments, and additional criteria are required to specify a unique probability distribution. One such criterion that is popular is given by the maximum entropy method. According to this criterion, one chooses that distribution which has maximum entropy compared to all distributions with the same moments. For example, for a random variable defined on the real line, and for specified values of mean and variance, the maximum entropy distribution is a Gaussian. In R^n, correspondingly if the mean and the covariance matrix are specified and the latter is positive definite, then the maximum entropy distribution is a multivariate Gaussian.

This procedure generalizes to continuous stochastic processes. However, as discussed earlier, the conditions for the existence of a continuous stochastic process and its associated probability distribution are nontrivial and must be taken into account. We will not go in to a detailed discussion of these issues here but will note that these problems are also encountered in statistical physics and quantum field theory. Usually, these problems can be addressed through discretization and the introduction of appropriate cutoffs.

The Gaussian stochastic process can therefore be uniquely specified in terms of its first two moments. The only condition is that the correlation function should be positive definite. For a univariate stationary Gaussian process, the condition is equivalent to choosing the power spectrum to be a real positive function. For a multivariate stationary Gaussian process, the condition is that the power spectral matrix should be positive definite at each frequency.

---

35. The moments have to exist—probability distributions that decay too slowly at infinity may not have defined moments. However, it is no great loss of generality to stick to distributions that possess moments, because this can always be achieved by altering the distribution at very large values of the variable that are not physically relevant.

Product Densities or Factorial Moments

In contrast with continuous processes, moments of point processes contain delta function pieces that have to be treated with care. Recall that point processes can be described in terms of delta function trains

$$\eta(t) = \sum_i \delta(t - t_i) \tag{5.219}$$

The moments of the process are defined analogously to continuous processes

$$m(t_1, t_2, \ldots, t_n) = E[\eta(t_1)\eta(t_2)\ldots\eta(t_n)] \tag{5.220}$$

There are delta functions if any two of the times coincide. Removing these gives the so-called product densities or factorial moments

$$\rho(\tau_1, \tau_2, \ldots, \tau_n) = E[\Sigma_{i_1 \neq i_2 \neq \ldots i_n} \prod_j \eta(\tau_j - t_{i_n})] \tag{5.221}$$

The relations between the first and second moments, and the corresponding product densities, are given by

$$\rho(t_1) = m(t_1) \tag{5.222}$$
$$\rho(t_1, t_2) = m(t_1, t_2) - \rho(t_1)\delta(t_1 - t_2) \tag{5.223}$$

For a translationally invariant process the rate is a constant

$$\rho(t_1) = \rho \tag{5.224}$$

The second order product density is given by

$$\rho(t_1 - t_2) = m(t_1 - t_2) - \rho\delta(t_1 - t_2) \tag{5.225}$$

For a Poisson process, points at distinct times are independent, so that the product densities are constants

$$\rho(t_1, t_2, \ldots, t_n) = \rho^n \tag{5.226}$$

These have a probabilistic interpretation as the joint density of finding points at $t_1, t_2, \ldots, t_n$, allowing for other points to occur at other times. Note the contrast with *sample function density* discussed earlier, which plays the role of point process likelihoods and gives the probability density of finding a set of time points, with no other points anywhere else. The product densities are what can be realistically measured or estimated (in particular the first and second order product densities) in experiments. This is the reason for interest in the method of specification in terms of moments.

The product densities are sometimes loosely referred to as "correlation functions," although this designation is not consistent with the fact that the product densities go to a constant value at large separation between the time points, whereas correlation functions would be expected to decay with separation of times. Therefore, it is preferable to use the designation "correlation function" or "connected correlation function" for the moments with the asymptotic values subtracted

$$c(t_1, t_2, \ldots, t_n) = E[(\eta(t_1) - \rho(t_1))(\eta(t_2) - \rho(t_2)) \ldots (\eta(t_n) - \rho(t_n))] \quad (5.227)$$

In particular, the second-order correlation function is related to the raw moments as follows:

$$c(t_1, t_1) = m(t_1, t_2) - m(t_1)m(t_2) \quad (5.228)$$

Second Moment for an Inhomogeneous Poisson Process

To explicitly exhibit the difference between the three quantities, consider the corresponding expressions for a rate modulated or inhomogeneous Poisson process, with time-dependent rate given by $\rho(t)$. All three quantities are expressible in terms of this time-dependent rate, which carries a full characterization of the process. The product density can be written down by inspection

$$\rho(t_1, t_2) = \rho(t_1)\rho(t_2) \quad (5.229)$$

The second moment contains an extra delta function piece

$$m(t_1, t_2) = \rho(t_1)\rho(t_2) + \rho(t_1)\delta(t_1 - t_2) \quad (5.230)$$

On the other hand, the correlation function contains only a delta function piece

$$c(t_1, t_2) = \rho(t_1)\delta(t_1 - t_2) \quad (5.231)$$

This is intuitively sensible, because the inhomogeneous Poisson process is not correlated from one time point to another.

Stationary Point Process Spectra

As in the case of continuous processes, the Fourier transform of the correlation function is defined to be the spectrum of the point process. For a stationary point process

$$S(f) = \int_{-\infty}^{\infty} dt e^{-2\pi i f t} C(t) \quad (5.232)$$

From the above discussion, the spectrum of a Poisson process is a constant, given by its rate

$$S_{Poisson}(f) = \int_{-\infty}^{\infty} dt e^{-2\pi i f t} \rho \delta(t) = \rho \quad (5.233)$$

This shows the formal correspondence between a Poisson process and white noise. More generally, the spectrum will not be a constant; however, for *any* stationary point process, the spectrum asymptotically goes to a constant value given by the rate of the process

$$\lim_{f \to \infty} S(f) = \rho \qquad (5.234)$$

The value of the spectrum at zero frequency $S(0)$ also has a simple interpretation. It is given in terms of the number variance as follows:

$$S(0) = \lim_{T \to \infty} \frac{V[N(T)]}{T} \qquad (5.235)$$

More generally, the spectrum is related to the number variance in a finite interval, as a function of the interval size, through an integral transform. In the neuroscience literature it is customary to define the so called "Fano factor,"

$$F(T) = \frac{V[N(T)]}{E[N(T)]} \qquad (5.236)$$

Note that for a Poisson process, the Fano factor is identically one for all time intervals. More generally, number variance in a given interval is related to the point process spectrum through an integral transform:

$$V[N(T)] = \int_{-\infty}^{\infty} \left(\frac{\sin(\pi f T)}{\pi f} \right)^2 S(f) df \qquad (5.237)$$

The Fano factor is therefore also given by an integral transform of the spectrum

$$F(T) = \frac{1}{\rho T} \int_{-\infty}^{\infty} \left(\frac{\sin(\pi f T)}{\pi f} \right)^2 S(f) df \qquad (5.238)$$

Noting that $\frac{1}{T} \left(\frac{\sin(\pi f T)}{\pi f} \right)^2$ becomes a delta function for large T, it is clear that the dependence of $F(T)$ on time at long times depends on the shape of the spectrum at low frequencies. In other words, the low-frequency behavior of the point process spectrum is determined by the number variance in long time windows.

Dynamic Spectra for Nonstationary Point Processes

One may define dynamic spectra or spectrograms for nonstationary point processes in the same way that one can define the analogous quantity for a continuous process

$$S(f, t) = \int_{-\infty}^{\infty} dt\, e^{-2\pi i f \tau} C\left(t + \frac{\tau}{2}, t - \frac{\tau}{2}\right) \qquad (5.239)$$

As an example, consider the inhomogeneous Poisson process with time-dependent rate $\rho(t)$. The correlation function for this process is given by

$$C(t_1, t_2) = \rho(t_1)\delta(t_1 - t_2) \qquad (5.240)$$

It follows that the dynamic spectrum of the inhomogeneous Poisson process is given by

$$S(f, t) = \rho(t) \qquad (5.241)$$

It should be noted that the spectrogram shows no frequency dependence: each time, one obtains a white spectrum, with a strength given by the time-dependent rate. This motivates the definition of the normalized spectrogram for a point process

$$S_n(f, t) = \frac{S(f, t)}{\rho(t)} \qquad (5.242)$$

For the inhomogeneous Poisson process, $S_n(f, t) = 1$. Therefore, departures of $S_n(f, t)$ from unity provides a useful practical measure the presence of non-trivial correlations in the process. The logarithm of this quantity may also be considered.

Specification of Point Processes via Moments

Point processes can be specified in terms of the moments in the same way as for continuous processes. There are some additional constraints on the moments, which make for some subtle considerations. The conditions under which stationary point processes exist for given forms of the correlation function are a topic of current research. Recent progress has been made in refining the relevant conditions.[36] Given the interest in the subject in the context of spike train spectra, we provide a brief discussion of the issues involved.

To understand the origin of such additional constraints, consider the number variance of the process $V[N(T)]$. As for a continuous process, this number variance has to be nonnegative. However, there is a stricter constraint. Let the rate of the process be ρ. Note that $E[N(T)] = \rho T$. If ρT is an integer, then there can be exactly ρT points in the interval, and the number variance can be zero. However, if ρT is not an integer, then $N(T)$ can never be equal to ρT, but must be an integer larger than, or less than, ρT. Because the average of $N(T)$ is ρT, $N(T)$ must take at least two values. From these considerations, it is easy to show that $V[N(T)] \geq \theta(1 - \theta)$, where θ is the fractional part of ρT. From the above

---

36. See the paper by Kuna, Lebowitz, and Speer available in preprint form from the physics preprint archive http://arxiv.org, preprint number math-ph-0612075.

expression for the variance, we obtain the following inequality for the spectrum ($\theta = \rho T - [\rho T]$, where $[x]$ denotes the integer just smaller than x)

$$\theta(1-\theta) \leq \int_{-\infty}^{\infty} \left(\frac{\sin(\pi f T)}{\pi f} \right)^2 S(f) df \tag{5.243}$$

This is an extra constraint compared to a continuous process, for which all that is required is that $S(f)$ be non-negative. There are other similar constraints that the point process spectra must satisfy. Note, however, that if the point process is given the spectrum can always be computed; the question here is whether an arbitrary function of frequency can serve as a point process spectrum, and the answer is in the negative.

Suppose that the spectrum (or equivalently the correlation function) is given, and also that at least one corresponding point process exists. What is the form of the maximum entropy process consistent with the spectrum or correlation function? Discretizing the process by binning time, a heuristic argument can be given that the form of the maximum entropy process, with given correlation function or spectrum, should have the Gibbs-Boltzmann form with only two body or pairwise interactions.

Consider the discretized approximation of a point process, where a configuration is given as a string of binary variables σ_i taking the values 0, 1. Define the correlation function to be

$$C_{ij} = E[\sigma_i \sigma_j] \tag{5.244}$$

Consider the probability distribution $p(\sigma_1, \sigma_2, \ldots, \sigma_n)$. The entropy of the distribution is well defined because it is a discrete and finite sample space, and it is given by

$$S = - \sum_{\sigma_1, \sigma_2, \ldots, \sigma_n} p(\sigma_1, \sigma_2, \ldots, \sigma_n) \log(p(\sigma_1, \sigma_2, \ldots, \sigma_n)) \tag{5.245}$$

Constraining the correlation functions to their desired values may be implemented using Lagrange multipliers J_{ij}, leading to the maximum entropy condition

$$\max\left(S + \sum_{ij} J_{ij}(C_{ij} - E[\sigma_i \sigma_j]) \right) \tag{5.246}$$

This leads straightforwardly to the maximum entropy distribution

$$p = \frac{1}{Z} e^{-\sum_{ij} J_{ij} \sigma_i \sigma_j} \tag{5.247}$$

Here Z is the partition coefficient or normalization constant. Making the identification $J_{ij} \sigma_i \sigma_j \leftrightarrow J(t_i, t_j)$, this is the Gibbs distribution with pairwise interactions. Note that this relation is formal, because the relation between

J_{ij} and C_{ij} is complicated and nonlinear. However, the argument establishes the Gibbs form with pairwise interactions as the maximum entropy distribution with given correlation functions.

Recall that for point processes confined to a finite interval, the process could be specified by giving the sample function densities or Janossy densities $p(t_1, t_2, \ldots, t_n)$ for all n. In this case one can explicitly write down the relationship between the product densities or factorial moments, and the sample function densities, which play the role of point process likelihood [54]:

$$\rho(t_1, t_2, \ldots, t_k)$$
$$= \sum_{n=0}^{\infty} \frac{1}{n!} \int_0^T \cdots \int_0^T p(t_1, t_2, \ldots, t_k, \tau_1, \ldots, \tau_n) d\tau_1 d\tau_2 \ldots d\tau_n \qquad (5.248)$$

$$p(t_1, t_2, \ldots, t_n)$$
$$= \sum_{k=0}^{\infty} \frac{(-1)^k}{k!} \int_0^T \cdots \int_0^T \rho(t_1, t_2, \ldots, t_n, \tau_1, \ldots, \tau_k) d\tau_1 d\tau_2 \ldots d\tau_k \qquad (5.249)$$

This concludes our discussion of point processes. Although a lot more can be said about stochastic processes, we have tried to cover some of the essential concepts that are relevant for understanding neurobiological signals.

6

Statistical Protocols

I have no data yet. It is a capital mistake to theorize before one has data. Insensibly one begins to twist facts to suit theories, instead of theories to suit facts.
— Sherlock Holmes, in *A Scandal in Bohemia*, by Sir Arthur Conan Doyle

In this chapter we provide a mini-review of classical and modern statistical methods for data analysis before moving onto the more specialised topic of statistical methods specific to time series analysis. Statistics is a complex and multifaceted subject, partly due to the many domains of application. Although neuroscientists in particular and biologists in general are exposed to statistical methodology, it is often in a somewhat narrow and specialised context, which may not always lead to a deep appreciation of the basic principles.

This leads to two problems. First, the more advanced techniques, such as those used in time series analysis, appear more complicated and esoteric than they really are. For example, in what gets called "decoding," the neural "code" is usually not much more than an application of the classical statistical methods of regression or function estimation to time series data. Depending on the application, a stimulus time series, or the time course of a behavioral output, is usually the dependent variable in the regression, and the spike train, or other measure of neural activity, is the independent variable. In principle, someone who has thoroughly understood simple linear regression of one scalar variable onto another should be able to understand the basic concepts involved in such "decoding." However, if regression has been encountered as part of a statistical package, without a good conceptual understanding of the statistical under-

148

pinnings, then these connections may not be apparent. Second, there is the old adage: if one is not aware of history then it is apt to be repeated: the same basic solution tends to be rediscovered in slightly different variations. This is wasteful and can also be avoided based on a firm grasp of existing statistical principles.

Producing a one-chapter introduction to statistical concepts with sufficient depth to ameliorate the two problems pointed to above is perhaps too ambitious a task. However, taking this material for granted and not covering it at all would leave too large a lacuna in our introduction to the methods of neural data analysis. We have therefore attempted to present such an introduction in this chapter. It is necessarily limited, particularly in the context of modern techniques. There are several excellent monographs which the reader can consult for more extensive discussion of modern statistical methodology [63, 107, 147, 195, 228].

6.1 Data Analysis Goals

Neuroscience is a complex subject, and the statistical analysis of neurobiological signals offers opportunities to use a broad variety of techniques. Unquestionably, technical developments form a subject of study in themselves; indeed, this book would perhaps not be written if it were not for specific technical developments that need exposition. However, this has an inherent element of danger, in the form of the instrumental fallacy, where the focus becomes the data analysis technique itself. It is important therefore to take the broader view and keep in mind *what* it is that one is trying to achieve with the technical tools.

One may classify data analysis goals in neuroscience into two broad categories, not necessarily mutually exclusive: advancing scientific knowledge and understanding, and biomedical applications in diagnostics and therapeutics. Scientific data analysis goals may be further subdivided into exploratory and confirmatory; these are often combined, but depending on the problem domain there may be more emphasis on one or the other. In data-driven empirical studies, the goal may be to discover patterns in the data and to formulate parsimonious hypotheses that distill the structure present in the observations. On the other hand, in situations where experiments have been carefully designed to test specific hypotheses, the analysis goals are to assess the evidence in the light of these hypotheses and to take appropriate actions.

Apart from exploratory and confirmatory analyses, another important set of goals in scientific data analysis concerns the communication of results. Science is a social enterprise, particularly in a rich area such as neuroscience, and effective means of communication are important; when reporting the results of data analysis, the usage of shared metrics and tools are critical to avoid a scientific Tower of Babel. Development of such shared metrics and tools are therefore an important part of the challenge.

Although biomedical data analysis has overlapping goals with scientific data analysis, the requirements are more of a pragmatic, engineering nature. In diagnostics, the goal could be to draw inferences about a disease state, to locate the site and understand the nature of a pathology, and so on. One may use the analogy of a microscope: in performing pathological analysis of tissue, one looks at a sample of the tissue under a microscope; the neural signal analyst has at his or her disposal a variety of mathematical microscopes with which to examine the signals and draw similar inferences. On the other hand, neural signal processing is playing an increasingly important role in therapeutics, in applications such as neural prosthetics, where electrical signals are read out of the brain and used to control, for example, an artificial limb, or even in closed loop brain stimulation applications. This is reminiscent of control engineering, with statistical estimation playing an important role in sensing the system output to generate appropriate control signals. Automation is clearly critical for such applications, and a thorough understanding of statistical methodology for handling neural signals will likely be needed in the future for a variety of biomedical applications.

6.2   An Example of a Protocol: Method of Least Squares

What do we mean by a statistical protocol? By this we are referring to a problem-solving technique or algorithm that may be applied to a data analysis problem. Before discussing statistical protocols in more detail we shall consider an example.

A statistical protocol that goes back to Gauss, Legendre, and Laplace, but still retains a central place in contemporary statistics, is the method of least squares. In its simplest form, the method applies to (possibly noisy) observations of pairs (y_i, x_i) where the underlying variable y is related to the variable x through a known (or postulated) functional form, $y = f(x, \beta)$, and the goal is to determine β. The method is to construct the sum of squared errors $\sum_i (y_i - f(x_i, \beta))^2$ and to minimize over β. The beauty of this procedure is its simplicity and generality. With a bit of care in pruning outliers and dealing appropriately with issues relating to the dimensionality of parameter space, this old method requires only elementary algebra to understand, yet still has much practical use—the hallmark of a good protocol. A more extensive treatment of the least square method will be given in the section on estimation.

It is interesting to note that Legendre and Gauss discovered the method while analyzing astronomical data dealing with planetary orbits. This shows the coevolution of statistical methodology with the scientific questions of the day. If the nineteenth century saw statistics protocols coevolve with the

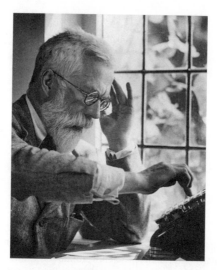

Figure 6.1: British statistician and geneticist Sir Ronald Aylmer Fisher (1890–1962), perhaps the key founding figure of modern statistics, made equally fundamental contributions to the mathematical study of population genetics and evolution.

analysis of astrophysical observations, the twentieth century saw the coevolution of biology and statistics, with leading statisticians like Fisher (fig. 6.1) also contributing fundamentally to population genetics. Further, the development of sophisticated mathematical methods in statistical physics has happened hand in hand with trying to understand complex interacting systems. Such systems include particles in a fluid or solid, with many more degrees of freedom than the planets in the solar system.

6.3 Classical and Modern Approaches

Currently, we are seeing another stage of development where the level of resolution and volumes of data in biology and in studies of complex physical phenomena (such as the weather) have increased greatly compared to mid-twentieth century levels, as has the ability to perform complex computations on these data. In this stage of growth, it is not so much the development of new mathematical tools but the implementation of mathematical tools on increasingly larger computers that is playing the most important role.

Given the exponential growth curves in processor speed and storage power that are yet to saturate, computational methods themselves are in some state of flux, and details of the current implementations could quickly become obsolete. However, the basic approaches to problem solving and the underlying mathematics is less prone to change. In discussing statistical protocols, we therefore

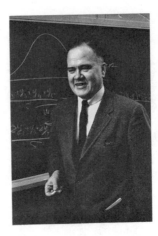

Figure 6.2: American statistician John W. Tukey (1915–2000) championed exploratory data analysis and had a significant impact on modern statistical practise. Among other things, Tukey is well known for having coined the word "bit," and introduced the widely used method of data display called the box plot. (The photo is dated 1965.)

concentrate on these and provide an introduction the classical areas of statistical estimation and inference.

The division between classical and modern is somewhat contrived; what we group under "classical" estimation and inference is of recent vintage (mid-twentieth century) and still basic to modern data analysis. The following are some of the differences between the "classical" and "modern" periods:

1. Greater emphasis on visualization and exploratory data analysis, as espoused by Tukey (fig. 6.2) among others.
2. The growing need as well as ability to handle larger data volumes.
3. A number of advances in machine learning or supervised learning (which corresponds to regression in the classical approach).
4. The increased ability to apply nonparametric procedures (such as the bootstrap and permutation procedures).
5. The increased application of Monte Carlo techniques to deal with probability distributions with many parameters.

6.3.1 Data Visualization

The importance of data visualization cannot be overemphasized [46]. Despite advances in computational technologies, for most interesting data sets data analysis tasks cannot be fully automated. A useful example to keep in mind is that of spike waveform classification in electrophysiology. Although a number of automated algorithms are available for clustering spike waveforms, a visual inspection step is required to check the output of the clustering algorithm and to correct it if necessary. That this is the case, even after a lot of effort has been applied to the automation problem for spike classification, is fairly typical.

This emphasis on visualization may be thought superfluous; after all, it seems obvious that one should look at one's data. Surprisingly enough, in the authors' experience, a number of errors in real-life data analysis have stemmed from a lack of adequate visualization of the raw data. In the context of neural signals, this may entail looking at spike rasters, plots of time courses, looking at spectrograms of time series, looking at movies of image data sequences, and so on. Details of visualization methods are of course very much problem dependent and will be discussed in the applications portion of the book.

6.4 Classical Approaches: Estimation and Inference

Later stages of data analysis typically involve statistical *estimation* and *inference*. Estimation comes in two broad flavors, depending on whether one is dealing with a single group of variables or multiple groups of variables. For a single group of observations one may be interested in characterizing that group with a probability distribution, and estimating parameters of the distribution, or estimating moments of the associated random variables, and so on, whereas for multiple groups one is in addition interested in estimating the functional relationship between the groups, which could also take the form of estimating the associated conditional probability distributions. *Point estimation* deals with obtaining a single estimate of some property of the underlying probability distribution, whereas in *interval estimation*, one looks for a set of point estimates with a desirable property (for example, that the probability measure of the set is close to one). Interval estimation usually takes the form of estimating confidence bands or error bars.

Inference involves choosing between alternatives. In practice, most uses of statistical protocols in the experimental neuroscience or biology involve hypothesis testing, or deciding between alternative hypotheses. In the simplest case, the investigator has designed the experiment with a specific binary hypothesis in mind that one of two alternatives is true. The hypothesis-testing protocol is the set of steps that lead from the data gathered in the experiment to adoption or rejection of the hypotheses. It is customary to qualify such a decision with appropriate probabilities that quantify the potential for error inherent in such a decision procedure. Different fields of research have different thresholds for deciding for or against hypotheses; in biology, it is customary to set this threshold at a 5% chance of error, whereas such a high error rate would hardly be tolerated in testing hypotheses in the context of physical law. Also, the relevant decisions cannot always be made based purely on probabilistic considerations, but additional information about the costs of making a mistake may need to be taken into account. This is the subject of study in decision theory.

The organization and choice of material in this section is inspired by the excellent monograph on *Statistical Inference* by Silvey [204].

6.4.1 Point Estimation

In the following discussion it will be assumed that we start from a set of data *samples*. In much of the discussion we also assume that these samples are independently and identically[1] distributed (conventionally abbreviated as i.i.d) random variables with an associated probability distribution, which is typically not fully known a priori. Note that the assumption of independence and identical distribution is a very strong one and needs to be checked. It will typically not be satisfied, and the procedures have to be suitably adopted. Further, the individual data point may be a complex object—in most of the analysis we are interested in, a whole time series will be regarded as a single sample of a high-dimensional object rather than a sequence of correlated samples from some distribution. However, for simplicity, we start with samples that are a finite collection of i.i.d real scalars or vectors. This is a good point to remind the reader that there are alternative descriptions of uncertainty other than probability theory, such as set-based methods or game theoretic approaches. However, we will not discuss these in the current section.

In point estimation one is usually interested in some property of the underlying distribution. This property may be a moment or cumulant of the distribution. Alternatively, the distribution may be characterized by one or more parameters that are not known and have to be estimated from the data. For example, suppose we are given a set of samples $N_1, N_2, \ldots, N_n$ that are i.i.d Poisson. Recall that the Poisson distribution is given by $P(N = \chi) = e^{-\lambda}\lambda^n/n!$. This sets the stage for the estimation problem: given the sample $N_1, N_2, \ldots, N_n$, estimate λ. One can imagine applying this trivial example to a neurobiological data set where N_i is the number of spikes recorded from a neuron during some fixed time window, in the ith trial of n repeated experiments. The considerations below of course carry over to more complicated probability distributions.

Estimator; Bias and Variance

The idea is to define an *estimator*, which is a function of the samples. Note that a function of the sample values is also referred to as a *sample statistic*, or simply, statistic. Not all sample statistics are used as estimators of parameters of the distribution—as we will see later, sample statistics are also useful in hypothesis testing. The *value* of the estimator function evaluated on the samples in question gives us an estimate of the parameter. It is sometimes easy to guess what such an estimator might be: for example, we know that for the Poisson dis-

---

1. This means that the random variables are drawn from the same distribution.

tribution, $E[N] = \lambda$. Therefore, we might guess that the sample mean might be a good estimator for λ. We therefore define the estimator

$$\hat{\lambda}(N_1, N_2, \ldots, N_n) = \frac{1}{n} \sum_{i=1}^{n} N_i \tag{6.1}$$

We naturally want the estimator to be "good" in an appropriate sense. Considerations of what are good estimators lead to a number of concepts, including bias, variance, and sufficiency, which we define and discuss in turn.

Because an estimator or a statistic is a function of random variables, it is in turn a random variable itself. It is therefore natural to consider the expectation value and variance of an estimator. We would like that the expectation value be equal to the parameter being estimated, and that the variance be small in some measure. This leads to the following definitions:

1. *Estimation bias*, or simply bias, for an estimator $\hat{\lambda}$ of a parameter λ is defined as the difference between the expected value of the estimator, and the true value, $Bias = E[\hat{\lambda}] - \lambda$.
2. Estimation variance is simply the variance $Variance = V[\hat{\lambda}]$. If a vector of parameters is being estimated, then one defines the covariance matrix of the vector $\hat{\lambda}$.

Note that both the bias and the variance are in general functions of λ. A trivial example of an estimator is to choose a fixed value of λ, say λ_0. This is of course a bad estimator, but note that both the bias and variance vanish when $\lambda = \lambda_0$. This is like the parable of a stopped clock being more accurate than a slow clock—the latter never tells the right time, but the former tells the right time twice a day. Of course, by any reasonable criterion, the stopped clock is the worse choice. Therefore, whether an estimator is good or bad has to be judged over a range of parameter values, not at a single parameter value.

The reader should verify as an exercise that the expected value of the mean square error when using an estimator $\hat{\lambda}$ has the so called bias-variance decomposition, $E[|\hat{\lambda} - \lambda|^2] = Bias^2 + Variance$. This shows that there can be a trade-off between bias and variance; ideally, one would like choose an estimator that is unbiased and also has minimal variance in an appropriate sense, although this is not always possible.

Returning to the Poisson example, we compute the bias and variance.

- Show that the bias is zero, namely $E[\hat{\lambda}] = \lambda$.
- Show that the variance is given by λ/n.

If the bias vanishes for all values of λ the estimator is said to be unbiased. The variance of the estimator described above goes to zero as the sample size goes to infinity. This means that as for large sample sizes, the value of the estimator converges to the true value, a property known as *consistency*. Now consider another estimator, which is also unbiased

$$\hat{\lambda}_1(N_1, N_2, \ldots, N_n) = N_1 \qquad (6.2)$$

The estimator is unbiased because $E[\hat{\lambda}_1] = \lambda$, but it is not a good estimator, because it has a variance $V[\hat{\lambda}_1] = \lambda$ that is n times larger compared with the previous estimator. This is of course not surprising because no averaging has been performed in constructing this estimator. A less trivial example is the sample variance

$$\hat{\lambda}_2(N_1, N_2, \ldots, N_n) = \frac{1}{n} \sum_{i=1}^{n} (N_i - \bar{N})^2 \qquad (6.3)$$

Here $\bar{N} = \hat{\lambda}$ is the sample mean, our first estimator. Because the variance of the Poisson distribution is the same as the mean, one might expect that this is also a good estimator for the Poisson parameter. However, this estimator is biased: $E[\hat{\lambda}_2] = (1 - 1/n)\lambda$. Note that the bias $B(\lambda) = -\lambda/n$ goes to zero as $n \to \infty$, so this estimator is *asymptotically unbiased*. Under conditions where it is not possible to construct an unbiased estimator, one may still construct asymptotically unbiased estimators.

Sufficient Statistics

Finally, let us write down the joint distribution of the random variables constituting the sample. This is given by

$$p(N_1, N_2, \ldots, N_n) = e^{-n\lambda} \lambda^{\sum_i N_i} \prod_{i=1}^{n} \frac{1}{N_i!} \qquad (6.4)$$

This joint distribution has the interesting property that the only interaction between the parameter λ and the sample is mediated by the sum $\sum_i N_i$, or equivalently the sample mean. If the sample mean is kept fixed, then the probability distribution factorizes into two parts, one of which depends on λ but not on the rest of the details of the sample, whereas the other part does not depend on λ. In other words, the sampling distribution has the form

$$p(N_1, N_2, \ldots, N_n) = f(\lambda, \hat{\lambda}(N_1, \ldots, N_n)) g(N_1, \ldots, N_n) \qquad (6.5)$$

For a sampling distribution that has this factorized form, $\hat{\lambda}$ is called a *sufficient* statistic for the parameter λ—it carries all the relevant information from the sample about the parameter in question. In a Bayesian formulation, one has $p(\lambda \,|\, Sample) = p(\lambda \,|\, \hat{\lambda})$. This can be generalized to multiple parameters.

Cramer-Rao Bound

How do we know whether our estimator has small variance compared to all other possible estimators? This question can be addressed through the *Cramer-*

Rao (CR) bound to the estimator variance. It can be shown that for any estimator $\hat{\lambda}$, the variance has a lower bound that can be computed from knowledge of the underlying probability distribution $p(x, \lambda)$[2]:

$$V[\hat{\lambda}] \geq B(\lambda)^2 + \frac{1}{nI(\lambda)} \tag{6.6}$$

$$B(\lambda) = E[\hat{\lambda}] - \lambda \tag{6.7}$$

$$I(\lambda) = E\left[\left(\frac{\partial \log (p)}{\partial \lambda} \right)^2 \right] \tag{6.8}$$

Here $B(\lambda)$ is the estimator bias defined earlier. $I(\lambda)$ is known as the Fisher information. For an unbiased estimator, this leads to a definition of the *efficiency* of an estimator

$$Efficiency(\hat{\lambda}) = \frac{(nI(\lambda))^{-1}}{V[\hat{\lambda}]} \tag{6.9}$$

Due to the CR bound, the efficiency is a number between zero and one.

- Show that for the Poisson distribution, the Fisher information for the parameter λ is given by $I(\lambda) = 1/\lambda$.
- Show that the estimator $\hat{\lambda}$ discussed above has a variance equal to the CR bound.

For a vector of parameters, there is an appropriate generalization to this result, which we state below for the unbiased case in matrix form. Because we are dealing with a vector, instead of a variance one needs to consider the covariance matrix, and the inequality takes the form that the difference matrix is positive definite. Define the covariance matrix for the estimator, $V_{ij} = E[(\hat{\lambda}_i - \lambda_i)(\hat{\lambda}_j - \lambda_j)]$, and the Fisher information matrix $I_{ij} = E[\frac{\partial \log (p)}{\partial \lambda_i} \frac{\partial \log (p)}{\partial \lambda_j}]$. Then the CR bound for the case of a vector estimator (assumed unbiased) is the condition that the matrix $V - I^{-1}/n$ is positive definite. This is the same as saying that for all vectors μ, $\sum_{ij} \mu_i V_{ij} \mu_j \geq \frac{1}{n} \sum_{ij} \mu_i (I^{-1})_{ij} \mu_j$.

Method of Maximum Likelihood

The sampling probability distribution, regarded as a function of the parameters of the distribution, is known as the likelihood function:

$$Likelihood(\theta) = p(x_1, x_2, \ldots, x_n; \theta) \tag{6.10}$$

---

2. The probability distribution for the random variables constituting the sample have to satisfy some regularity conditions for the CR bound to hold.

Because we are dealing with the case where the sample consists of i.i.d random variables, the likelihood function is a product of the individual likelihoods, $Likelihood(\theta) = \prod_i p(x_i, \theta)$. The likelihood function can be used to define a very useful class of estimators, the maximum likelihood estimator (MLE):

$$\hat{\theta}_{MLE}(x_1,..., x_n) = argmax_\theta \; p(x_1,..., x_n; \theta) \qquad (6.11)$$

The MLE estimator is obtained by maximizing the likelihood function for a fixed data set; we have emphasized the fact that this is an estimator (a function of the samples) by explicitly exhibiting the dependence on the sample values. Typically, it is more convenient to consider the log likelihood, $L(\theta) = \log(p(x_1,..., x_n; \theta))$. Assuming that the likelihood function is sufficiently smooth and that the maximum does not occur at the boundaries of the parameter space, the MLE is given by the equation

$$\sum_i \frac{\partial \log p(x_i, \theta)}{\partial \theta} = 0 \qquad (6.12)$$

For the Poisson example above, $\log p(N_i, \lambda) = -\lambda + N_i \; \log(\lambda) - \log(N_i!)$. Therefore, it follows that the maximum likelihood estimator for λ is given by the sample mean.

- Suppose n samples $x_1, x_2, \dots, x_n$ are drawn from the Gaussian or normal distribution with mean μ and variance σ. Find the MLEs of the mean and the variance.
- Show that the MLE of the variance is biased (but asymptotically unbiased).

Asymptotic Properties of MLE

Maximum likelihood estimators have some nice properties; under suitable conditions, they are asymptotically unbiased and efficient. This means that for large sample sizes they converge to the true parameter values. However, it should be noted that in a lot of practical cases one does not have a sufficiently large number of samples for these asymptotic properties to hold.

The asymptotic properties of the MLE can be understood using the law of large numbers. Let $x_1, x_2, \dots, x_n$ be i.i.d with a distribution $p(x, \theta_0)$. The log likelihood divided by the number of sample points, considered as a function of θ, is given by

$$l(x_1,..., x_n, \theta) = \frac{1}{n} \sum_{i=1}^{n} \log \; (p(x_i, \theta)) \qquad (6.13)$$

It is important to keep in mind that the x_i have the distribution $p(x, \theta_0)$, and $p(x, \theta)$ corresponds to the distribution from which the samples are drawn *only* when $\theta = \theta_0$. Now $\log(p(x_i, \theta))$ are themselves random variables, and by the law of large numbers, the sample mean of these random variables tends to the expectation value, so that for large n, $l(\{x_i\}, \theta) \approx \lambda(\theta)$, where

$$\lambda(\theta) = E[\log(p(x, \theta))] = \int dx p(x, \theta_0) \log(p(x, \theta)) \qquad (6.14)$$

Now recall the definition of the Kullback-Leiber divergence between two probability distributions, $D(p\|q) = \int dx p(x) \log(p(x)/q(x))$, and that $D(p\|q) \geq 0$, equality being achieved when $p = q$. Applying this equation to the above equation, we obtain the inequality

$$\lambda(\theta_0) \geq \lambda(\theta) \qquad (6.15)$$

Equality is achieved when $p(x, \theta) \equiv p(x, \theta_0)$, which in general will imply that $\theta = \theta_0$. Therefore the function $\lambda(\theta)$ has a unique maximum at θ_0. In the large sample limit, the log likelihood function divided by the number of samples, $l(x_1, \ldots, x_n, \theta)$ is close to $\lambda(\theta)$, and can therefore be expected to have the same property. This shows that for large samples the MLE will be close to θ_0, the true value of the parameter.

Identifiability

Now it may be the case that $\lambda(\theta)$ has multiple maxima, or does not depend on θ in some region around the maximum. In this case, the parameter θ is not identifiable. It is not difficult to construct a situation where this is the case. For example, consider the Poisson likelihood, and let the parameter λ be the sum of two parameters $\lambda = \theta_1 + \theta_2$. Now we can formally write the likelihood function as a function of two parameters, $l(\theta_1, \theta_2) = l_{Poisson}(\theta_1 + \theta_2)$. It is clear that this function has the same value for a number of different values of θ_1 and θ_2, as long as $\theta_1 + \theta_2 = \lambda$. Therefore the parameters are not separately identifiable.

This was clearly an artificially constructed example. However, when dealing with a vector of parameters it may be the case that some combination of the parameters is close to being not identifiable. As we will see in the following discussion, it is convenient to regard the expected value of the negative log likelihood as an "energy landscape" or energy function for the vector of parameters. The minimum of this energy landscape corresponds to the true value of the parameters, and non-identifiable combinations of parameters correspond to flat directions in the energy landscape.

Asymptotic Normality of MLE

The MLE is a function defined on the samples and is therefore a random variable in its own right, as pointed out earlier. It can be shown using the central limit theorem and the law of large numbers that under appropriate regularity conditions, the MLE $\hat{\theta}$ has an asymptotically normal distribution, with mean θ (the true value of the parameter) and variance $(nI(\theta))^{-1}$, where θ is the Fisher information defined earlier, $I(\theta) = E[(\partial \log(p(x, \theta)) / \partial \theta)^2]$. Note that in practice, the true value of the parameter θ is not known and therefore has to be approximated by the MLE itself in estimating the Fisher information. This introduces an error, but for large n the correction appears at a subleading order.

Fisher Information Matrix

This scalar result generalizes to the vector case, and highlights the importance of the Fisher information matrix. For a vector of parameters θ_i, the MLE is a vector $\hat{\theta}_i$ that is asymptotically Gaussian distributed for large n, with mean θ and a covariance matrix given by

$$E[(\hat{\theta}_i - \theta_i)(\hat{\theta}_j - \theta_j)] = \frac{1}{n} I_{ij}^{-1} \tag{6.16}$$

$$I_{ij} = E\left[\frac{\partial \log (p)}{\partial \theta_i} \frac{\partial \log (p)}{\partial \theta_j}\right] \tag{6.17}$$

Therefore, the eigenvalue spectrum of the Fisher information matrix carries information about the identifiability of parameters. In particular, small eigenvalues correspond to linear combinations of parameters that have large estimation variance, and they are therefore more difficult to identify.

Because the likelihood is a non-negative function of the parameters, it is tempting to normalize it (assuming this is possible), to obtain a probability distribution over the parameters. This is close to the Bayesian approach and corresponds to the adoption of a uniform prior. In analogy with statistical physics, this likelihood-based probability distribution can also be thought of as a Gibbs-Boltzmann distribution with an energy function given by the negative log likelihood. This sort of approach is useful if one wants to assign probabilities to regions in parameter space, namely for interval estimation, which will be discussed in a later section.

Difficulties When $p >> n$

In all of the discussion above, it has been tacitly assumed that the sample size n becomes large while the number of parameters p is held finite. Unfortunately, this is not the case for most of the time series analysis that is of interest to us in this book. Rather, one has the opposite extreme, where p is much greater than n, or even infinite (because an infinite number of parameters may be needed to determine a particular function of time or to determine the spectrum of a stochastic process). Clearly, there is no hope of a direct application of MLE in this case, because the number of things to be estimated exceeds the number of available independent variables, and the system is underconstrained.

One may try to get around this predicament by putting strong constraints on the parameter space in the form of priors, which effectively reduce the number of degrees of freedom to be estimated to a number smaller than the number of available data points. There is something unsatisfying about this procedure, however; in trying to estimate an infinite number of parameters from a finite data set, one necessarily needs an infinite number of constraints. Combining a finite amount of data with an infinite number of constraints seems like a rather strange procedure.

An argument that is often advanced is that one can *check* the results of the procedure by asking if some appropriate model residuals show the behavior one expects from applying the model. However, because the likelihood is *uninformative* about certain parameter combinations, *any prior* placed on those combinations will still be fully consistent with the data.

An alternative approach, which we will pursue in dealing with time series, is to estimate only some properties of the original infinite dimensional distribution, rather than trying to obtain a full estimate of the distribution. In particular we will be interested in *moments* of the distribution, although we will find that it is in general hopeless to go beyond the second moment. Alternatively, it is sometimes possible to reduce the original problem to a low-dimensional one through appropriate feature extraction; in this case, one can still take advantage of the power of the likelihood based approach.

As an aside, if one does estimate some properties of the distribution, such as its moments, one can define the so-called maximum entropy distribution, one that is consistent with the constraints provided by the estimated properties but otherwise has maximal entropy among all distributions defined on the sample space. This is an attractive procedure but does not necessarily get rid of the problems associated with an ill conditioned Fisher information matrix (or the associated need to regularize by inserting prior information). We will not present a detailed discussion of the maximum entropy method but will refer to it in specific instances.

6.4.2 Method of Least Squares: The Linear Model

The linear model plays a central role in statistical estimation and inference. We first discuss the scalar and then the vector case. The setting is that there is an independent variable x with n sample values x_i (typically these are under experimental control) and an outcome or dependent variable y with the corresponding values y_i; the assumption is that these are related through a linear equation, allowing for measurement noise ε_i:

$$y_i = \beta x_i + \varepsilon_i \qquad (6.18)$$

The goal is to estimate the parameter β. The idea behind the least squares method is to minimize the mean squared error (MSE)

$$MSE(\beta) = \frac{1}{n} \sum_{i=1}^{n} (y_i - \beta x_i)^2 \qquad (6.19)$$

- Show that minimizing the MSE leads to the equation $\langle xy \rangle = \beta \langle x^2 \rangle$ (angle brackets denotes the sample mean [e.g., $\langle x^2 \rangle = (1/n) \sum_i x_i^2$]; for simplicity we use this notation on quantities involving x_i although x_i are fixed in advance and not samples in the same sense as y_i). Therefore, obtain the least square estimate $\hat{\beta}$ of the parameter β.
- Evaluate the minimum value of the squared error by substituting the estimate $\hat{\beta}$ into the equation for MSE.

Now one could take any set of pairs y_i, x_i that are not necessarily related, and find the best β that relates them using the least squares procedure. At this point, one may ask whether it was a good idea to fit a nonzero β to the data in question or whether it would be more parsimonious to set β to zero, given that there is measurement noise. This is a simple example of model selection. On the other hand, if we decide that β is nonzero, we might still want to estimate the uncertainty for the estimate itself. Both questions have systematic answers if the probability distribution of the noise ε_i is known.

The noise model that goes along with the least squares method is that of uncorrelated Gaussian noise. Although the least squares method can still be applied if the noise distribution is not Gaussian and can be suitably modified if the noise is correlated, the answers are simpler for the uncorrelated Gaussian noise and we will only consider that case here. Therefore, we assume ε_i are i.i.d Gaussian with mean zero and variance σ^2. Of course, σ is usually not known a priori and has to be estimated from the data. Now we are in a position to assess the variability of the least mean square (LMS) estimator $\hat{\beta} = \langle xy \rangle / \langle x^2 \rangle$.

Estimator Variance and Model Assessment

Because $\hat{\beta}$ is a linear combination of Gaussian distributed variables y_i, $\hat{\beta}$ is itself Gaussian distributed. It is straightforward to show that $V(\hat{\beta}) = \sigma^2 / \langle x^2 \rangle$. We now need to estimate σ^2. This can be achieved by considering the residuals, $y_i - \hat{\beta} x_i$. If the estimate was perfect, then these should equal the noise variables ε_i. We consider the residual sum of squares (RSS) $RSS = \sum_i (y_i - \hat{\beta} x_i)^2$. One can show that $E[RSS] = (n-1)\sigma^2$. Therefore, one can obtain an estimator for the variance given by $\hat{\sigma}^2 = RSS/(n-1)$.

We thus have an estimator for the variance of β given by $RSS/((n-1)\langle x^2 \rangle)$. To assess the "fit," it is natural to consider the statistic $(n-1)\hat{\beta}^2 \langle x^2 \rangle / RSS$, which is the ratio of the squared estimator for the mean, divided the estimator for the variance—a sort of signal-to-noise ratio. The upshot of this discussion is that we define the F statistic to assess whether there is evidence for a nonzero β:

$$\hat{F} = (n-1) \frac{\hat{\beta}^2 \langle x^2 \rangle}{\langle (y - \hat{\beta} x)^2 \rangle} \qquad (6.20)$$

Note that the estimator $\hat{\beta}$ will in general be nonzero even if the true value of β is zero. If $\beta = 0$, under the Gaussian assumption for ε_i, and also assuming that x_i are known accurately a priori,[3] the statistic defined above has a so-called F distribution with $(1, n-1)$ degrees of freedom (fig. 6.3). These are tabulated and are available as part of standard software packages. If the variables x_i and y_i are complex (this will be the case for the frequency F-ratio test to be encountered in the section on harmonic analysis), then the degrees of freedom are $(2, 2n-2)$.

The way this distribution is used is as follows: $\hat{F}$ is computed and the compared with some percentage point of the cumulative $F(1, n-1)$ distribution. For example, for $n = 10$, $P(F) = 0.95$ for $F = 5.12$. This means that if $\beta = 0$,

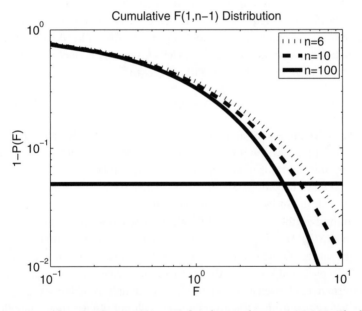

Figure 6.3: The cumulative $F(1, n-1)$ distribution for $n = 6,10,100$. The horizontal line corresponds to the 0.05% point, at which $P(F) = 0.95$ and therefore $1 - P(F) = 0.05$. This is a common threshold adopted in biological applications.

---

3. Measurements errors in the independent variables x_i lead to more complicated considerations, because these extra noise variables have to be now modeled and explicitly accounted for.

then with 95% probability, $\hat{F} < 5.12$. If the estimated $\hat{F}$ exceeds 5.12, one may wish to examine the alternative hypothesis that β is nonzero. We will consider this further in the section on hypothesis testing.

Multivariate Case

We now move on to the case of a linear model where there are multiple explanatory variables of the form $y_i = \sum_j x_{ij}\beta_j + \varepsilon_i$. This can also be written in matrix form $Y = X\beta + \varepsilon$, where Y and ε are $(n \times 1)$ column vectors, X is a $(n \times p)$ matrix (sometimes called the design matrix), and β is a $(p \times 1)$ column vector. Notice the difference from the first case studied, which may be regarded as the single parameter case.

This model has widespread usage. In the case of neural time series, this model is applied (for example, for functional magnetic resonance imaging data analysis) to explain voxel time series $y(t)$, where we make the identification $y_i \equiv y(t)$. The explanatory variables x_{ij} correspond to predetermined time courses $x_j(t)$ that are either expected stimulus response waveforms, or so-called "nuisance variables," used to model and remove noise sources with known waveform but unknown amplitudes. In our considerations below we will assume all variables are real. The complex case is also of interest and can be recovered from the real case by multiplying the degrees of freedom by two.

The LMS estimator for the linear model satisfies the *normal equations* obtaining the differentiating the MSE with respect to β

$$X^\dagger Y = X^\dagger X \beta \tag{6.21}$$

We can solve this equation if the matrix $X^\dagger X$ is invertible. Recall that X is a $(n \times p)$ matrix; if $n > p$ (the number of samples exceed the number of parameters), then this matrix is in general invertible, as can be seen by considering the singular value decomposition of X. If $n < p$ then the matrix is not invertible. Even if $n > p$ it might be the case that it is ill conditioned, and care must be exercised in inverting the matrix. In both of these cases (noninvertible or ill-conditioned $X^\dagger X$), the way to proceed is to reduce the dimensionality of the parameter space; one way to do this is to perform a singular value decomposition (SVD) on X and keep only the larger singular vales. A similar procedure is to perform a regularized inversion of $X^\dagger X$, for example by adding a multiple of identity before performing the inversion. We will not discuss these complications in detail here but will return to them in a later section. For the present, we assume that $X^\dagger X$ is invertible and well conditioned.

In this case, the LMS estimate of β is explicitly obtained as

$$\hat{\beta} = (X^\dagger X)^{-1} X^\dagger Y \tag{6.22}$$

In the linear model $E[Y] = X\beta$. The estimate for the mean value of Y is therefore given by $X\hat{\beta}$, which we can write as

$$\hat{Y} = X(X^\dagger X)^{-1} X^\dagger Y = HY \tag{6.23}$$

Where the matrix $H = X(X^\dagger X)^{-1} X^\dagger$ is called the hat matrix. This is a projection matrix—it can be verified that $H^2 = H$. The matrices are in fact somewhat of a distraction from the underlying model, and we will simplify things by working in a basis described by the singular vectors of X. We begin by writing X in terms of its SVD,

$$X_{ij} = \sum_{\alpha=1}^{p} x_\alpha u_{i\alpha} v_{j\alpha} \tag{6.24}$$

We can express all the quantities in terms of this basis[4]: $Y_i = \sum_{\alpha=1}^{n} y_\alpha u_{i\alpha}$, $\varepsilon_i = \sum_{\alpha=1}^{n} \varepsilon_\alpha u_{i\alpha}$ and $\beta_i = \sum_{\alpha=1}^{p} \beta_\alpha v_{i\alpha}$. In terms of these expansions, the MSE has a simple form,

$$MSE = \sum_{\alpha=1}^{p} (y_\alpha - x_\alpha \beta_\alpha)^2 + \sum_{\alpha=p+1}^{n} y_\alpha^2 \tag{6.25}$$

The LMS estimator of β_α can now be read off by simple inspection, $\hat{\beta}_\alpha = y_\alpha / x_\alpha$, and the residual sum of squares is simply given by $RSS = \sum_{\alpha=p+1}^{n} y_\alpha^2$.

Training Error and Generalization Error

These expressions allow us to study the important concepts of training error and generalization error. The training error is given by RSS and quantifies the failure of the model to fit the training data exactly. The generalization error (GE), on the other hand, is the squared error obtained when we try to predict a new observation Y_{new} using the estimated parameter $\hat{\beta}$. This is given by

$$GE = \sum_{\alpha=1}^{p} (y_{\alpha, new} - x_\alpha \hat{\beta}_\alpha)^2 + \sum_{\alpha=p+1}^{n} y_{\alpha, new}^2 \tag{6.26}$$

Note carefully that $\hat{\beta}_\alpha = y_\alpha / x_\alpha$ and $x_\alpha \hat{\beta}_\alpha = y_\alpha - \varepsilon_\alpha$. Therefore, the terms in the first sum contain both the noise in the training set, and the noise in the test set.

These errors (GE and RSS) are random variables and will show stochastic fluctuations; therefore, we look at their expected values. We need to assume a noise model, and we will do this by assuming that ε_i (and consequently ε_α) are

---

4. Because the rank of X is p, we need only p left singular vectors u_α in the expression for X. However, Y is n dimensional and according to our assumptions $n > p$. We therefore need $n - p$ other vectors; these can be any orthonormal set, orthogonal to the space spanned by u_α, $\alpha = 1 \ldots p$.

i.i.d Gaussian with zero mean and variance σ^2. The reader should show that $E[RSS] = (n-p)\sigma^2$, whereas $E[GE] = (n+p)\sigma^2$. Thus, the RSS or the training error is an overoptimistic estimate of the generalization error, with the "optimism" given by $E[GE] - E[RSS] = 2p\sigma^2$. Given the expectation values above, it is clear that we can estimate the generalization error by

$$\widehat{GE} = RSS \frac{n+p}{n-p} \tag{6.27}$$

Model Selection

We are now in a position to discuss model selection in the simple setting of the linear model. We have assumed the model $Y = X\beta$ with p parameters or degrees of freedom. However, not only do we not know the parameter values β in advance, we may not even know the model order, namely the value of p: we could start with the matrix X being full rank and the number of nonzero parameters given by $p = p_0 < n$. Is there are way of estimating p_0 from the data? One way to proceed is to estimate the model for arbitrary p and study the behavior of the generalization error as a function of p. If $p < p_0$, we may expect this quantity to decrease with increasing p, because we get a better model fit. For $p > p_0$, on the other hand, we expect that GE will increase, as a signature of overfitting. This is precisely the behavior shown by the expected value of the generalization error for the above scenario. For notational simplicity, we assume that $x_\alpha\beta_\alpha = \mu$ for $\alpha = 1\ldots p_0$, and $\beta_\alpha = 0$ otherwise.

$$p < p_0 \quad E[GE] = (p_0 - p)\mu^2 + (n+p)\sigma^2 \tag{6.28}$$
$$p \geq p_0 \quad E[GE] = (n+p)\sigma^2 \tag{6.29}$$

Assuming $\mu > \sigma$ (a reasonable assumption; for the signal to be detected, it has to be larger than noise), $E[GE]$ declines with p until $p = p_0$ and increases afterward. Therefore, by looking for the minimum of the GE curve, we can try to estimate the model order p_0. Of course, we do not know $E[GE]$; we could try to estimate it as above, $\widehat{GE} = RSS(n+p)/(n-p)$, to obtain a *model selection* criterion based on the data. In practice, unfortunately, it is rare to obtain a well-defined minimum in the GE curve; it tends to initially decline, but then have a flat region, susceptible to stochastic fluctuations. It is customary to look for a change in slope of the GE curve to detect the onset of this flat part and choose the model order conservatively according to this criterion. At this point we are back to visual inspection, symptomatic of the fundamental difficulties of the model selection problem.

For the same setting, the average training error is given by

$$E[RSS] = (p_0 - p)\theta(p_0 - p)\mu^2 + \sigma^2(n-p) \tag{6.30}$$

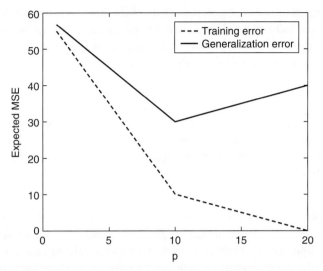

Figure 6.4: The expected values of the training and generalization errors for the linear model discussed in the text, with $\mu = 2$, $sigma = 1$, and $p_0 = 10$. MSE, mean square error.

E[RSS] continuously declines with p, showing a change in slope at $p = p_0$. These behaviors are illustrated in figure 6.4.

6.4.3   Generalized Linear Models

We have discussed the linear model as an application of the least squares method while noting the likelihood perspective as an aside. From the latter perspective, the following is true for the linear model as discussed above:

1. The dependent variables are y_i, and the independent variables are vectors $\mathbf{x}_i$, with components $x_{i\alpha}$. The model seeks to predict the dependent variables in terms of the independent variables. The components of the independent variables enter into the prediction as a linear combination $\theta_i = x_{i\alpha}\beta_\alpha$.
2. Once the independent variables are fixed, the dependent variable y_i is a random variable with a probability distribution with a mean μ_i that depends on the independent variable and a variance that does not depend on the $\mathbf{x}_i$.
3. The mean μ_i depends linearly on the linear combination of the independent variables, $\mu_i = \theta_i = \sum_\alpha x_{i\alpha}\beta_\alpha$.
4. The probability distribution describing the variability of y_i for given $\mathbf{x}_i$ is Gaussian, $y_i \sim N(\mu_i, \sigma)$.
5. The cost function, which is minimized in the method, is the log likelihood of the probability distribution, apart from a constant term.

An important class of generalizations of the linear model is obtained by relaxing the third and the fourth conditions. Crucially, vector of dependent variables is still combined linearly to produce the predictive combination $\theta_i = \sum_\alpha x_{i\alpha}\beta_\alpha$. However, we now allow two things:

1. The probability distribution describing the variability of y_i for given $\mathbf{x}_i$ is arbitrary, $y_i \sim P(\mu_i, \lambda)$, with the mean depending on $\mathbf{x}_i$ through the parameter μ_i (parameters in addition to the mean are allowed, but assumed not to depend on the dependent variable).
2. The mean μ_i depends on the linear combination of the independent variables $\theta_i = \sum_\alpha x_{i\alpha}\beta_\alpha$, through a function which is in general nonlinear, $\mu_i = f(\theta_i)$.

The parameters β_α are still unknown a priori and need to be estimated from the data. We still minimize the likelihood function of the random variables y_i. However, this likelihood function is no longer the squared error. More importantly, the dependent variable y_i no longer has to range over the entire real line; it could be restricted to some subset of the real line. In particular, we could even go to the extreme case of having a discrete dependent variable, $y_i = \pm 1$.

GLM Example: Logistic Regression

To illustrate the procedure, we consider the particular case of a binary dependent variable, with the Bernoulli probability distribution $P(y_i = 1 | \mu_i) = \mu_i$ and $P(y_i = 0 | \mu_i) = 1 - \mu_i$ (note that $E[y_i] = \mu_i$). This could be written as

$$P(y_i | \mu_i) = \mu_i^{y_i}(1 - \mu_i)^{1 - y_i} \qquad (6.31)$$

Supposing that we have a vector of dependent variables $\mathbf{x}_i$. It is tempting to apply a linear model to the mean $\mu_i = \sum_\alpha x_{i\alpha}\beta_\alpha$. However, if we do this, we will need to introduce constraints on the parameters $\beta\alpha$, because we need to constrain the Bernoulli probabilities $0 \le \mu_i \le 1$. Because these are hard constraints, this will lead to a difficult optimization problem. A different approach is to introduce the intermediate parameter $\theta_i = \sum_\alpha x_{i\alpha}\beta_\alpha$, and to let the mean μ_i be a nonlinear function of θ_i.

$$\mu_i = f(\theta_i) = \frac{e^{\theta_i}}{1 + e^{\theta_i}} \qquad (6.32)$$

Now μ_i is automatically constrained to be between zero and one. Also, the function $\mu = f(\theta)$ is invertible, with the inverse function being given by

$$\theta = g(\mu) = \log\left(\frac{\mu_i}{1 - \mu_i}\right) \qquad (6.33)$$

The negative log likelihood, which is minimized in order to estimate the model parameters β_α, is given by

$$-\sum_i \log\left(P(y_i|\mu_i)\right) = -y_i \log\left(\frac{\mu_i}{1-\mu_i}\right) - \log\left(1-\mu_i\right) \qquad (6.34)$$

$$= \sum_i -y_i\theta_i + \log\left(1+\theta_i\right) \qquad (6.35)$$

The log likelihood function is no longer a quadratic function of the parameters β_α, so the minimization has to be performed numerically. The procedure outlined above is known as *logistic regression*. As with a number of procedures discussed in this book, high performance algorithms to perform such numerical optimization are available as part of standard software packages for a large class of models, including the case just discussed.

After we have performed the model fit, given a new value of the prediction vector $\mathbf{x}_i$, instead of predicting the value of y_i we now predict the probability $P(y_i|\hat{\mu}_i)$. This can be turned into a predictor for y_i by choosing the value of y_i that maximizes this probability.

Logistic Regression and Classification

How can such a procedure be used in practice? The above example is in fact the case of *binary classification*, because we attach a discrete class label 1 or 0 to the independent vectors $\mathbf{x}_i$. This could be applied to a data set where some labeled pairs y_i, $\mathbf{x}_i$ are given and the task is to fit the logistic regression model described above. From the parameter β_α thus estimated, one could predict the class of a new, unlabeled example.

One application could be to categorize neural activity measured in an experiment into two classes corresponding to two output behaviors (e.g., movement to the left or to the right), labeled 1 and 0. During the training phase, one would gather experimental data in which the neural activities and the behaviors are both measured and the parameters of the logistic regression model are estimated. Later, one could measure the neural responses and use these to generate a prediction for the motor movement. One can imagine an application to a neural prosthetic application, where the predicted movement is used to drive an artificial limb. Although the present example is a bit too simple, the case should be clear for the generalized linear model in which the output or dependent variable has a restricted range, and a straightforward linear model fit is inappropriate.

Link Function

In specifying the generalized linear model, we need to fix the probability distribution, $P(y_i|\mu_i)$, and the relation between the mean and the linear sum of the dependent variables, $\mu = f(\theta)$. The inverse function $\theta = g(\mu)$ is assumed to be unique and is called the *link* function. Note that for a fixed probability distribution, multiple link functions are possible. Note that the role of the link function is to remove restrictions on the range of the independent variables and to allow arbitrary linear combinations. Another potential role of the link function is *variance stabilization*, a property that ensures that the variance of an estimator does not depend on the value of the corresponding parameter, a useful property when constructing confidence intervals. We have already seen the link function appropriate for the Bernoulli distribution, $\theta = \log(\mu/(1 - \mu))$. This is known as the logistic link or the logit link function. If y_i are assumed to be distributed according to a Poisson distribution, an appropriate choice of link is the log link function, $\theta = \log(\mu)$.

Note that the link function does not have to necessarily be nonlinear; a generalized linear model could have a linear link function but a non-Gaussian likelihood function reflecting non-Gaussian variability of the noise variables. For example, for data with a bell-shaped probability density but with long tails, one could use the Cauchy distribution, with a Lorentzian density function $p(y \mid \mu,\sigma) \sim 1/(\sigma^2 + (y - \mu)^2)$. Note that the Cauchy distribution does not have a variance, and σ is a scale parameter. This distribution can be used to perform robust regression.

Model Assessment and Model Selection

Let us consider the analogs of the RSS, generalization error, and model assessment. The negative log likelihood is the "energy function" that is used to fit the model:

$$\hat{\beta} = argmin_\beta \left[- \sum_i l(y_i \mid \mu_i(\hat{\beta})) \right] \tag{6.36}$$

So a natural choice would be to use this as a loss function. However, if this were used directly with the Gaussian likelihood, we obtain an extra constant term, which can be eliminated as follows. Note that $\hat{\beta}$ is obtained by minimizing the sum, not individual terms in this expression. Now consider a single observation pair y_1, $\mathbf{x}_1$ and consider minimizing the corresponding negative likelihood with respect to the parameter β. Clearly, this cannot produce a larger result, because a single term is being minimized. The difference between the minimum of a single term and its value when $\hat{\beta}$ is substituted is a measure of the *prediction error* of the model for this observation. Twice this difference is known as the deviance:

$$D(y_i \mid \mu_i(\hat{\beta})) = 2(max_\beta l(y_i \mid \mu_i(\beta)) - l(y_i \mid \mu_i(\hat{\beta})) \tag{6.37}$$

The reason for the factor of two is clear if one looks at the log likelihood of the Gaussian model (the reader should verify that the above definition yields the sum of squares familiar from the last section, scaled by the variance). The sum of the deviances over all observations is one possible definition for a *loss function* generalizing the RSS

$$D_{tot} = \sum_i D(y_i|\mu_i(\hat{\beta})) \tag{6.38}$$

It can be shown that asymptotically, the total deviance has a chi-squared distribution with $n - p$ degrees of freedom, thus showing the analogy with RSS. An estimate for the generalization error can therefore be obtained by adding $2p$ to the deviance, and this can be used to perform model selection. This is closely related to the criterion Akaike's information criterion for model selection, $AIC = 2p - 2 \log(Likelihood(\hat{\beta}))$.

6.4.4 Interval Estimation

In point estimation, the basic tool is an *estimator*, which is a random variable and therefore subject to stochastic fluctuations from sample to sample. We have already started characterizing these fluctuations by studying the variance of the estimator. However, if one is not in an asymptotic limit, the distribution of the estimator is not in general Gaussian. Knowledge of this distribution tells us precisely what variability to expect of the distribution, and in particular allows for interval estimation, where the goal is to determine a set of parameter values, such that the parameter estimate for a given sample lies in this *confidence set* with high probability. Such confidence sets or confidence bands are the standard method employed in the biomedical literature to report parameter values.

We start with the simplest case: let the observations x_i be given by a Gaussian distribution with mean μ and variance σ, both unknown. Unbiased estimates of the mean and variance are given by $\hat{\mu} = \langle x \rangle = \frac{1}{n}\sum_{i=1}^{n} x_i$, and $\hat{\sigma}^2 = \frac{1}{n-1}\sum_{i=1}^{n} x_i^2 - \langle x \rangle^2$. To construct confidence intervals for $\hat{\mu}$ one starts from the statistic

$$\hat{t}(x_1, \ldots, x_n; \mu) = \sqrt{n}\frac{-(\hat{\mu} - \mu)}{\hat{\sigma}} \tag{6.39}$$

The crucial point is that for $x_i \sim N(\mu, \sigma)$, the distributional assumption for the samples, $\hat{t}$ has a distribution, the so-called student's t-distribution with $n - 1$ degrees of freedom, that *does not* depend on any parameters except n. The distribution is a bell-shaped, symmetric distribution centered around zero. Now let us define t_α such that the tails of the distribution beyond t_α have probability α (which is chosen to be a small value, for example $\alpha = 0.05$),

$$P[-t_\alpha < t < t_\alpha] = 1 - \alpha \tag{6.40}$$

Therefore, with probability $1 - \alpha$, the estimator $\hat{t}$ lies in the interval $-t_\alpha < t < t_\alpha$. This pair of inequalities can be rewritten as

$$-t_\alpha < \sqrt{n}\frac{(\hat{\mu} - \mu)}{\hat{\sigma}} < t_\alpha \tag{6.41}$$

$$\hat{\mu} - t_\alpha \frac{\sigma}{\sqrt{n}} < \mu < \hat{\mu} + t_\alpha \frac{\sigma}{\sqrt{n}} \tag{6.42}$$

This provides the desired interval $\hat{\mu} \pm t_\alpha \frac{\sigma}{\sqrt{n}}$ for the estimate of the sample mean.

Note that the above procedure is contingent on finding a statistic that does not depend on the parameters μ and σ. Although this cannot always be achieved, it is still a useful procedure for many cases of interest, as shown by its widespread applicability.

How does one obtain confidence intervals if the underlying distribution is unknown? One way to proceed is to estimate the variance of the estimator using a resampling procedure, such as the bootstrap or the jackknife, to be discussed in a later section. If the sample size is large and a maximum likelihood procedure is used to obtain the estimator, it will be asymptotically Gaussian distributed. This asymptotic result can be combined with the estimated variance to obtain approximate confidence bands.

6.4.5 Hypothesis Testing

Both in scientific and biomedical applications, one of the major roles of statistical analysis is to help choose between alternative courses of action based on incomplete or partial evidence. This is the domain of hypothesis testing and decision theory. In the statistical setting, the incomplete information is in the form of a statistical sample drawn from an underlying distribution that is not completely known. In the simplest case, the samples are drawn from one of two distributions, which are otherwise known, and the task is to determine which of those distributions the samples came from. The alternative distributions are known as hypotheses and are typically differentiated into a null hypothesis, which is the default choice unless the sample presents strong evidence otherwise, and an alternative hypothesis, to which the null hypothesis is compared in making the decision. More generally, the two alternatives may be two nonoverlapping sets of probability distributions, or one may consider multiple alternatives.

Making choices of this sort have their merits and demerits. If the evidence is overwhelming one way or the other, a choice may not particularly require statistical machinery. Such examples do in fact appear in the scientific literature in the form of astronomically small probabilities; in such cases, using the machinery of hypothesis testing serves little purpose. On the other hand, if the evidence is not completely one-sided, there is always the possibility that the wrong alternative will be chosen, and the evidence has to be weighed more carefully. It is in this gray zone that the statistical theory of hypothesis testing plays a role. Given that variability is a deeply rooted characteristic of biological phenomena, it is no surprise that the usage of hypothesis testing has become a standard feature of most biology papers. Of course, sometimes it may be a better alternative not to make any decisions at all but simply to report all the evidence without choosing one of the alternative hypotheses; however, this is not always practical.

Another thing to keep in mind is that the standards of evidence differ from community to community; although a 1 of 20 chance of error may be acceptable in the biological community (where 5% probability thresholds are common), such large possibilities of error would not be tolerated when testing the laws of physics. With these caveats, we proceed to discuss the important subject of statistical hypothesis testing.

Binary Hypotheses

We first consider the simple case of a single binary choice described above, which will be labeled H_0 and H_1. Based on a sample, one of two alternatives is to be selected; thus, what is required is a function from the space of samples to the set H_0, H_1. Such a *decision* function can be constructed in different ways, and without necessarily invoking underlying probability distributions, as we will see later. For the present discussion, however, we make the assumption that the sample (which we will denote x) is drawn from one of two probability distributions, $p_0(x)$ and $p_1(x)$, but we do not know which. H_0 will denote the "hypothesis" that x is drawn from distribution $p_0(x)$, and H_1 the hypothesis that x is drawn from distribution $p_1(x)$.

The task is to decide whether x was drawn from $p_0(x)$ (a situation which is referred to as "H_0 is true", or "accept H_0," which can be taken as shorthand for the statement that "the decision is that the underlying distribution was $p_0(x)$)"), or the alternative that x was drawn from $p_1(x)$ (which is referred to as "reject H_0"). Let us introduce the *decision* variable y, where $y = 0$ if we decide x was drawn from $p_0(x)$ and $y = 1$ for the converse decision. The decision rule $y(x)$ associates a value of y with any observation x, namely it is a function from the space of samples to the set 0, 1. This induces partition on the sample space. Let R be the region in sample space for which $y = 0$, namely $R = \{x \in \Omega \mid y(x) = 0\}$, also called the *critical region*. Specifying the region R is equivalent to specifying the function $y(x)$. The complementary region to R in the sample space Ω is denoted $R^c = \Omega - R$, so that $R^c = \{x \in \Omega \mid y(x) = 1\}$. Since y is a function defined on the sample space, it is a random variable. The function $y(x)$ or region R specifies the "hypothesis test."

Type I and Type II Errors

The basic idea is that there are two types of errors that have to be controlled:

1. Type I error (or errors of false rejection): we choose $y = 1$ but H_0 is true.
2. Type II error (or errors of false acceptance, or false alarm): we choose $y = 0$ but H_1 is true.

The corresponding error probabilities are defined as follows:

- $\alpha = \int_{R^c} p_0(x)dx = E[y|H_0]$, referred to as the probability of type I error or the false rejection rate. It is also referred to as the *size* of the test.
- $\beta = \int_R p_1(x)dx = 1 - E[y|H_1]$, referred to as the probability of type II error or the false alarm rate. $1 - \beta$ is called the *power* of the test.

Clearly, it is desirable to choose a test (or correspondingly, a critical region) that minimize both errors as much as possible. If $p_0(x)$ and $p_1(x)$ are nonoverlapping probability distributions, then it is possible to have a decision criterion so that both errors are zero. This is however, precisely the uninteresting case where statistical analysis plays no role, because it means that once we know x we know unambiguously which alternative was true. More generally, there will be some values of x for which both alternatives are possible, and α and β cannot be simultaneously zero.

It is instructive to study this trade off for a simple model. Let $p_0(x)$ and $p_1(x)$ be Gaussian distributions with means 0 and μ, and standard deviation σ. There is a single parameter in this problem, namely the signal-to-noise ratio μ/σ. Because the two means are different, it makes sense to compare x to some threshold value in order to make a decision. This corresponds to a simple critical region of the form $x < x_c$. Figure 6.5 shows the tradeoff curves between α and β for decision rules of the form $y(x) = \theta(x - x_c)$, where H_0 is chosen if $x < x_c$. The different curves correspond to different choices of the parameter μ/σ. The different points on each curve, correspond to different values of the threshold x_c. Two questions arise. First, how should we choose x_c? Second, we are considering one family of decision criteria parameterized by x_c; is this better than other more complicated critical regions?

Likelihood Ratio Test

Neyman-Pearson theory attempts to provide a systematic set of answers to these questions. The basic idea is to fix α at some small value, and then choose the decision criteria to minimize β. For the two alternative case discussed above, the Neyman-Pearson lemma gives a simple decision criterion that minimizes β for fixed α, the *likelihood ratio test* (LRT). This is given by the decision rule

$$y(x) = \theta\left(\frac{p_1(x)}{p_0(x)} - k\right) \qquad (6.43)$$

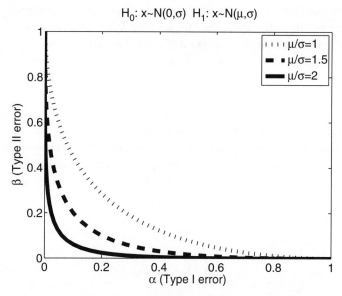

H_0: x~N(0,σ) H_1: x~N(μ,σ)

Figure 6.5:   Tradeoff curves between type I and II errors for two simple alternatives. The distributions $p_0(x)$ and $p_1(x)$ are Gaussian distributions with different means but equal variance. The critical region is of the form $x < x_c$.

The rule says, in words, reject H_0 if the likelihood ratio $p_1(x)/p_0(x)$ exceeds a constant k. The constant k is obtained by setting the type I error to be equal to α.[5] Under general conditions, the lemma guarantees that for fixed α, there is no decision criterion that will have a smaller value of β than given by the LRT.

$$E[y(x)|H_0] = \int \theta\left(\frac{p_1(x)}{p_0(x)} - k\right) p_0(x)dx = \alpha \tag{6.44}$$

So far, we have considered simple alternatives. However, this is too simple for practical applications. One might consider generalizations in two directions: more than two input distributions from which the sample is potentially chosen and more than two outcomes or decisions. In the current section, we will restrict ourselves to the first generalization, where the hypothesis space consists of two families of probability distributions, but the outcome is still binary. At least in principle, more complex choices may be built up from binary choices.

---

5. In case the sample space is discrete, the type I error will also take discrete values as the parameter k is varied and cannot be chosen arbitrarily. This can be handled using a randomization procedure or more pragmatically by simply fixing α to one of the discrete values bracketing the desired value [204].

We assume that the sample in question is drawn from a parameterized probability distribution $p(x|\theta)$, where the parameter is in general a vector. The sample x is meant to represent one or more sets of random variables gathered during an experiment. For simple hypotheses discussed earlier, there were two possible parameter values. We now consider the more general case where the two alternatives correspond to the parameters taking their values in two disjoint sets Θ_0 and Θ_1. Given the sample x, we have to decide whether the probability distribution that generated it came from the set Θ_0, or Θ_1. We first reduce this problem to the case of two simple alternatives. This can be done if we select a representative parameter value from each set; the natural parameter value to choose is the maximum likelihood estimate of the corresponding parameter *restricted* to the set Θ_0 or Θ_1. This leads us to the decision rule

$$\lambda(x) = \frac{p(x|\hat{\theta}_1)}{p(x|\hat{\theta}_0)} \tag{6.45}$$

$$y(x) = \theta(\lambda(x) - k) \tag{6.46}$$

Where $\hat{\theta}_i = argmax_{\theta i \,\in\, \Theta i} p(x\,|\,\theta_i)$ are the restricted maximum likelihood estimates. The parameter α is now no longer uniquely defined. It could conservatively be chosen as the worst false rejection rate over the family of parameterized distributions with $\theta \in \Theta_0$,

$$\alpha = \max_{\theta_0 \in \Theta_0} E[y(x)|\theta_0] \tag{6.47}$$

In some special cases, α does not depend on θ_0, in which case there is no ambiguity. The false alarm rate β can be defined similarly. However, in general defining and computing these quantities for the situation described above poses analytical and numerical difficulties, and the utility of the LRT stems from asymptotic, large-sample results that lead to chi-square distributions for $2\log(\lambda(x))$ and approximations of the corresponding values for the size and power of the test.

Chi-Square Distribution of Log Likelihood Ratio

Consider a vector of parameters θ with d components, and let the null hypothesis space be specified by r constraints on the parameters. For example, if samples were drawn from two real Gaussian distributions in N-dimensional space, the most general parameterized form of the distributions need two means and two covariance matrices, leading to a total of $d = 2N + N(N-1) = N^2 + N$ parameters. Now consider the null hypothesis that the two means are equal; this requires $r = N$ constraints on the parameters. The asymptotic result referred to states that for large enough sample sizes, $2\log(\lambda(x))$ has a χ^2 distribution with r degrees of freedom. The threshold parameter $k(\alpha)$ can therefore be chosen to be the upper α point of the chi-square distribution function with r degrees of freedom.

Now even the LRT $\lambda(x)$ may involve a nontrivial computation, because one has to obtain both the restricted and unrestricted maximum likelihood estimates of the parameter θ; there is a further simplification that leads to the so-called *chi-square statistic* for hypothesis testing. Let the sample contain n i.i.d observations x_i, with the likelihood $L(\theta) = \prod_{i=1}^{n} p(x_i|\theta)$ and Fisher information matrix $I_{ij}(\theta) = -E[\frac{\partial}{\partial\theta_i}\frac{\partial}{\partial\theta_j}p(x|\theta)]$. Let $\hat{\theta}_r$ be the restricted MLE for θ incorporating the r constraints defining the null hypothesis. Without any restrictions, the MLE satisfies the equations $\frac{\partial}{\partial\theta_i}L(\theta) = 0$. The idea is that if the null hypothesis is true, then the unrestricted MLE for θ should be close to the restricted MLE, and one should therefore have $\frac{\partial}{\partial\theta_i}L(\hat{\theta}_r) \approx 0$. Moreover, we know that the covariance matrix of the vector $\frac{\partial}{\partial\theta_i}L(\theta)$ is given in terms of the Fisher information matrix. This motivates the following definition:

$$\hat{\chi}^2 = \frac{1}{n}\sum_{ij}\frac{\partial}{\partial\theta_i}L(\hat{\theta}_r)I_{ij}^{-1}(\hat{\theta}_r)\frac{\partial}{\partial\theta_j}L(\hat{\theta}_r) \qquad (6.48)$$

It can be shown that under the null hypothesis, and for large n, under appropriate conditions the statistic defined above is asymptotically the same as $2\log(\lambda)$, and has a *chi-squared* distribution with r degrees of freedom.[6] Given the unrestricted likelihood and the constraint equations, one proceeds as follows: the restricted MLE $\hat{\theta}_r$ is computed and substituted in the above expression to obtain the test statistic. The threshold parameter $k(\alpha)$ and the corresponding values of α and β are obtained from a chi-square distribution with r degrees of freedom. It should be kept in mind that the justification for this procedure is asymptotic and based on the availability of large samples.

Chi-Square Test

The most common usage of this test (and the usual situation when the chi-square test is referred to) is that observations belong to one of K classes, and the sample consists of the number of observations n_i in the ith class. The class labels are i.i.d random variables, and the likelihood is given by a multinomial distribution. The unknown parameters are the relative fractions of the classes $E[n_i/n] = p_i$. The restrictions are constraints on the p_i; for example, the null hypothesis might be that some of the p_i have predetermined values, $p_i = p_i^0$ for $i = 1 \ldots r$. Another example is the constraint that $r + 1$ of the p_is are equal, also

---

6. Note that we have used the same name for the statistic and the distribution in keeping with common usage. This can be confusing in the beginning and it is desirable to keep the distinction between the two in mind.

leading to r constraint equations. Note that $\sum_i p_i = 1$, so that the number of restrictions has to be less than K. Let the restricted MLEs of the parameters be designated $\hat{p}_i$. The test statistic constructed above reduces to

$$\hat{\chi}^2 = \sum_i \frac{(n_i - n\hat{p}_i)^2}{n\hat{p}_i} = \sum_i \frac{(observed - expected)^2}{expected} \qquad (6.49)$$

Under the null hypothesis, this quantity is asymptotically distributed as chi-squared with r degrees of freedom, and α and β are again computed using the chi-square probability distribution.

6.4.6 Nonparametric Tests

In the previous discussion of hypothesis testing, the focus has been on parameterized classed of probability distributions. However, this is not necessarily always a useful approach: it may be the case that one wants to consider two hypothesis distributions which do not fall into simple parametric classes. A simple example is where two samples of scalar random variables x_i and y_i are available, and the question is whether these are drawn from the same distribution, without specifying the shapes of the distributions.

This could be converted into a parametric hypothesis-testing problem, for example, by grouping the data into bins and applying the chi-squared test. However, this introduces the extra complication of choosing an appropriate bin size; if the bin size is too large, then the structure of the distributions is lost, and this may also reduce the possibility of discovering the difference between the two distributions. On the other hand, one cannot make the bin size too small, because that will make the number of parameters close to the sample size, thus violating the asymptotic requirements that make the chi-square test generally useful.

Kolmogorov Smirnov Test

One approach to this problem is to obtain estimates of the density functions (using local likelihood methods, for example; these method will be discussed in a later chapter), and then compare these estimates. Another approach is to apply a nonparametric test such as the Kolmogorov Smirnov (KS) test that does not depend on the details of the two distributions. In this section we discuss some of the commonly used nonparametric procedures to perform statistical testing.

We take the example given above, of the two-sample KS test. We are given two samples of i.i.d real variables of size n and m, where n is not necessarily equal to m. The test is based on the empirical cumulative distribution functions $F_n(t)$ and $G_m(t)$, defined as sums over unit step functions ($\theta(t - x_i) = 1$ if $t > x_i$ and zero otherwise)

$$F_n(x) = \frac{1}{n}\sum_{i=1}^{n}\theta(x-x_i) \tag{6.50}$$

$$G_n(x) = \frac{1}{m}\sum_{i=1}^{m}\theta(x-y_i) \tag{6.51}$$

The two-sided KS test statistic is defined as

$$\hat{D}_2 = \sqrt{\frac{mn}{m+n}}max_x|F_n(x)-G_m(x)| \tag{6.52}$$

The procedure is therefore to approximate the two distributions by their corresponding empirical cumulative distribution functions and to measure the largest departure between the two curves, appropriately normalized. The null hypothesis is that both samples are drawn from the same underlying probability distribution $F(t)$, assumed to be continuous. The interesting point is that the distribution of the statistic D_2 does not depend on the form of the distribution $F(t)$, but is universal or distribution independent.

The reason for this becomes clear if we perform the *probability transform*, given by the equation $z(x) = F(x)$. The probability density function of z is given by $p(z)dz = p(x)dx$; because $dz \, / \, dx = dF \, / \, dx = p(x)$, it follows that $p(z) = 1$. Therefore, z_i are i.i.d with a uniform distribution in the interval $[0 \; 1]$. The collection $z_1, z_2, \ldots z_n$ can therefore be treated as a sample path of a Poisson process, conditioned on a total count of n points in the interval $[0 \; 1]$.

The empirical cumulative distribution $F_n(x)$ can be rewritten in terms of the variable z, and it can be expressed in terms of the counting process $N(z) = \sum_i \theta(z-z_i)$ as $F_n(z) = (N(z)-nz) \, / \, n$. Recall from the section on stochastic process theory that if $N(t)$ is the counting process for a Poisson process, then $x(t) = (N(t)-\lambda t)/\sqrt{\lambda}$ is a Wiener process or diffusion process starting at the origin. One can exploit this, and in the limit of large m, n one can obtain an analytical expression for the asymptotic distribution of the statistic $\hat{D}_2$

$$P(D_2 < M) = 1 - 2\sum_{k=1}^{\infty}(-1)^{k+1}e^{-k^2M^2} \tag{6.53}$$

Note, however, that even if one is not in this asymptotic limit, the distribution of D_2 does not depend on the form of the distribution $F(x)$; it has been tabulated. The KS approach using the empirical distribution function is in fact the precursor of an important set of developments in modern machine learning due to Vapnik [228].

Wilcoxon and Mann-Whitney Test

We consider two more nonparametric approaches to the two sample problem. It may be that the distributions have the same shape but are shifted with respect to each other. One way to approach this problem would be to look at the difference in the sample means and compare with some measure of the variance, which will lead to a t-statistic as before. A nonparametric approach to this problem is provided by the Wilcoxon rank sum test (or equivalently the Mann-Whitney test). To perform this test, the observations are pooled together, and the resulting $n + m$ numbers are ordered. The rank of the first set of observations is then determined; these are n numbers $r_1, r_2, \ldots, r_n$ that range from 1 to $m + n$. The rank sum $R = \sum_i r_i$ is the test statistic of interest.

If the distribution of the xs is entirely to the left of ys, then R takes its smallest value given by $n(n + 1)/2$, and conversely the maximum value of R is $mn + m(m + 1)/2$. The number of possible values of R is $(m + n)!/(m!n!)$, and under the null hypothesis, each configuration is equally likely. Therefore, a test of size α can be constructed by arranging the possible rank sums in order and choosing an upper and lower cutoff such that the fraction of ranks within these cutoffs is a fraction $(1 - \alpha)$ of the total number of possible values.

Similarly, one can construct a one-sided test to determine whether the first distribution is to the left of the second distribution, and so on. The critical region for the statistic R are also tabulated for small n, m, and for large n, m the distribution of R (after an appropriate shift and rescaling) is a standard Gaussian. This test provides a nonparametric alternative to the usual t-test and is more robust to outliers.

Permutation Test

Yet another approach of considerable generality is that of permutation tests. The general idea here is that the sampling distribution has a larger set of permutation symmetries under the null hypothesis as opposed to the alternative hypothesis. Suppose we still start from the two sample problem and are also interested in the locations of the two distributions as earlier. Let the sample means be $\langle x \rangle = \frac{1}{n} \sum_i x_i$ and $\langle y \rangle = \frac{1}{m} \sum_i y_i$. A natural statistic is the difference between the two means $\langle x \rangle - \langle y \rangle$. In the parametric case, where the underlying distributions are assumed to be Gaussian, the critical region for the test, corresponding to appropriate thresholds for the difference in sample means, is given by the t-distribution as discussed earlier.

The permutation test in this context works as follows: the two samples are pooled together to obtain $n + m$ values, which are then subjected to a permutation. After each permutation, a new pair of "samples" is obtained by taking the first n permuted values and assigning them to the first group. The difference between the two means is now computed for this new sample generated by permutation. All $(n + m)!$ permutations are assigned equal probability in order to empirically obtain the distribution of $\langle x \rangle - \langle y \rangle$ under the null hypothesis. The threshold appropriate for a value of α can be determined from this distribution. In practice, of course, it is prohibitively expensive to apply all permutations exhaustively, and a random sampling of the permutations are used.

The permutation procedure offers a bridge between parametric and non-parametric tests: one can start with a test statistic constructed under distributional assumptions, but determine the critical region for the test empirically, based on a permutation procedure. Other applications of the permutation procedure lead to confidence bands for parametric estimates. Related to the permutation procedure are the bootstrap and jackknife procedures, which will be discussed in a later section.

6.4.7 Bayesian Estimation and Inference

In this section we provide a brief introduction to the ideas behind Bayesian inference. Bayesian inference is sometimes associated simply with the usage of Bayes theorem, namely $p(x|y)p(y) = p(y|x)p(x)$. However, this is misleading. The statement about conditional probabilities follows from the axiomatic framework of probability theory, and as such is not differentiated from the mathematical theory of probability. Rather, the key idea in Bayesian inference is to treat the parameters of a probability distribution as random variables themselves and to regard the likelihood function $p(x|\theta)$ as a conditional probability.

In order to make any progress, one has to specify the probability space for the parameters θ and a corresponding probability measure $\pi(\theta)$, also known as the prior probability distribution. Given these, one can obtain the joint distribution of the random variables that form the statistical sample of interest and the parameter random variables, $p(x, \theta) = p(x|\theta)\pi(\theta)$. The starting point for Bayesian inference is the conditional probability $p(\theta|x)$, also referred to as the posterior probability,

$$p(\theta|x) = \frac{p(x|\theta)\pi(\theta)}{p(x)} = \frac{p(x|\theta)\pi(\theta)}{\int d\theta p(x|\theta)\pi(\theta)} \tag{6.54}$$

The interpretation of the above equation is as follows: one starts before making the observation x with the prior probability $\pi(\theta)$; inclusion of the observation x and the likelihood $p(x|\theta)$ leads to the posterior distribution $p(\theta|x)$.

Maximum A Posteriori Estimate

The rules for inference are fairly straightforward. For example, consider point estimation. The MLE of the parameter θ can be replaced by the maximum a posteriori (MAP) estimate

$$\hat{\theta}_{MAP} = argmax_\theta p(\theta|x) \tag{6.55}$$

Note that the MAP estimate differs from the MLE estimate only if $\pi(\theta)$ is *informative*, namely provides a constraint on the maximization; if $\pi(\theta)$ does not depend on θ we are back to the MLE estimator. There is a tension here: if the sample size n is sufficiently large compared to the number of parameters, the likelihood becomes strongly peaked, and the prior distribution becomes relatively uninformative. As long as the parameter space has finite volume, one can define a uniform distribution on this space. The posterior distribution is simply the likelihood function multiplied by a parameter independent normalizing constant, and one is more or less back to likelihood-based inference.

On the other hand, if n is small and the prior is constraining, then the parameter estimate may become strongly dependent on the nature of the prior distribution. Errors in formulating the prior distribution will propagate to the results; having a consistent mathematical machinery will not ensure that the resulting output will be meaningful. Therefore, the utility of the approach is contingent on whether the parameters can be meaningfully treated as random variables with well-defined probability distributions, which in turn have to be estimated.

Assigning Prior Probabilities

If one adopts a subjective view of probability, then there may not be any difficulty, at least conceptually, in ascribing probabilities to anything and everything. On the other hand, if one adopts an objective perspective, then probability measures are used to describe real phenomena that can be measured and follow physical laws rather than the investigator's psychological state.

With an objective view of probability, it is still possible to use the machinery of Bayesian inference. It could make sense to divide a set of random variables into two subsets, one of which shows relatively little change during an experiment, and can therefore be treated as a set of constant parameters. It may be that these parameters show stochastic variations in *other* circumstances, and their *probability distributions* could therefore be determined using the classical approach. Alternatively, the parameters could have bona fide probability distributions characterized by physical law or previous empirical knowledge about the world. As long as the parameter space has finite volume, one can define a uniform distribution on this space. This corresponds to normalizing the likelihood function and is largely similar to likelihood based inference.

There may, however, be other cases where such prior probability assignments are not made (or are possible to make) on any empirical grounds whatsoever; the best that can be said about such a situation is that the prior probability is being used to quantify the assumptions about the parameters. As long as this does not lead to any false sense of security about the conclusions then drawn, no great harm is done. However, completely arbitrary choices made about the prior, which cannot be empirically verified, could still have a strong determinative effect on the outcome. In scientific practice, letting un-verifiable biases play a strong role in the conclusions drawn is clearly fraught with danger.

Inference Based on Posterior Probabilities

Returning to Bayesian estimation, note that because the entire probability distribution of θ is now known conditional on the observations, interval esti-mation is also straightforward: for example, one may determine the desired parameter set using a threshold criterion on the posterior density, $p(\theta|x) > c$, where the constant c is chosen to control the probability measure of the confidence interval according to the posterior distribution, at some predeter-mined level (e.g., 95%). Of course, because the complete posterior distribution is known, any desired property of the distribution can be computed; it may even be considered superfluous to separately report these properties. However, point and interval estimates still make sense, especially because the distribu-tions in question can be multidimensional and need to be summarized.

The likelihood ratio is naturally replaced by a ratio of the posterior densities. The simple two alternative test now has the criterion function λ

$$\lambda = \frac{p(\theta_1|x)}{p(\theta_2|x)} = \frac{p(x|\theta_1)\pi(\theta_1)}{p(x|\theta_2)\pi(\theta)} \qquad (6.56)$$

In contrast with the LRT, the threshold for the criterion is now 1, namely we choose alternative 1 if $p(\theta_1|x) > p(\theta_2|x)$. This corresponds to comparing the likelihood ratio to the inverse ratio of the prior probabilities, as the reader can easily show. The procedure may be regarded as being more objective because we no longer have to choose the threshold and the corresponding error probabilities as earlier; of course, the reality is that the choice has simply been relegated to a choice of the prior probabilities. In fact, this procedure is not completely satisfactory, because it does not account for the different costs that may be associated with making type I or type II errors. Such costs are extra-neous information about the problem and are not contained anywhere in the probabilistic framework. This is the subject of decision theory, which we will not treat in detail here.

7

Time Series Analysis

...since you desire it, we will not anticipate the past—so mind, young people—our retrospection will all be to the future.
—Mrs. Malaprop, in Act IV, *The Rivals*, by Richard Sheridan

Time series analysis or signal processing is a very big field. Many books have been written and remain to be written about the subject, and a single chapter cannot do justice to all the material that would need to be covered even in the relatively narrow context of neural signals. The present chapter has been kept short for two reasons. First, time series analysis is an applied subject; like surgery, it is difficult to gain a good feeling for it from dry theoretical material, without practical applications. These applications are the bulk of the third part of the book, which provides detailed accounts of time series analysis methods applied to multiple types of neural signals. Second, the subject can be very confusing without some focus. The choice of focus in this chapter is dictated by a set of core ideas that form the basis for much of the analysis presented later in the book.

In addition, we have already provided extensive preparatory overview in the chapters on mathematical preliminaries and statistical protocols. Probability theory and stochastic process theory were covered in the first of those chapters, along with detailed considerations regarding Fourier analysis, which provide background material for this chapter. The general statistical material covered in the second of the two chapters is also directly applicable to this chapter—neural signals may simply be treated as multidimensional random variables, and considerations about multivariate statistics apply to time series as well.

This chapter has an emphasis on spectral analysis, for reasons discussed in the next section. Many volumes have been written on spectral analysis itself, and again our coverage is by no means intended to be comprehensive. We have been strongly influenced in our choice of methodology by the multitaper framework for spectral analysis, which was developed at Bell Laboratories by David J. Thomson. Other influences include the emphasis on exploratory data analysis espoused by John Tukey and the work of David Brillinger in applying spectral analysis methods to spike train data.

7.1   Method of Moments

As we have emphasized in the section on stochastic process theory, time series should be regarded as random variables drawn from a high-dimensional space. The fundamental difference between doing statistical analysis with one- or two-dimensional random variables and very high-dimensional random variables is that estimating the underlying probability distribution is practical in the former case but a virtual impossibility in the latter case. This follows from a simple counting argument: if the sample space is D dimensional,[1] and k levels are retained in each dimension, then the number of "histogram bins" are k^D. If one does not make prior assumptions about the smoothness of the distribution, then the number of data samples required to estimate this histogram soon becomes astronomical and beyond practical reach. To make matters worse, strictly speaking one only has *one* sample of a stochastic process. Independently and identically drawn samples of time series segments are theoretical fictions, especially in neurobiology, where no two brains are quite the same and experimental conditions cannot be exactly replicated. Deriving a histogram estimate in a high-dimensional space from one sample is a tall order indeed.

Density estimation always requires assumptions, even in one dimension; without any smoothness assumption, the empirical estimate of the density would be a series of delta functions at the sample points. The issue, however, is that the smoothness requirements become more and more severe as the dimensionality increases for a fixed sample size. It is of course possible to put in sufficiently strong prior constraints and obtain a density estimate or likelihood estimate, and one can make the case that theoretical progress is always contingent on making simplifying assumptions. There is a big difference, however, between applying such inductive methodology in physics, say to the motion of the planets, and in biology, to neurobiological time series data. In the latter case, the procedure is more akin to smoothing and fitting regression lines than

---

1. Recall that a time series of length T and bandwidth $2W$ lives in a $2WT$ dimensional space. Taking the spectral bandwidth of electroencephalography (EEG) data to be conservatively 10 Hz, without making further assumptions, an hour of EEG data lives in a space of dimensionality $D = 36,000$.

to finding some deep-seated simplicities expressed parsimoniously in a few equations of motion.

The way out of this conundrum is to adopt a pragmatic approach. Ultimately, one is not really interested in the probability distribution of the stochastic process underlying a neural signal. The investigator has some concrete goal in mind, either to decide between alternative courses of action based on the outcome of an experiment, or to estimate some quantity that is not the probability distribution itself, but some derivative quantity. For example, one may want to know if two neural time series are correlated in any way and what the nature of the correlations is. It is possible to first derive a density estimate and then estimate the correlations from this density, but it may be possible to estimate the correlations directly from the data. Another frequent example is the determination of the functional relation between a neural time series and a stimulus or a motor action, usually referred to as a "neural code." Again, it is possible to determine such a functional relationship through an intermediate step of likelihood estimation, or such a functional relationship could be estimated directly using machine learning methods. The form of the functional relationship could of course be chosen with input of knowledge about the system, but the parameters of the relationship could be determined using a cross validation procedure, without the intervention of a density estimation step.

The method of moments provides an intermediate strategy to the full estimation of underlying stochastic process likelihood functions, and a purely black box, machine learning approach. The idea is to estimate low-order moments of the process (typically only the first and the second moment), and then carry out the decision procedure or estimation of functional relationships in terms of these moments. Although these moments do not fully characterize the underlying probability distribution, they do constrain the distributions and therefore provide some information about the densities. For a single scalar random variable, the method of moments consists of evaluating the mean, variance, skewness, and so on. The decision procedure could be to distinguish between two random variables in terms of statistics constructed out of these moments. For two variables, one can evaluate the correlation and regression coefficients to characterize the relationship between the variables.

For time series data, the first and second moments are themselves already functions of time, and present nontrivial estimation problems. However, having obtained these moments, one can then carry out decision procedures, hypothesis tests, or estimation of functional relationships between the time series in terms of these estimated moments. There are two further steps that can make this method quite powerful. First, the data can be transformed appropriately before moment estimation, to make the moment computations more suited to the application. Second, the moment estimates can themselves be taken as inputs to downstream statistical procedures. One of the most sophisticated contemporary signal processing applications is that of speech recognition. In this application, one starts with a second-moment estimate (spectra computed with a moving window), performs Fourier transformation of the log spectrum (to obtain cepstral coefficients), and then uses the cepstral coefficients as feature vectors in a hidden Markov model (HMM) used to model speech at a phonetic level. This procedure is ultimately more successful than attempting to fit a likelihood model to the entire speech signal at once.

The basic idea is that "simple local models when stitched together can help build complicated global models." This is similar in spirit to the description of physical phenomena in terms of differential equations encoding local laws: integrating these equations along with boundary conditions can reproduce complicated global phenomena. In the present instance, the method of moments can be used to construct simple local descriptions of the time series. These can then be pieced together or further processed at a coarse-grained level to provide a flexible methodology for achieving the pragmatic goals of data analysis.

7.2   Evoked Potentials and Peristimulus Time Histogram

In the context of neural signals, *first moments* appear in the forms of evoked potentials or event related potentials, spike rate functions, peristimulus time histograms (PSTHs), and so on. The unfamiliar reader may want to read this section together with the brief review of basic neuronal biophysics and electrophysiology in the next chapter. Recall that for a continuous stochastic process $x(t)$ the first moment is given by $E[x(t)]$. For a stationary stochastic process, $E[x(t)]$ is a constant independent of time. However, in presence of a nonstationarity, usually in the form of a fixed external event (such as the start of a stimulus presentation), the first moment will in general be time dependent. One usually considers the first moment of the series *conditioned on* some variable (e.g., a stimulus), $E[x(t)|S]$. This is known as the regression estimate of the process given S. It can be shown that $E[x(t)|S]$ provides the best approximation (in a least square sense) to the process given the condition S.

In an experimental setting (where $x(t)$ may denote, for example, the voltage time course measured at an electrode), the recorded waveforms $x_i(t)$ (obtained under nominally identical repeats of the same experimental protocol) are considered to be samples of a stochastic process with an underlying probability distribution. The simple estimator of the first moment of this distribution is given by the arithmetic average over trials, $\langle x(t) \rangle = \frac{1}{N} \sum_i^N x_i(t)$. This is sometimes referred to as an *evoked potential*. Typically there is scope for further smoothing the evoked potential or first moment estimate, which could be accomplished using frequency filtering, spline smoothing, local regression, and likelihood methods, and so on.

Neuronal spike trains are modeled using point processes. The first moment of a point process (in general conditional on a stimulus) is known as the *rate function*.[2]

$$r(t) = E[x(t)] = E[\sum_i \delta(t - t_i)] \qquad (7.1)$$

The nomenclature *rate function* does not imply that the process has a Poisson distribution. The rate or first moment may be computed for processes that are non-Poisson. Stationary processes having a constant rate and stimulus-driven nonstationarity will in general lead to a time-dependent rate function.

For estimating the rate function of spike trains, one can start with a delta function train consisting of all spikes as the empirical rate estimate. This is not very useful numerically but provides visualizations in the form of *raster plots*. A slightly refined elementary estimate is provided by pooling spikes from all trials, and to each time point associating the instantaneous rate given by the inverse of the interspike interval surrounding that time point. This, too, can be subjected to further smoothing.

Therefore, in either case the problem of estimating first moments reduces to a smoothing problem. One elegant framework in which to perform such smoothing, is that of local regression and local likelihood.[3] This method is described in more detail in chapter 13, and illustrated with examples in part III of the book. We will therefore not discuss this further here.

A specific case of first moment estimation that we will treat in a later section of this chapter is that of harmonic analysis, where periodic components are present in the time series and have to be estimated. This is relevant to frequently used experimental protocols involving periodic presentations of stimuli. Even if the stimuli are not presented periodically, such an approach may be used by creating a periodic train through the assembly of identical trials into a single time series. If the stimulus is presented periodically, the first moment will in general have a "stimulus locked" periodic component. The extraction of such periodic components falls naturally into a spectral analysis setting known as harmonic analysis or sinusoidal estimation.

---

2. The distinction between the moments of the underlying stochastic process models and empirical estimates of these moments should be kept in mind. It should normally be clear from the context if we are talking about the moment of the process, or an *estimate* of the moment. The terms *rate* or *evoked potential* are somewhat ambiguous in this context, although they are typically applied to the estimates of the first moment.

3. For point processes, one may employ a local Poisson likelihood. The idea is not that the original process has a Poisson likelihood function, but that the rate function can be estimated using a Poisson assumption in a small time window. Under suitable regularity conditions, when there are enough trials to produce a sufficiently large number of points in a small enough local neighborhood, the local statistics become Poisson even if the process itself is not.

7.3 Univariate Spectral Analysis

Second moments appear in the neurobiology literature in the form of correlation functions, joint (PSTHs), spectra and cross coherences; the time-dependent dynamic counterparts of these quantities; and multivariate versions. These measures can be applied to a "spontaneous activity" setting, or applied to neural activity in the presence of an applied stimulus or a motor output. The estimation of such second moments is the subject of spectral analysis.

We start with univariate spectral analysis for a stationary stochastic process. While neural time series are often nonstationary, stationarity is a reasonable starting assumption when the brain state and external context are relatively stable over some controlled period. As we will see later, the degree of nonstationarity can be assessed to check the stationarity assumption. We will, however, discuss the problem in a theoretical setting, where sample segments are drawn from a stationary stochastic process with a given spectrum. Note that the process need *not* be assumed to be Gaussian, non-Gaussian processes also have well defined spectra. However, the statistical variance of the estimate *will* depend on the probability distribution of the process.

Recall that a bandlimited stochastic process is fully characterized by samples on a discrete grid with sufficiently fine spacing of the grid points. Because experimental data are gathered on discrete grids, we will consider the spectral estimation problem for such processes only. Consider that we are given a segment of a sample of a stochastic process x_t of length $T+1$, so that $t = -T/2 \ldots T/2$ (we assume T is even for simplicity) with $\Delta t = 1$. The full sample can be specified by giving all time points x_t. We will also assume that the process has a Fourier representation, so that it could be specified instead in terms of the frequency domain version of the process $X(f)$.[4] Keeping in mind the subtleties discussed earlier in the section on the convergence of Fourier series in chapter 5, x_t are the Fourier coefficients of $X(f)$:

$$x_t = \int_{-\frac{1}{2}}^{\frac{1}{2}} e^{2\pi i f t} X(f) df \tag{7.2}$$

The process is assumed stationary with power spectrum $S(f)$, so that

$$E[X^*(f)X(f')] = S(f)\delta(f - f') \tag{7.3}$$

---

4. Note that because the time interval has been chosen to be unity, the frequency range can be chosen to be $[-1/2 \ 1/2]$. We will comment on the matter of units in a separate section later in this chapter. Care must be exercised in analyzing actual neurobiological time series to maintain consistency in terms of units. For notational simplicity we will not carry around explicit time or frequency grid spacings.

Note that

$$E[x_t^2] = \int_{-\frac{1}{2}}^{\frac{1}{2}} S(f)df \tag{7.4}$$

Consider the discrete Fourier transform (DFT)

$$\tilde{x}(f) = \sum_{t=-T/2}^{T/2} x_t e^{-2\pi i f t} \tag{7.5}$$

This is often the starting point of a spectral estimation exercise, computed using a padded fast Fourier transform (FFT) on a discrete frequency grid. The DFT of a data segment, is clearly a *truncated* sum of the Fourier series for $X(f)$. At this point, the reader might want to revisit the discussion about narrow-band and broadband bias in the section on Fourier transforms and recall that this truncated sum is given by

$$\tilde{x}(f) = \int_{-\frac{1}{2}}^{\frac{1}{2}} D_T(f - f')X(f')df' \tag{7.6}$$

Where the Dirichlet kernel $D_T(f)$ is given by

$$D_T(f) = \frac{\sin(\pi f(T+1))}{\sin(\pi f)} \tag{7.7}$$

Recall that the Dirichlet kernel has large, slowly decaying sidelobes. The function $\tilde{x}(f)$ is computed from the data segment, whereas $X(f)$ carries information about all time points x_t. Thus, the effect of having a finite data segment is to smear (with the Dirichlet kernel) the underlying frequency domain representation of the stochastic process. This smearing causes loss of information; $X(f)$ has an infinite number of degrees of freedom corresponding to the infinite sequence x_t, whereas $\tilde{x}(f)$ only has $T+1$ degrees of freedom.

7.3.1 Periodogram Estimate: Problems of Bias and Variance

A simple spectral estimate that is still in use (but not recommended) is the periodogram estimate, given by

$$S_{Per}(f) = |\tilde{x}(f)|^2 \tag{7.8}$$

The problem with this estimator is twofold. First, note that

$$E[S_{Per}(f)] = \int_{-\frac{1}{2}}^{\frac{1}{2}} |D_T(f - f')|^2 S(f')df' \tag{7.9}$$

This is the problem of *bias*, because $E[S_{Per}(f)] \neq S(f)$. The bias arises from the departure of the Dirichlet kernel from a delta function, and can be broken up into two components. The first is *narrowband* bias, corresponding to the width of the central lobe. This width is given by the inverse of the data segment length. The second component is *broadband* bias, corresponding to the slowly decaying sidelobes. The bias problem goes away as $T \to \infty$, so that the estimator is asymptotically unbiased, but due to nonstationarity and other practical considerations one is seldom in such asymptotic ranges of T. Moreover, the approach to the asymptotic value is highly oscillatory due to the Gibbs's phenomenon, captured by the oscillatory nature of the Dirichlet kernel.

Second, note the problem of variance. Consider the case in which x_t is a Gaussian stochastic process. Because $\tilde{x}(f)$ is a sum of Gaussian variables, it has a Gaussian distribution itself. This means that $S_{Per}(f) = |\tilde{x}(f)|^2$ has a distribution with the chi-squared form (with two degrees of freedom, because $\tilde{x}(f)$ is complex). More precisely, $S_{Per}(f)/E[S_{Per}(f)]$ is distributed as χ_2^2, independently of T. This means that the estimator is *inconsistent*, namely its variance does not decrease in the limit of large T. As one increases T, one obtains faster and faster oscillations in $S_{Per}(f)$, with a conserved amplitude. The variance of the estimator is given by

$$V[S_{Per}(f)] = E[S_{Per}(f)]^2 \tag{7.10}$$

So that the variance remains finite for large T, the limiting value being the process spectrum squared

$$\lim_{T \to \infty} V[S_{Per}(f)] = S(f)^2 \tag{7.11}$$

Spectra are usually shown on a logarithmic scale, and the logarithm of a χ_2^2 variable has an exponential distribution. The most probable value of $S_{Per}(f)$ is therefore zero. This explains why an unsmoothed or unaveraged periodogram estimate fluctuates rapidly and resembles "grass."

7.3.2 Nonparametric Quadratic Estimates

The cures for the bias and variance problems of the periodogram are well established. As noted earlier in the section on Fourier analysis in chapter 5, the broadband bias can be reduced by the introduction of a *data taper* w_t,[5] to obtain the tapered spectral estimate

$$S_w(f) = |\tilde{x}_w(f)|^2 \tag{7.12}$$

$$\tilde{x}_w(f) = \sum_{t=-T/2}^{T/2} w_t x_t e^{-2\pi i f t} \tag{7.13}$$

---

5. The word *taper* is used to distinguish the function w_t from the data window or segment.

The reduction of broadband bias by tapering corresponds to the replacement of the Dirichlet kernel with the Fourier transform of the taper

$$D_w(f) = \sum_{t=-T/2}^{T/2} w_t e^{-2\pi i f t} \qquad (7.14)$$

As discussed in the section on Fourier analysis, the taper w_t can be chosen to suppress the sidelobes at the expense of broadening the central lobe. Because one is typically concerned more with suppressing leakage from distant frequencies than with the local spread of frequencies, this tradeoff is beneficial. Recall also the discussion on optimal choice of tapers. We will use the Slepian tapers, which maximize the concentration of the Fourier energy of the taper within a specified bandwidth.

Tapering does not, however, reduce the variance problem; the single tapered estimate is still distributed as χ_2^2. This can only be reduced by further averaging. There are two popular ways of performing such averaging.[6] The first is to break the data segment up further into subsegments and average the corresponding single tapered estimates. To minimize data loss due to tapering, the segments are allowed to overlap, and the corresponding estimates are known as *overlap-add* estimates or Welch estimates. These estimators have the form (n is the number of overlapping segments, each of length T, and with starting points τ_l)

$$S_{WOSA}(f) = \frac{1}{n} \sum_{l=1}^{n} |\tilde{x}_w^l(f)|^2 \qquad (7.15)$$

$$\tilde{x}_w^l(f) = \sum_{t=-T/2}^{T/2} w_t x_{t+\tau_l} e^{-2\pi i f t} \qquad (7.16)$$

where τ_l is incremented at some fraction of the window size T, and WOSA stands for weighted overlapped segment averaging. A different kind of estimator is obtained by applying smoothing procedures directly to a single tapered estimate. For example, one may perform the kernel smoothing operation,

$$S_{LW}(f) = K(f)*S_w(f) \qquad (7.17)$$

Noting that a convolution in the frequency domain is a product in the time domain, and that the Fourier transform of the spectrum is the autocorrelation function, it can be seen that the kernel smoothing operation on the spectral estimate is equivalent to *tapering an estimate of the autocorrelation function in*

---

6. In repeated trials of an experiment, one can obtain independent samples of process segments, which provide a further source of averaging. We are mostly concerned with methods for a single data segment. However, these methods can be extended in a straightforward way with averaging over trials.

the time domain (hence the name "lag window" estimate, as denoted by the subscript LW).

Quadratic Estimates as Multitaper Estimates

Both the overlap-add and the lag window estimators are special cases of *quadratic* spectral estimators, because both are given by quadratic forms of the data. By inspection, both of these estimators have the form

$$S_Q(f) = \sum_{t=-T/2}^{T/2} \sum_{t'=-T/2}^{T/2} M_{t,t'} x_t x'_{t'} e^{2\pi i f(t-t')} \tag{7.18}$$

The matrix M (assumed to be real, symmetric, and non-negative) is cumbersome to write down, but the reader is invited to construct these matrices for the WOSA and LW methods from the above definitions. The important point for our discussion is that the two fall into a general family, and the question naturally arises as to what choices of this matrix are optimal. To gain insight into this problem, consider the eigenvalue decomposition of the matrix

$$M_{t,t'} = \sum_k \mu_k w_t^{(k)} w_{t'}^{(k)} \tag{7.19}$$

Because the matrix has been considered to be symmetric and non-negative, such an eigenvalue decomposition exists, and further $\lambda_k \geq 0$. In terms of these eigenvalues and eigenvectors, the most general quadratic spectral estimator can always be written in the form

$$S_Q(f) = \sum_k \mu_k |\tilde{x}_k(f)|^2 \tag{7.20}$$

where

$$\tilde{x}_k(f) = \sum_{t=-T/2}^{T/2} w_t^{(k)} x_t e^{-2\pi i f t} \tag{7.21}$$

An estimator of this form is called a *multitaper spectral estimator*, with the family of taper functions being given by $w_t^{(k)}$. Therefore, although the multitaper spectral estimation methodology postdates the more classical nonparametric estimates such as overlap add and lag window methods, it should be clear that the multitaper method conceptually encompasses *all* these methods (for specific choices of tapers). The multitaper *form* of the quadratic estimator is most useful if one can select the matrix M to be of low rank, so that only a few taper functions need to be kept in the estimation procedure.

Multitaper Spectral Estimator Using Slepians

From our earlier discussion in the section on the spectral concentration problem, the Slepian functions form a family of functions that are well suited for use in the multitaper estimate described above. Recall that the Slepian functions are characterized by two parameters, the sequence length T and the bandwidth parameter $2W$. Note that in the earlier sections we have taken the sequences to be of length $T+1$, with T being odd, to avoid cumbersome phase factors in the definition of the convolution kernel. In this section and the following ones, we adopt instead the convention that the sequence length is T, for notational simplicity. For these choice of parameters, there are $K = [2WT]$ tapers $w_t^{(k)}$ that are well concentrated in the frequency range $[-W\ W]$. The simple multitaper spectral estimate using Slepian tapers is then given by

$$S_{MT}(f) = \frac{1}{K} \sum_k |\tilde{x}_k(f)|^2 \qquad (7.22)$$

where $\tilde{x}_k(f)$ are the tapered Fourier transforms of the data segment using Slepian tapers and

$$\tilde{x}_k(f) = \sum_{t=1}^{T} w_t^{(k)} x_t e^{-2\pi i f t} \qquad (7.23)$$

It is easy to show that the expected value of the estimate is given by

$$E[S_{MT}(f)] = \int_{-\frac{1}{2}}^{\frac{1}{2}} H(f - f') S(f') df' \qquad (7.24)$$

where the smoothing kernel is given by

$$H(f) = \frac{1}{K} \sum_{k=1}^{K} |U_k(f)|^2 \qquad (7.25)$$

This is a "square-topped" (or boxcar-shaped) function that is small outside the interval $[-W\ W]$. Therefore, the expected value of the multitaper estimator is the original spectrum, smoothed by convolution with a boxcar-like function with a smoothing width of $2W$. Note that the smoothing is achieved within the band $[-W\ W]$ without causing excessive sidelobe leakage outside of the band, as would be caused by a simple boxcar smoothing of the periodogram. Further, the same effect cannot be achieved by a boxcar smoothing of a single tapered estimate using the first Slepian, because such a procedure would broaden the smoothing bandwidth beyond the bandwidth parameter for the first Slepian, whereas the multitaper procedure does not introduce such extra broadening.

Usage of the Slepian functions control broadband bias. In addition, however, averaging over K Slepian functions reduces the variance of the spectral estimate by a factor of K, as can be seen from the following discussion.

Estimation Variance

In this section we consider the estimation variance of the multitaper estimator using K tapers. The degrees of freedom of the estimator is $2m$, where $m = K$ if a single data segment is being considered, and $m = KN_{Tr}$ if one also averaging over N_{Tr} trials. Assuming that the original process is Gaussian, the spectral estimate $S_{MT}(f)$ has a chi-square distribution with $2m$ degrees of freedom.[7] From this, it follows that

$$V[S_{MT}(f)] = \frac{1}{K} E[S_{MT}(f)]^2 \qquad (7.26)$$

Two salient points can be noted from this expression. First, the variance of the MT estimator is reduced by a factor of K. Note that the chi-square distribution makes it possible to derive local confidence bands for the spectra, rather than just reporting the variance. Second, the variance depends on the expected value of the spectrum. This makes it difficult to judge the estimation variance by looking at a plot of $S_{MT}(f)$ because the estimation variance depends on frequency for general spectral shapes.

A remedy for this problem is to use the log transform of the spectrum, which makes the estimation variance constant and independent of frequency:[8]

$$E[\ln (S_{MT}(f)] = \ln[E(S_{MT}(f))] + \psi(m) - \ln(m) \qquad (7.27)$$
$$V[\ln (S_{MT}(f)] = \psi'(m) \qquad (7.28)$$

where $\psi(m)$ is the so called digamma function, $\psi(m) = \Gamma'(m)/\Gamma(m)$. For large m, $\psi'(m) \approx \frac{1}{m}$. Therefore, the estimation variance of the logarithm is also reduced approximately linearly with the number of tapers, independently of frequency.

Jackknife Method For Estimation Variance

If the process is strongly non-Gaussian, and the data window is not long enough for the central limit theorem arguments to apply, the above formulas may not provide an accurate estimate of the variance. The "jackknife" procedure provides a way to obtain an estimate of the variance without such distributional assumptions. Basic to the jackknife procedure is the computation of *pseudo-values* corresponding to some statistic to be estimated. These are obtained by leaving out one sample in turn.

---

7. Even if the original process is *not* Gaussian distributed, the central limit theorem ensures that $\tilde{x}_k(f)$ tend to have Gaussian distributions for large T. Therefore, the assumption of Gaussianity for the original process can be relaxed somewhat in these considerations.

8. This is called a *variance stabilizing* transformation.

The multitaper approach facilitates the application of the jackknife to a single data segment. The usual leave-one-out procedure employed for computing jackknife variances cannot be applied to time series data by leaving out one time series sample in turn, because the samples may be correlated. However, the jackknife procedure may be applied by leaving out *one taper* in turn from a multitaper estimate [221]. This may be applied equally well to spectra and to other quantities for which multitaper estimates may be computed. For spectra that are constant within the band $[-W \ W]$, the quantities $\tilde{x}_k(f)$ may be shown to be uncorrelated, thus justifying the usage of the jackknife procedure. Spectra that are strongly varying within the band may be made approximately constant by prior application of a prewhitening procedure to be discussed in a later section.

Units in Spectral Estimation

The units of time and frequency are relatively straightforward: if the digitization rate is R Hz, then the frequencies range from $-R/2$ to $R/2$ Hz. For unpadded FFTs when the data series is N samples long, each frequency bin is therefore R/N Hz. Similarly, if the data series is padded to a total length N_{pad}, then the frequency grid spacing is R/N_{pad}. The units of the spectral estimate have to be accounted for more carefully. A simple way to do this is to equate the total power as computed in the frequency and time domains. For example, consider the direct spectral estimate

$$S_D(f) \propto |\tilde{X}(f)|^2 \tag{7.29}$$

where

$$\tilde{X}(f) = \sum_{j=1}^{N} w_j x(j\Delta t) e^{-2\pi i f j \Delta t} \tag{7.30}$$

Note that f is evaluated on a discrete grid using a padded FFT. One should ensure that the normalization of the FFT routine corresponds to the above equation. Factors of N or N_{pad} may appear in some implementations of the FFT routine, which have to be accounted for. If a different normalization is in use, then the result should be multiplied by a suitable factor to conform to the above. We can determine normalization by assuming that the original discrete time process was white noise with variance σ. The spectral power density is therefore given by σ^2/R, where R is the digitization rate. For the white noise case, a straightforward computation shows that

$$E[|\tilde{X}(f)|^2] = \sigma^2 \sum_{j=1}^{N} |w_j|^2 \tag{7.31}$$

If we take the taper function w_j to be normalized so that $\sum_j |w_j|^2 = 1$, then it follows that the appropriate proportionality constant that will give the spectral density in the right units is given by:

$$S_D(f) = \frac{1}{R}|\tilde{X}(f)|^2 = \Delta t|\tilde{X}(f)|^2 \qquad (7.32)$$

The spectral power density for an EEG time series can therefore be evaluated in appropriate units of $\mu V^2/\text{Hz}$, and so on.

Often, we are interested in the changes in the spectral power density rather than absolute spectral power; these changes are best measured in decibel units. If $S_B(f)$ is the spectral power density in a baseline or reference condition, then the relative change in spectral power is given in decibels by

$$10\log_{10}\left(\frac{S(f)}{S_B(f)}\right) \qquad (7.33)$$

Sometimes $S_B(f)$ is standardized—in this case it is enough to cite the relative power in decibels. Otherwise, the baseline spectral density should be supplied in absolute units, along with a report of the changes in decibel units.

For point process spectra to be discussed later, the spectral power density has units of Hz^2/Hz or simply Hz. It can be initially confusing to see frequency units along both axes in a plot of a point process spectrum, but one way to remember this is that for point processes, the asymptotic value of the spectrum at large frequencies is given by the rate of the process, which is of course measured in units of frequency.

7.3.3 Autoregressive Parametric Estimates

So far, we have discussed nonparametric spectral estimates, because no explicit assumption has been made about the form of the underlying stochastic process. A different approach is to fit a parametric model of the likelihood of the stochastic process, and then to evaluate the spectrum of the parameterized process. The simplest and most widely used example is the autoregressive approach. We will provide only a brief description of this approach, before commenting on the relative merits of autoregressive spectral estimates and the quadratic estimates described earlier.

First consider the moving average model MA(q) given by

$$x_t = \sum_{k=0}^{q-1} b_k n_{t-k} \qquad (7.34)$$

It is assumed that n_t is an uncorrelated Gaussian stochastic process (Gaussian white noise) with variance $E[n_t^2] = \sigma^2$. Note that the process x_t is obtained from n_t by the application of a finite length filter (also called an FIR or finite impulse response filter). It is easy to verify that

$$X(f) = b(f)N(f) \qquad (7.35)$$

Here $b(f) = \sum_{k=0}^{q-1} b_k e^{-2\pi i f k}$, and $X(f)$ and $N(f)$ are the Fourier transforms of the series x_t, n_t. The power spectrum of x is therefore given by

$$S_X(f) = \sigma^2 |b(f)|^2 \qquad (7.36)$$

In contrast, an autoregressive Gaussian AR(p) model is described by the equation,

$$x_t = \sum_{k=1}^{p} a_k x_{t-k} + n_t \qquad (7.37)$$

The equation can be Fourier transformed to obtain

$$X(f) = a(f)X(f) + N(f) \qquad (7.38)$$

Here $a(f) = \sum_{k=1}^{p} a_k e^{-2\pi i f k}$. This equation can be solved to obtain the power spectrum as

$$S_X(f) = \frac{\sigma^2}{1 - |a(f)|^2} \qquad (7.39)$$

The a_ks define an IIR or infinite impulse response filter; the reader is invited to verify this by iterating the defining equation through a substitution of x_{t-k} in terms of its AR description to obtain a filter acting on the noise process n_t.

The two equations above can be combined to obtain the ARMA(p,q) model with power spectrum given by

$$S_X(f) = \frac{\sigma^2 |b(f)|^2}{1 - |a(f)|^2} \qquad (7.40)$$

AR and ARMA processes are in use to model spectra. To fit an autoregressive model, one proceeds by multiplying both sides of the defining equation for the AR model by $x_{t-\tau}$ for $0 < \tau \le p$ and taking an expectation of the resulting equation. Because $x_{t-\tau}$ does not depend on n_t, it follows that $E[n_t x_{t-\tau}] = 0$. One therefore obtains the so-called Yule-Walker equations ($k = 1 \ldots p$)

$$C(\tau) = \sum_{k} a_k C(\tau - k) \qquad (7.41)$$

Here $C(\tau) = E[x_t x_{t-\tau}]$ is the correlation function of the stochastic process x_t. Consider for example the AR(1) process

$$x_t = a_1 x_{t-1} + n_t \qquad (7.42)$$

There is only one Yule-Walker equation, $C(0) = a_1 C(1)$. As long as $C(1)$ is nonzero, this equation can be used to estimate a_1 from estimates of $C(0) = E[x_t^2]$ and $C(1) = E[x_t x_{t-1}]$.

The idea behind autoregressive spectral estimation is to estimate the correlation functions $C(\tau)$ from data and to then substitute in the above equation to obtain the AR coefficients a_k. The spectral estimate is then obtained using Equation 7.39. The model order p is typically not known in advance and provides a bias-variance tradeoff. For small p, the spectrum may not be well estimated (larger bias) but has lower variance. For large p, the spectrum will exhibit less bias but may suffer from overfitting (larger variance). Thus, p plays the role of a smoothing parameter.

Cautions Related to AR Spectral Estimates

The AR spectral estimates appear attractive because they are discrete versions of ordinary differential equations (with stochastic forcing) and lead to a parametrization of the underlying dynamical system in terms that are familiar from physics. There are significant problems with these estimates, however, that require care. If the spectra are smooth and with relatively small dynamical range, then only a low-model order is needed to fit the spectrum, and the AR procedure works reasonably well. The AR model can also work well to model narrowband processes that correspond to sharp spectral peaks. However, one often obtains mixed spectra, containing both broadband and sharp line components. These are not well approximated by AR models, particularly from small samples.

The source of the difficulty is that the parameters a_k are *nonlocal* in frequency (i.e., they can depend on the entire frequency range). This means that the estimate at one frequency can depend on the estimate at a quite different frequency, and there is no obvious parametric way of isolating the different frequency bands. It should also be noted that in some sense, the AR estimate assumes the result: the inputs to the estimation procedure are correlation coefficients, and knowledge of the correlation coefficients is *equivalent* to knowledge about spectra. There is some circularity to this procedure. Finally, the parameter values become highly ill conditioned as model order increases, so that even when the spectrum is well estimated, the underlying parameters may not be. This reduces the real utility of a parametric model.

One way to improve the estimation of the coefficients a_k is to use improved estimates of the correlation function $C(\tau)$ by starting from a nonparametric spectral estimate. This of course is not useful if the desired end result is the spectral estimate. However, it is a more robust way to proceed if the AR parameters themselves are of intrinsic interest, as might be the case in making a black box model from data.

Prewhitening

AR spectral estimation has an important use, which is to "prewhiten" a stochastic process. The procedure is as follows. Obtain a fixed, low-order (say $p < 5$) AR fit to the process, and then construct the "innovations" process

$$\varepsilon_t = x_t - \sum_{k=1}^{p} a_k x_{t-k} \tag{7.43}$$

The low-order AR fit models the overall shape of the spectrum, which is helpful in reducing the dynamic range of the spectrum. A nonparametric estimate is then obtained of the innovations process using a multitaper estimate. Whitening of the original process improves the multitaper estimate, because the condition of "local whiteness" is better met. The spectrum of the original process can be reconstructed from the estimate of the spectrum of the innovations process, using the equation

$$S_X(f) = \frac{S_\varepsilon(f)}{1 - |a(f)|^2} \tag{7.44}$$

When used with care, this procedure combines the strengths of the parametric and nonparametric approaches.

7.3.4 Harmonic Analysis and Mixed Spectral Estimation

A special case of first moment analysis is given by a deterministic sinusoid in the signal, corresponding to a line component in the power spectrum. Such components are visible in preliminary estimates as sharp peaks in the spectrum, which for multitaper estimation with Slepians appear with flat tops.[9] Consider one such sinusoid embedded in colored noise

$$x_t = A \cos(2\pi f_0 t + \phi) + n_t \tag{7.45}$$

It is customary to apply a least square procedure to obtain A and ϕ by minimizing the sum of squares $\sum_t [x_t - A \cos(2\pi f_0 t + \phi)]^2$. However, this is a nonlinear procedure that must be performed numerically; moreover, it effectively assumes a white noise spectrum. Thomson's F-test offers an attractive alternative within the multitaper framework that reduces the line-fitting procedure to a simple linear regression. Multiplying both of the sides of the equation by a Slepian taper $w_t^{(k)}$ with bandwidth parameter $2W$, and Fourier transforming, one obtains

$$X_k(f) = \mu U_k(f - f_0) + \mu^* U_k(f + f_0) + N_k(f) \tag{7.46}$$

---

9. The flat-topped peaks correspond to the square shaped convolution kernel of the multitaper estimator using Slepian tapers.

Here $\mu = Ae^{i\phi}$ and $U_k(f)$ is the Fourier transform of $w_t^{(k)}$. If f_0 is larger than W, then $f+f_0$ and $f-f_0$ are separated by more than $2W$, and $U_k(f-f_0)$ and $U_k(f+f_0)$ have minimal overlap.[10] In that case one can neglect one of the terms, and set $f=f_0$ to obtain the linear regression equation

$$X_k(f_0) = \mu U_k(0) + N_k(f_0) \tag{7.47}$$

This has the solution

$$\hat{\mu}(f_0) = \frac{\sum_{k=1}^K U_k^*(0) X_k(f_0)}{\sum_{k=1}^K |U_k(0)|^2} \tag{7.48}$$

The goodness of fit of this model may be tested using an F-ratio statistic with $(2, 2K-2)$ degrees of freedom, which is usually plotted as a function of frequency to determine the position of the significant sinusoidal peaks in the spectrum,

$$F(f) = \frac{(K-1)|\mu(f)|^2 \sum_k |U_k(0)|^2}{|X_k(f) - \mu(f) U_k(0)|^2} \tag{7.49}$$

The frequency of a sinusoid embedded in noise can be determined to an accuracy *better* than the Raleigh resolution $\Delta f = 1/T$. It can be shown that for long window length T, the standard deviation of the frequency estimate for a sinusoid with amplitude A embedded in noise with spectral power density $S_n(f)$ is given by

$$\sigma^2(f_0) = \frac{1}{T^2} \frac{6 S_n(f_0)}{\pi^2 A^2 T} \tag{7.50}$$

Notice that $\sigma(f_0) \sim 1/T^{3/2}$ rather than $1/T$. This does not mean, however, that the limits set by the uncertainty principle have gone away. This can be seen by looking at *two* sinusoids embedded in noise; in that case, the determination of the two frequencies becomes ill posed when the frequencies come closer than the Raleigh frequency $1/T$.

Peaks deemed significant may be removed from the original process, to obtain a *reshaped* estimate of the smooth part of the spectrum

$$S_{reshaped}(f) = \frac{1}{K} \sum_{k=1}^K \left| X_k(f) - \sum_i \mu_i U_k(f - f_i) \right|^2 \tag{7.51}$$

This reshaped estimate may be augmented with the previously determined line components, to obtain a "mixed" spectral estimate. This provides one of the more powerful applications of the multitaper methodology, because the estimation of such mixed spectra is in general difficult.

---

10. This is because $U_k(f)$ is concentrated on the interval $[-W\ W]$.

7.3.5 Dynamic Spectra

So far we have confined our attention to a spectrum estimate, with the default assumption of a stationary power spectrum. This is of course an untenable assumption in most applications. The presence of external stimuli, sources of drift, or slow state changes on the scale of the data segment require explicit treatment of the potential nonstationarities present in the process.

Armed with Slepian sequences and the associated careful treatment of time and frequency resolution, we are already well equipped to deal with such nonstationarities. The simplest solution is to obtain a dynamic spectrum estimate or spectrogram estimate, using a moving analysis window. Such a procedure is governed by three parameters: the moving window length T, the step size ΔT, and the total bandwidth $2W$. Assuming that ΔT is small compared with T, one then obtains an estimate of the dynamic spectrum $S(f, t)$, where the resolution of the estimation procedure determined by a time-frequency tile $T \times 2W$. If the features in $S(f, t)$ are coarser than this tiling, then we obtain an adequate estimate (apart from variance issues).

If there are finer features than set by these resolution parameters, one can vary T and $2W$. Note, that good spectral concentration cannot be obtained unless $2TW > 1$ (the "uncertainty principle"). This sets the area of the smallest feasible tile in the time-frequency plane. One may choose tall skinny tiles or short, fat tiles, but the area is effectively bounded below. Moreover, one typically wants to stay away from the lower bound, so as to obtain better sidelobe suppression and to be able to accommodate more than one Slepian function per tile. Accommodating K Slepian functions requires $2WT \geq K$; this in turn provides a variance reduction by a factor of $1/K$. Note that further variance reduction is possible when trial averaging is included.

In this approach, the frequency resolution is left constant throughout the frequency plane. Another popular approach is to use wavelets, which allow for finer time resolution at high frequencies. Because the area of the time-frequency resolution tile has to be conserved, this comes at the price of coarser frequency resolution. The justification provided for such an approach is that natural processes have coarser spectral features at higher frequencies. This assumption may not, however, be true, and the a priori imposition of different point spread functions in different regions of the time-frequency plane builds in a certain bias into the estimation procedure. Rather than look like rectangular bricks the point spread functions of wavelets are typically asymmetric and resemble teardrops. This causes "flame"-like artifacts to appear in under-smoothed estimates of the dynamic spectrum. An alternative approach is to use the constant bandwidth approach described in the previous sections, but split the frequency range so as to accommodate changes in the widths of spectral peaks at different frequencies.

Wigner Transform

Yet another approach to estimating the dynamic spectrum is through the so-called Wigner transform. For a continuous function of time $x(t)$, the Wigner transform is defined as

$$A(f, t) = \int d\tau x\left(t - \frac{\tau}{2}\right) x\left(t + \frac{\tau}{2}\right) e^{-2\pi i f \tau} \qquad (7.52)$$

Note that if $x(t)$ is a stochastic process, then $E[A(f, t)] = S(f, t)$, so it is tempting to associate $A(f, t)$ with an estimate of the dynamic spectrum. There are some potential problems with this approach. First, $A(f, t)$ as defined is not guaranteed to be positive definite, something that is required for a spectral estimate. Secondly, so-called "cross terms" may appear. For example, if the original signal is a single "chirp" or frequency-modulated sweep, the Wigner transform provides a good estimate of this sweep in the time-frequency plane. Unfortunately, when more than one such sweep is simultaneously present in the data, spurious sweeps may appear in intermediate regions.

A variety of fixes are available for these ills, but our experience is that a good estimate of the dynamic spectrum may be obtained by choosing appropriate parameters T and $2W$ for the multitaper estimates described above, without worrying about these extra issues. If high resolution is required and trial averaging is possible, one can keep $2WT$ close to one. However, there are cases where a refined estimate of the dynamic spectrum may be obtained using variants of the Wigner transform. In order to keep track of such fine features in $S(f, t)$, we prefer a somewhat different approach, namely to directly estimate the *changes* in $S(f, t)$ in the form of the time and frequency derivatives of the spectrogram.

Time and Frequency Derivatives

Recall that the simple (nonadaptive) multitaper spectrum estimate is given by

$$S_{MT}(f) = \frac{1}{K} \sum_k |\tilde{x}_k(f)|^2 \qquad (7.53)$$

This can be rewritten in the form

$$S_{MT}(f) = \tilde{x}_k^*(f) M_{kk'} \tilde{x}_{k'}(f) \qquad (7.54)$$

where the matrix M is proportional to the identity matrix, $M_{ij} = \frac{1}{K} \delta_{ij}$. The question naturally arises, as to what happens when the matrix M is of more general form and *not* an identity matrix. Interestingly, by judiciously selecting the matrix M, one may in fact obtain estimates of *derivatives* of the spectrum with respect to frequency or with respect to time (in case of dynamic spectra). The corresponding theoretical considerations are fairly involved, but the resulting formulas are quite simple. For example, define the following *off-diagonal* sum, which is perhaps the simplest generalization of the diagonal form that gives the spectral estimate.

$$Z(f) = \frac{1}{K-1} \sum_{k=1}^{K-1} \tilde{x}_{k+1}^*(f)\tilde{x}_k(f) \tag{7.55}$$

For reasons that have to do with the form of the time and frequency "operators" expressed in the Slepian basis,[11] it turns out that $Im[Z(f)]$ resembles $\partial S(f, t)/\partial f$ and $Re[Z(f)]$ resembles $\partial S(f, t)/\partial t$. Note that we have not explicitly written $Z(f)$ as a function of t, the location of the data segment in time, but this dependence is understood. More generally, we have found that

$$Re[e^{i\phi}Z(f)] \tag{7.56}$$

provides an approximate *directional derivative* of $S(f, t)$ in the time-frequency plane at an angle ϕ to the time axis. The quantity defined above is of interest because it provides a simple algorithm to estimate the derivatives of the dynamic spectrum in the time frequency plane *directly*, without first estimating $S(f, t)$ and then taking a derivative using a convolution procedure (which can further broaden the estimate).

This is a *heuristic* result, but the quadratic inverse theory of spectral estimation developed by Thomson [219] provides a rigorous procedure to estimate the frequency derivative of the spectrum and the time derivative of the dynamic spectrum. To understand the basic idea, consider the matrix of correlations between the tapered Fourier transforms, $C_{kk'}(f) = \tilde{x}_k^*(f)\tilde{x}_{k'}(f)$. Noting that $\tilde{x}_k(f) = \int df' U_k(f - f')X(f')$, where $U_k(f)$ is the Fourier transform of the kth Slepian function $w_t^{(k)}$, the expectation value of this matrix can be shown to be

$$E[C_{kk'}(f)] = \int_{-1/2}^{1/2} df' U_k^*(f')U_{k'}(f')S(f - f') \tag{7.57}$$

Now note that $U_k(f')$ is small outside the interval $[-W, W]$. Therefore, the integral can be restricted to this interval to provide an approximation for the above expression. Making the further assumption that $S(f)$ varies slowly inside the interval $[f - W, f + W]$, within that interval one can use the first-order Taylor approximation, $S(f - f') \approx S(f) - f'S'(f)$. Assembling these together, one obtains the expression

$$E[C_{kk'}(f)] \approx S(f)\delta_{kk'} - F_{kk'}S'(f) \tag{7.58}$$

---

11. This argument can be made more precise by noting the relation between the Slepian functions and Hermite functions familiar in quantum mechanics, as well as noting that time and frequency (for a time series) play a mathematically similar role to position and momentum (for a wave function). The position and momentum operators, as expressed in the basis of Hermite functions, have a simple, bidiagonal form. Similarly, the time and frequency operators expressed in the Slepian basis have an approximately bidiagonal form. This is the origin of the heuristic expression for $Z(f)$.

where the matrix $F_{kk'}$ is given by

$$F_{kk'} = -\int_{-W}^{W} fU_k^*(f)U_{k'}(f)df \tag{7.59}$$

Because $|U_k(f)|^2$ is even, $F_{kk} = 0$ and the diagonal terms of F are zero. An explicit computation shows that F is approximately bidiagonal, with the largest terms above and below the main diagonal. It follows that $Tr(F) = 0$, so that

$$E[Tr(F^\dagger C)] = Tr(F^\dagger F)S'(f) \tag{7.60}$$

This leads to the following estimate for the frequency derivative of the spectrum

$$\hat{S}'(f) = c\sum_{kk'} \tilde{x}_k^*(f)F_{kk'}^*\tilde{x}_{k'}(f) \tag{7.61}$$

Here the normalization constant c is given by $c = Tr(F^\dagger F)^{-1}$. A more refined procedure [219] is to expand $S(f - f')$ in terms of a set of special functions $B_l(f)$, which are defined through the eigenvalue equation

$$g_l B_l(f) = \int_{-W}^{W} |P(f,f')|^2 B_l(f') \tag{7.62}$$

The matrix $P(f, f')$ is the projection operator into the band $[-W, W]$, given by

$$P(f,f') = \sum_l \tilde{x}_k^*(f)\tilde{x}_k(f') \tag{7.63}$$

The functions $B_l(f)$ are normalized over the interval $[-W, W]$. It can be shown that approximately $4TW$ of the eigenvalues g_l are nonzero and fall off approximately linearly with l. The spectrum is expanded in terms of these functions, with the expansion coefficients (which correspond to the Taylor coefficients) denoted by $b_l(f)$

$$S(f - f') = \sum_l b_l(f)B_l(f') \tag{7.64}$$

Approximately, $b_0(f)$ is the spectrum $S(f)$, and $b_1(f)$ is the first derivative, $b_1(f) \approx S'(f)$. Define matrix $B_{kk'}^{(1)}$ as

$$B_{kk'}^{(1)} = -\int_{-W}^{W} B_1(f)U_k^*(f)U_{k'}(f)df \tag{7.65}$$

Note that this resembles the definition of the matrix F above, with f replaced by $B_1(f)$. In terms of this matrix, the coefficient $b_1(f)$ is estimated from the data as

$$\hat{b}_1(f) = \frac{1}{g_1}\sum_{kk'} \tilde{x}_k^*(f)B_{kk'}^{(1)*}\tilde{x}_{k'}(f) \tag{7.66}$$

The frequency derivative estimate $S'(f)$ can then be approximated by this quantity, $S'(f) \approx \hat{b}_1(f)$.

Time Derivative Estimate

A similar set of considerations lead to the estimate of the time derivative of the dynamic spectrum [221], $\partial S(f, t)/\partial t$. We will not describe the details here but simply present the estimation formulas. Corresponding to the expansion functions $B_l(f)$, one defines time domain functions $A_l(t)$ that are used instead of a simple Taylor expansion in terms of powers of t. The dynamic spectrum $S(f, t)$ is therefore expanded around a given time as

$$S(f, t) \approx \sum_l a_l(f)A_l(t) \tag{7.67}$$

The functions $A_l(t)$ are eigenfunctions of the Fejer kernel, which we encountered in chapter 5,

$$\alpha_l A_l(t) = \sum_{t'=1}^{T} \left[\frac{\sin(2\pi W(t - t'))}{\pi(t - t')} \right]^2 A_l(t') \tag{7.68}$$

The time derivative of the dynamic spectrum $\partial S(f, t)/\partial t$ is approximated by $a_1(f)$

$$\frac{\partial S(f, t)}{\partial t} \approx \hat{a}_1(f) \tag{7.69}$$

$$\hat{a}_1(f) = \frac{1}{\alpha_1} \sum_{kk'} \tilde{x}_k^*(f) A_{kk'}^{(1)*} \tilde{x}_{k'}(f) \tag{7.70}$$

where the matrix $A_{kk'}^{(1)*}$ is given in the same way as the matrix $B_{kk'}^{(1)*}$ with $B_l(f)$ replaced by $A_l(f)$, the Fourier transform of the series $A_l(t)$.

Test for Nonstationarity

The estimates $\hat{a}_l(f)$ can be used to provide a test for the nonstationarity of the series [221], as follows. Define the numbers e_l as the sums of $A_l(t)$. These are the coefficients of expansion of a time-independent constant in terms of $A_l(t)$

$$e_l = \sum_{t=1}^{T} A_l(t) \tag{7.71}$$

Also, define the average of the estimated dynamic spectrum over the time range, obtained by computing a multitaper estimate with a moving window and averaging over time,

$$S_{av}(f) = \frac{1}{T} \sum_t \hat{S}(f, t) \tag{7.72}$$

In terms of the quantities defined above, the test statistic for nonstationarity is defined as

$$\zeta(f) = \sum_{l=0}^{L-1} \alpha_l \left[\frac{\hat{a}_l(f)}{S_{av}(f)} - e_l \right]^2 \qquad (7.73)$$

This quantity has an approximately χ^2_{L-1} distribution. By plotting $\zeta(f)$ as a function of frequency and studying excursions beyond thresholds chosen according to the χ^2_{L-1} distribution, one can assess the degree of nonstationarity in the time series.

7.4 Bivariate Spectral Analysis

We have discussed univariate spectral analysis in detail, and many of the same considerations carry over to multivariate spectral analysis for several time series. Our treatment of bivariate and multivariate spectral analysis will therefore be relatively short. The basic idea in multivariate spectral analysis is that for multiple time series $x_i(t)$, once we have moved to the frequency domain, $X_i(f)$ are uncorrelated for different frequencies for stationary processes

$$E[X_i^*(f)X_j(f')] = S_{ij}(f)\delta(f - f') \qquad (7.74)$$

Thus, after Fourier transformation, one may fix f and perform ordinary multivariate analysis. In the case of bivariate spectral analysis, the covariance function between two processes at a given frequency is known as the cross-spectrum, and the correlation coefficient is known as the coherency

$$E[X_1^*(f)X_2(f')] = S_{12}(f)\delta(f - f') \qquad (7.75)$$

$$C_{12}(f) = \frac{S_{12}(f)}{\sqrt{S_1(f)S_2(f)}} \qquad (7.76)$$

The cross-spectrum is the Fourier transform of the time domain cross-correlation function, but the cross-coherence does not have a simple interpretation in terms of a time domain quantity. We have assumed that the processes are zero mean; if there is a nonzero mean or first moment then this has to be subtracted first (this is particularly important for nonstationary processes, although we are discussing stationary processes right now).

The multitaper estimate of the cross spectrum can be obtained in the same way as the estimate for the spectrum

$$\hat{S}_{ij}(f) = \frac{1}{K} \sum_k \tilde{x}_i^{(k)*}(f)\tilde{x}_j^{(k)}(f) \qquad (7.77)$$

This is the basis for the estimates of the other quantities in the following sections, and we will not repeat the equations for the estimate in this discussion.

7.4.1 Cross-Coherence

The complex cross-coherence is sometimes referred to as the coherency. It plays a fundamental role as a measure of association between two processes and has a number of notable properties:

1. The coherency is a *function* of frequency rather than being a single number. This is not surprising because time series can be regarded as multivariate objects themselves, and the cross-covariance is a *matrix*, which gives a frequency-dependent function when diagonalized. It is not in general possible to quantify the strength of association between two series by a single number in an informative way. If the magnitude of the coherency is relatively constant with respect to frequency over some frequency range of interest, then that magnitude can be taken to be the summary measure of association.

2. The magnitude of the coherency (usually referred to as the coherence), as a function of frequency, lies between zero and one. It is a normalized measure of association between two processes, which can be *pooled* across pairs of time series. This is particularly important, because the time domain correlations cannot be easily averaged in this manner; a negative correlation between one pair may cancel a positive correlation between another pair, which may be undesirable.

3. The phase of the coherency carries information about the temporal relationship between the two processes. In particular, if two processes are otherwise identical but shifted with respect to each other by a time delay τ, then the coherency is given by

$$C(f) = e^{2\pi i f \tau} \tag{7.78}$$

Due to this reason, the frequency derivative of the phase may be used to *define* the time delay between two processes (this quantity is known as the *group delay* in physics). If $C(f) = e^{i\phi(f)}|C(f)|$, then the group delay $\tau(f)$ is defined as

$$\tau(f) = \frac{1}{2\pi}\frac{d\phi}{df} \tag{7.79}$$

The estimate for the coherency is obtained by dividing the corresponding cross-spectral estimate by the spectrum estimates for the individual processes

$$\hat{C}_{12}(f) = \frac{\hat{S}_{12}(f)}{\sqrt{\hat{S}_1(f)\hat{S}_2(f)}} \tag{7.80}$$

The statistical properties of this estimate are more complicated than that of the spectrum estimate. The distribution function of the squared coherence estimate is given in terms of a hypergeometric function when the true coherence is nonzero. When the true coherence is zero, then the distribution of the estimator has a simpler form. If the estimator has m degrees of freedom, the distribution is given by

$$p(|C|^2) = \frac{1}{m-1}(1 - |C|^2)^{m-2} \tag{7.81}$$

so that

$$P(|C|^2 > \theta) = (1 - \theta)^{m-1} \tag{7.82}$$

If the population or true coherence is nonzero and given by γ, then asymptotically (for large degrees of freedom m) the distribution is approximately Gaussian, especially if the variance stabilizing *Fisher* transform is first applied, $q = \sqrt{2m - 2}\tanh^{-1}(|C|)$:

$$E[q] = \sqrt{2m - 2}\tanh^{-1}(\gamma) + \frac{1}{\sqrt{2m - 2}} \tag{7.83}$$

$$V[q] = 1 \tag{7.84}$$

These may be used to estimate confidence limits for the estimate of the coherence, or a jackknife procedure may be used to estimate the variance of the estimator.

7.5 Multivariate Spectral Analysis

Multivariate spectral analysis generalizes the above considerations to more than two time series. When dealing with many time series, it becomes important to summarize the correlations across variables or to reduce dimensionality in some way. One way to do this is to perform an eigenvalue decomposition of the cross spectral matrix.

7.5.1 *Singular Value Decomposition of the Cross-Spectral Matrix*

The cross-spectral matrix $S_{ij}(f)$ can be factorized using a singular value decomposition (SVD)[12] to obtain the *eigenspectra* $\sigma_\alpha(f)$

$$S_{ij}(f) = \sum_\alpha \sigma_\alpha(f)u_\alpha^*(i\,|\,f)u_\alpha(j\,|\,f) \tag{7.85}$$

This reduces an $N \times N$ matrix of cross-spectra to N eigenspectra $\sigma_\alpha(f)$. These eigenspectra can be further condensed into an *global* coherence $C_G(f)$ by

---

12. Because the cross-spectral matrix is Hermitian, this is equivalent to an eigenvalue decomposition. However, the SVD is a more robust algorithm.

taking the fractional energy captured by the leading eigenspectrum as a fraction of the total energy at a given frequency

$$C_G(f) = \frac{\sigma_0(f)}{\sum_\alpha \sigma_\alpha(f)} \qquad (7.86)$$

This is a number between zero and one. If $C_G(f)$ is one, this means that the cross-spectral matrix $S_{ij}(f)$ is rank one, and at that frequency, all the processes are multiples of a single process, so that there is perfect correlation. The multitaper approach provides a fast algorithm to estimate this global coherence and the leading eigenspectra without having to first compute the cross-spectral matrix. $S_{ij}(f)$ is $N \times N$, and N can become large especially in applications with image time series. One performs an SVD directly on the tapered Fourier transforms $\phi(y|f)$ of the individual time series,[13] $x_i(t)$:

$$\tilde{x}_{ik}(f) = \sum_\alpha \lambda_\alpha(f) u_\alpha^*(i|f) v_\alpha(k|f) \qquad (7.87)$$

This involves an $N \times K$ matrix instead of an $N \times N$ matrix, which may take the computation from being intractable to being tractable. This computation is repeated for all frequencies on a grid to obtain the eigenspectra $\lambda_\alpha(f)$. The leading eigenspectra are then estimated as

$$\hat{\sigma}_\alpha(f) = |\lambda_\alpha|^2(f) \qquad (7.88)$$

The estimate of the global coherence is then obtained as

$$\hat{C}_G(f) = \frac{|\lambda_0|^2(f)}{\sum_\alpha |\lambda_\alpha|^2(f)} \qquad (7.89)$$

Traveling Waves

So far, we have not discussed the eigenmodes from the above decompositions. Some of this discussion is to be found in the applications sections. However, one case is of particular interest, namely where the original time series are from the individual voxels in an image, $I(\mathbf{y}, t)$. The eigenmodes obtained from the decomposition described above are complex numbers and have phases. Consider the leading eigenmode of the decomposition at a given frequency, $I_0(\mathbf{y}|f) = e^{i\phi(\mathbf{y}|f)} |I_0(y|f)|$. Just as the gradient of the phase of the coherency may be used to define group delays, the *spatial* gradients of the phases obtained

---

13. If there are multiple trials of the time series, these are included along with the taper indices and SVD performed on the combined matrix.

from the mode decomposition may be used to define the wave vectors of any traveling waves present in the data (at the frequencies of interest):

$$k(\mathbf{y}\,|f) = \nabla\phi(\mathbf{y}\,|f) \tag{7.90}$$

More generally, rather than compute the gradients of the phase, the spatial modes may be further subjected to spatial Fourier analysis. Alternatively, spatial Fourier analysis may be combined with temporal Fourier analysis. This will not be discussed here further, but this combination of temporal and spatial Fourier analysis is promising for optical imaging data in which complex traveling waves are present.

7.6   Prediction

Prediction of a given time series is a problem in extrapolation. This need not always involve stochastic process concepts. For example, if $x(t)$ is approximately linear, then the best way to extrapolate it might be to fit a straight line and extrapolate using this fit (similar comments hold for more complicated, but deterministic functions). If $x(t)$ is a stationary Gaussian process with a nontrivial correlation function, on the other hand, the prediction problem involves a regression that is somewhat more complicated.

The power spectrum of a stochastic process is an indicator of how predictable the process is. For linear predictors, the predictability is entirely governed by the shape of the spectrum. This makes intuitive sense; for Gaussian white noise (where there is no predictability), the spectrum is flat. On the other hand, if the process consisted of a single sinusoid, then the power spectrum is a delta function and the process is completely predictable. Similarly, cross coherence between two time series is an indicator of the predictability of one time series from another.

Given two stationary stochastic processes $x(t)$ and $y(t)$, the problem of linear prediction simplifies considerably because one needs only to consider time-invariant linear filters,

$$y(t) = \sum_{\tau} k(\tau)x(t - \tau) \tag{7.91}$$

In the frequency domain, the convolution becomes a product, so the prediction equation is

$$Y(f) = K(f)X(f) \tag{7.92}$$

This resembles univariate linear regression. If no causal restrictions are placed on the filter, then the best filter in a least squares sense is given by the *transfer function* between the two series,

$$K(f) = \frac{S_{XY}(f)}{S_{XX}(f)} \tag{7.93}$$

The cross spectra and spectra can be estimated as described earlier. In practice, this ratio has to be regularized, because $S_{XX}(f)$ can approach zero due to stochastic sampling fluctuations and cause large errors in the estimate of the transfer function.

This method of time series prediction is useful in trying to remove the effects of one time series from another, in a context where the corresponding filters do not have to be causal. For example, one may have a neural time series $y(t)$ corrupted by an artifact, which can be measured separately in the form of an auxiliary time series $x(t)$. The component of $y(t)$ predictable from $x(t)$ can be removed using the transfer function. This can be done directly in terms of the tapered Fourier transforms to obtain the residual coefficients

$$\Delta \tilde{y}_k(f) = \tilde{y}_k(f) - \hat{K}(f)\tilde{x}_k(f) \tag{7.94}$$

This can be then used to compute spectra and cross-spectra involving $y(t)$, with the effects of $x(t)$ removed.

7.6.1 Linear Prediction Using Autoregressive Models

It might be desirable to predict the future values of a given series from the current and past values of the same series or other series. In the framework of linear prediction using the method of least squares, this amounts to an auto-regressive modeling of the data. Recall that an AR(p) process satisfies the equation

$$x_t = \sum_{k=1}^{p} a_k x_{t-k} + n_t \tag{7.95}$$

Once the parameters a_k have been estimated as described earlier, they can be used to perform prediction for future values of the process. The one-step prediction is given by

$$x_{t+1} = \sum_{k=1}^{p} \hat{a}_k x_{t+1-k} \tag{7.96}$$

The same procedure generalizes to multiple time series, except that one has to estimate a matrix of prediction coefficients

$$x_{i,t+1} = \sum_{k=1}^{p} \hat{a}_{ij}(k)x_{j,t+1-k} \tag{7.97}$$

The same cautions as presented earlier for estimation of mixed spectra apply here as well. If the process contains identifiable line noise components, these can be estimated and removed, to be predicted separately from the broadband part. The resulting predictions can be added to obtain the prediction for the full process.

7.7   Point Process Spectral Estimation

As indicated in the section on the method of moments for point processes, correlation functions and spectra can be defined for point processes as well as for continuous processes. Here we are concerned with the corresponding estimation issues. The considerations presented above for spectral estimation for continuous processes largely apply [125], so we will only indicate the areas where there are some differences.

First, a segment of point process belonging to a time window $[0, T]$ may be represented by a collection of time points, $t_1, t_2, \ldots, t_n$. Note that the time window is defined in terms of the *observation* interval rather than by the first and last time points. To proceed, one first discretizes the time window into sufficiently fine bins so that each bin contains only one point; for spike trains, bins finer than a millisecond are sufficient for this purpose, although finer binning could be used. One straightforward way to proceed is to discretize the point process as a binary, zero-one process defined on these bins, and then to treat the resulting process using the methods described above. The alternative is to deal directly with the list of times.

In our discussion of multitaper spectral analysis, the basic quantity that enters into all calculations is the tapered Fourier transform $\tilde{x}_k(f)$. If the list-of-times approach is used to describe the segment of the point process, one can evaluate $\tilde{x}_k(f)$ directly as

$$\tilde{x}_k(f) = \sum_j w_k(t_j)e^{-2\pi i f t_j} \tag{7.98}$$

If there are only a few points, then this might be faster than using a discretized description and applying the FFT algorithm. However, note that the taper function $w_k(t)$ has to be evaluated on a discrete grid. In practice, we have found in applications to neural point process data that the direct summation method does not lead to a large time saving over the approach where discretization is followed by an FFT.

Second, the subtraction of the first moment before computation of spectra is an issue. For continuous processes, this involves the removal of the estimated first moment (which is in general time dependent) from the original process. For point process data, one has to remove the first moment as well. For a constant rate process, if the rate is estimated to be $\hat{\lambda}$, then one replaces $\tilde{x}_k(f)$ with the subtracted quantities $\delta\tilde{x}_k(f)$ in the formulas for estimating spectra and cross-spectra.

$$\delta\tilde{x}_k(f) = \sum_j w_k(t_j)e^{-2\pi i f t_j} - \hat{\lambda}\Delta t \sum_t w_k(t)e^{-2\pi i f t} \tag{7.99}$$

Failure to perform this subtraction will cause distortions to appear around zero frequency, in the range $[-W, W]$.

7.7.1 Degrees of Freedom

One additional subtlety of point process spectral estimation is that the number of degrees of freedom is different from the nominal degrees of freedom given by the number of trials and the number of tapers in the case of multitaper estimation. The reason for this has to do with the finiteness of the number of points in the sample. If there are only a total of ten spikes in the entire sample, the number of degrees of freedom in the estimator cannot be more than ten (although it can be less). Thus, if one were to perform multitaper spectral estimation with the time bandwidth product $2WT = 20$, then in the continuous process case the estimator might have 20 degrees of freedom but in the point process example given above it cannot exceed 10.

This means that one should not attempt to obtain spectral estimates with only a few points in the sample. One way to deal with this problem is to try to correct for the number of degrees of freedom in the presence of a relatively small number of points in the sample. This was attempted in [125], where an approximate correction formula is given for the effective number of degrees of freedom. For N_T trials of a homogeneous Poisson process, the effective degrees of freedom v is given (for the periodogram estimate) by the equation [125]

$$\frac{1}{v} = \frac{1}{N_T} \left(1 + \frac{1}{\langle N_{sp} \rangle} \right) \tag{7.100}$$

where $\langle N_{sp} \rangle$ is the average number of spikes in a given trial. Thus, if the number of spikes per trial is larger than 10, then the correction to the number of degrees of freedom is less than 10%.

7.7.2 Hybrid Multivariate Processes

One of the advantages of the multitaper spectral estimation methodology described in this chapter is that it applies with almost equal facility to the spectral estimation of continuous processes, point processes, and also to hybrid multivariate processes. By a hybrid multivariate process we refer to the situation where some of the processes are continuous and some are point processes.

A typical example relevant to neural signals is a spike train paired with a voltage time series recorded from a microelectrode. Suppose the spike times are given by t_i, $i = 1, 2, \ldots, n$ and the voltage time series is $V(t)$. How to measure the association or correlation between these processes? The conventional answer is to use the *spike-triggered average* (STA)

$$\bar{V}(t) = \frac{1}{n} \sum_{i=1}^{n} V(t - t_i) \tag{7.101}$$

Adopting the delta function description of the point process corresponding to the spike train,

$$x(t) = \sum_i \delta(t - t_i) \tag{7.102}$$

it is easy to see that the STA is simply the cross correlation function between the spike train and the voltage time course

$$\bar{V}(t) = \langle V(t - t')x(t') \rangle \tag{7.103}$$

The STA is not a normalized quantity and cannot be easily pooled or compared across conditions. A more fruitful approach if such pooling or comparison is to be performed is to use the *cross-coherence* between the spike train and the voltage time course

$$C_{Vx}(f) = \frac{S_{Vx}(f)}{\sqrt{S_V(f)S_x(f)}} \tag{7.104}$$

In this equation, the cross-spectrum $S_{Vx}(f)$ is equal to the Fourier transform of the STA, $S_V(f)$ is the spectrum of the voltage time course, and $S_x(f)$ is the spectrum of the point process corresponding to the spike train. This example will be further elaborated in the applications section.

7.8 Higher-Order Correlations

One measure of higher-order correlations is given by the bispectrum, which is a third-order correlator. The bispectrum can only be nonzero for a non-Gaussian process, and it can be defined (for a stationary stochastic process) as

$$E[X(f_1)X(f_2)X(f_3)] = S(f_1, f_2)\delta(f_1 + f_2 + f_3) \tag{7.105}$$

A multitaper estimator for the bispectrum is given by

$$S_{MT}(f_1, f_2) = \frac{1}{K}\sum_{k=1}^{K} \tilde{x}_k^*(f_1 + f_2)\tilde{x}_k(f_1)\tilde{x}_k(f_2) \tag{7.106}$$

Note that trial averages can be performed in addition to the averages over tapers. Other higher-order correlations may be estimated in the same way. The curse of dimensionality limits the utility of these estimation procedures. The nth order correlation function for a stationary stochastic process requires $n - 1$ frequencies to be specified, and if each frequency direction is discretized to keep m levels, then the number of frequency "bins" are m^{n-1}. This grows exponentially with the degree of the correlation function, and one again does not have enough data to fill these bins.

7.8.1 Correlations Between Spectral Power at Different Frequencies

One way to obtain estimates of higher-order correlations is to treat the estimated dynamic spectrum as a multivariate time series. Suppose we start with a spectrogram estimate

$$\hat{S}(f, t) \tag{7.107}$$

It is to be understood in this discussion that $\hat{S}(f, t)$ is estimated with some choice of window parameters T, ΔT, and $2W$, and the quantities defined below all depend on these choices. The idea is to treat the spectral power at each frequency as a time series in its own right. A log transformation makes the spectrogram estimate have a distribution that is closer to being Gaussian. Define the mean subtracted log spectrogram

$$\delta \log\left(\hat{S}(f, t)\right) = \log\left(\hat{S}(f, t)\right) - \frac{1}{N_t} \sum_t \log\left(\hat{S}(f, t)\right) \tag{7.108}$$

We define the *spectral correlations*

$$C_4(f, f', t, t') = \langle \delta \log\left(\hat{S}(f, t)\right) \delta \log\left(\hat{S}(f', t')\right) \rangle \tag{7.109}$$

Note that the angle brackets denote an average over trials. If trials are not available, or if the process is to be treated as a stationary process, then in the usual way we consider dependence only on a time difference, by averaging over the time t in addition to averaging over trials

$$C_3(f, f', \tau) = \langle \delta \log\left(\hat{S}(f, t+\tau)\right) \delta \log\left(\hat{S}(f', t)\right) \rangle \tag{7.110}$$

The simplest case of this is the *instantaneous* spectral correlations at $\tau = 0$.

$$C_2(f, f') = C_3(f, f', 0) \tag{7.111}$$

In contrast with the dependence on time difference for a stationary process, there is no reason in general to assume that $C_3(f, f', \tau)$ is a function only of the *frequency difference* $f - f'$. An example of the instantaneous spectral correlations will be considered in the applications part of the book.

Because our focus in this chapter has been spectral estimation, our treatment of higher-order correlations has been quite cursory. The example of spectral correlations was included to illustrate the general point, that second moment estimates can be *nested* in order to build up estimators for higher-order correlations present in the underlying stochastic process.

PART III

APPLICATIONS

8

Electrophysiology: Microelectrode Recordings

8.1   Introduction

In the previous tutorial part of the book, we have presented mathematical and statistical methods for the analysis of time series data. This part of the book is devoted to applications of these methods to specific examples of neural signals.

Experimental methods for acquiring neural signals span a wide range of temporal and spatial resolutions (table 8.1) and have different sources of signal as well as noise. In addition, unless the activity of single neurons are being measured, the observed signals have a complex relationship to the underlying neural activity.

Microelectrode recordings are acquired from implanted electrodes. Although invasive, and hence of limited use in human research, such recordings offer the finest temporal and spatial resolution possible (table 8.1) among neurophysiological measurements. We therefore begin by discussing the analysis of data gathered using microelectrodes. Subsequent chapters address indirect measurement techniques, including electroencephalography (EEG) and magnetoencephalography (MEG), optical imaging and functional magnetic resonance imaging (fMRI).

In the current chapter, we first discuss common experimental paradigms or approaches employed for electrophysiological recordings. We then present a brief review of neuronal biophysics related to microelectrode recordings followed by a discussion of different measurement techniques and their associated noise sources. Finally, we discuss analysis methods for voltage time series recorded from microelectrodes. A good discussion of different electrophysiological techniques along with some history may be found in Chapter 2 of Steriade's *The Intact and Sliced Brain* [214].

Table 8.1: Spatiotemporal Resolutions of Different Experimental Techniques

Experimental Technique	Temporal Resolution (s)	Spatial Resolution (mm)
Patch clamp	10^{-4}	10^{-3}
Single unit	10^{-4}	10^{-2}
EEG/MEG	10^{-3}	10
fMRI	1	1
PET	10^{2}	1
Voltage sensitive dyes	10^{-3}	10^{-2}
Intrinsic optical imaging	1	10^{-1}

For comparison, some relevant neuroanatomical scales are dendrites, 10^{-3} mm; neurons, 10^{-2} mm; cortical layer, 10^{-1} mm; cortical column, 1 mm; map, 10 mm.

8.2 Experimental Approaches

A variety of experimental preparations are used in neuroscience research. In vitro preparations, including isolated single neurons, cell cultures, brain slices, explants, and occasionally whole brain preparations allow high-resolution measurements and the ability to control and directly manipulate conditions such as ionic concentrations and ion channel activity. These advantages have enabled significant progress in our understanding of processes in individual cells, synapses, and small neuronal networks. However, important physiological properties may be dramatically altered in vitro [214].

In contrast, in vivo experiments in the intact animal preserve physiological conditions; allow for studies at a higher level of organization; and in the case of recordings in awake behaving animals, provide a means to directly relate neural activity to behavior. In vivo experiments tend to fall into the two broad classes of approaches discussed in the fourth chapter: controlled experimentation versus empirical or purely observational, with the former predominating in current neuroscience research.

Examples of controlled experimentation include electrophysiological recordings in anesthetized or otherwise passive animals, usually in a "stimulus-response" paradigm, in which controlled stimuli are presented to the animal during recording. Recordings in awake, behaving animals performing carefully designed behavioral or cognitive tasks also fall into the category of controlled experimentation. The aim in these experiments is often to determine the functional relationship between a given stimulus or behavior and a measured neuronal response, sometimes referred to as a neuronal code. We emphasize that learning such functional relationships from data[1] is nothing other than

---

1. This relationship is usually stochastic, which can be captured through the inference of conditional probabilities.

regression, a familiar method in classical statistics. So it is not clear that the concept of a "code" is appropriate. The methods used to establish and analyze such relationships are a major part of modern statistical learning theory.

In vivo experiments taking an empirical approach usually involve more naturalistic behaviors and have closer ties to ethology. Although difficult, both in implementation and analysis, there is increasing interest in moving away from the constrained behavioral paradigms of traditional experimental psychology and toward more natural behaviors. This is in part because new technologies and computational power have made such approaches more feasible.

8.3   Biophysics of Neurons

Here we describe some basic aspects of neuronal biophysics. We do not intend for this material to provide a complete overview but rather hope it will encourage the reader from a non-neuroscience background to consult one of the many textbooks available [20, 128, 133, 163, 183].

8.3.1   Transmembrane Resting Potential

Neurons maintain a negative potential difference across the cell membrane that reflects different ion concentrations in the intracellular and extracellular space and the different selective permeabilities of the membrane to these ions. The intracellular concentrations of sodium (Na^+) and chloride (Cl^-) ions are lower than extracellular concentrations, and the reverse is true for potassium (K^+) ions. The resting potential, reflecting a balance between the steady state conductances and the ion pumps, is typically between -50 and -90 mV.

8.3.2   Action Potentials and Synaptic Potentials

The specialized electrical excitability of neurons is mediated by ion channels in the cell membrane. The conductance of these channels can be altered by electrical or chemical means. Voltage-gated ion channels have conductances that show a sensitive dependence on the transmembrane voltage. Ion channel conductances may also be altered directly or indirectly via chemical means, through the direct binding of ligands to the channels or to other transmembrane proteins that indirectly influence ion channels through biochemical intermediates.

Electrical signaling within a neuron is mediated via action potentials, which are large, stereotyped excursions in the transmembrane potential. In a series of classic papers [113–117] that remain exemplary in combining experiment

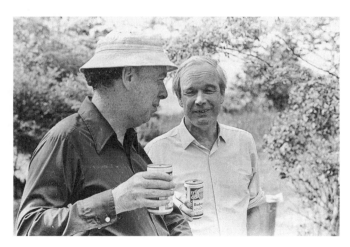

Figure 8.1: Alan Lloyd Hodgkin (1914–1998), right, with James D. Watson, left, at the 1975 Symposium on The Synapse at Cold Spring Harbor Laboratory. British physiologists and biophysicists Hodgkin and Huxley formulated a set of differential equations to mathematically describe the action potential from measurements they made on the giant squid axon. Their work postulated the existence of ion channels, which was confirmed experimentally years later. Hodgkin and Huxley shared the Nobel Prize in Physiology or Medicine in 1963 with John Carew Eccles.

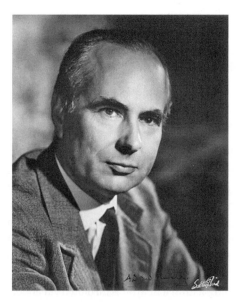

Figure 8.2: Andrew Fielding Huxley (1917–). Huxley shared the Nobel Prize in Physiology or Medicine in 1963 with Alan Hodgkin and John Carew Eccles.

with theoretical work, Hodgkin (fig. 8.1) and Huxley (fig. 8.2) elucidated the mechanism of action potential generation. A brief history of these developments may be found in [108].

The rapid (less than 1 msec) rising phase of the action potential is due to voltage-gated Na^+ channels that open in a positive-feedback process initiated above a certain threshold of membrane depolarization. After peaking, the action potential self-limits as Na^+ channels inactivate and voltage-gated K^+ channels, activated at positive membrane potentials, open. The influx of K^+ ions quickly repolarizes the membrane, usually leading to a transient hyperpolarized "undershoot" before the K^+ channels close and the neuron returns to its resting potential. Action potential propagation along an axon can reach speeds of 120 m/sec., and successful propagation triggers neurotransmitter release at synaptic terminals.

Neurotransmitter released from a presynaptic neuron binds to receptors on the postsynaptic neuron and evokes transient changes in the conductances of the postsynaptic neuron. This causes transient postsynaptic currents and potentials. Summation of excitatory postsynaptic potentials can raise the transmembrane voltage of the postsynaptic neuron to exceed the threshold for initiating action potentials, and the cycle then repeats. Note that although action potential firing, or spiking, predominates, some types of neurons do not fire action potentials (for example, bipolar cells in the retina), and instead control transmitter release through graded changes in membrane potential. Neurons can also be directly or electrically coupled through "gap junctions."

8.3.3   Extracellular Potentials

Microelectrodes placed in the extracellular space measure voltage changes with respect to an appropriately placed reference. These voltage changes originate in small charge imbalances across the membrane generated by currents flowing across the membrane. The currents arise both from action potentials and from synaptic activity. Correspondingly, the voltages recorded from a microelectrode typically contain two kinds of activity: action potential–generated spikes with high-frequency content (millisecond timescales), and so-called "local field potential" (LFP) with lower frequency content (typically tens of milliseconds or longer).

The origin of the LFP signal is complex and continues to be a subject of current research. The conventional wisdom is that this is due largely to synaptic currents and to a lesser extent to the summation of action potentials from far away neurons. The amplitudes of extracellular spike waveforms depend on a number of factors, including electrode geometry and proximity to a cell body, but are typically of the order of about 1 mV. LFP signals are usually at least an order of magnitude smaller (~ 10–$100\,\mu V$) under ordinary circumstances.

8.4   Measurement Techniques

8.4.1   Intracellular Measurements

Most of our understanding of the electrical properties of neurons comes from intracellular recordings. Sharp electrode intracellular measurements typically use glass micropipettes with tip diameters between 0.1 and 2 µm. When a micropipette with a sharp tip (with diameter 0.1–1 µm and resistance up to hundreds of MΩ) is made to penetrate the cell membrane, the voltage (or the current) across the membrane can be measured relative to a reference electrode in the extracellular space. If instead, a larger micropipette (diameter 1–2 µm), filled with a solution that has the same osmolarity as the cytoplasm, is attached to a patch of neuronal membrane to form a tight seal, the dynamics of the ion channels contained in that patch can be recorded. These are known as patch-clamp recordings.

Although glass micropipettes can give exquisite measurements of single channel or single neuron activity (including subthreshold membrane oscillations), they require contact between the pipette and the neuron being recorded. Respiratory and cardiac pulsation as well as behavior-related movements, combined with fragility of the electrodes, all make intracellular measurements difficult in vivo, particularly in awake, behaving animals [142]. Thus, extracellular measurements remain the standard approach for recording from awake, behaving animals. The remainder of this chapter deals exclusively with extracellular microelectrode recordings.

8.4.2   Extracellular Measurements

Although intracellular electrodes are used to measure either the voltage or the currents across the membrane, extracellular electrodes are used to measure the voltage with respect to some reference. As mentioned above, this voltage may be broken up into a high-frequency component that contains the action potentials (spikes) of neurons in the vicinity of the electrode, and a lower frequency LFP component (up to a few hundred Hz). Fine-tipped metal microelectrodes (tip diameter 1–2 µm) positioned close to a cell body provide the best extracellular measurements of the action potentials of that cell.

Extracellular measurements increasingly use arrays of electrodes in a variety of forms. In contrast to individual sharp metal electrodes, these arrays allow simultaneous recordings from multiple neurons. In addition, such arrays may be implanted chronically, enabling long-term recordings. Microwire electrodes with diameters 10–50 µm and resistance in the range 0.5–1 MΩ, are often used in stereotrode (two wires) or tetrode (four wires) configurations. In recent years, chronic implants of arrays of microwires and silicon probes have increasingly come to be used in awake, behaving animal studies. Although they typically pick up the activity of multiple neurons, this activity can often be clustered into distinct groups of putative single units using the techniques for classifying extracellular spike waveforms described in the next chapter.

8.4.3 Noise Sources

Important sources of noise in extracellular recordings include thermal noise in the electrodes (Johnson noise) and amplifier noise, effects of digitization on the analog voltage, and various forms of electrical and magnetic interference. Additional effects, such as thermal fluctuations due to dielectric properties of the micropipette glass, fluctuations in the seal between the membrane and micropipette, and various capacitive effects also appear in intracellular measurements. Most of these factors have little influence on analysis, either because they are small relative to the signals being measured or because they are easily controlled experimentally. For example, the root mean square fluctuation in voltage due to electrode Johnson noise [127, 168] is typically small even for the highest resistance electrodes.[2]

A more common cause of concern from the standpoint of data analysis is noise arising from electromagnetic interference. This includes line noise at 50 or 60 Hz that occurs due to radiative electrical pickup from lights and power sockets, currents due to ground loops, and currents induced by magnets in power supplies.

Electrical interference can be minimized by correctly shielding the recording setup, using shielded cables, moving magnetic sources as far away as possible, and careful grounding. Despite such care, it is possible to get some electrical interference, particularly 50–60 Hz of line noise. Fortunately, these can be removed using harmonic analysis techniques, and we present an example in chapter 10.

8.5 Analysis Protocol

It is useful to recall that there are two basic stages to data analysis, which may be iterated. Exploratory data analysis includes data conditioning, hypothesis generation and model discovery, whereas confirmatory analysis involves hypothesis testing and model validation.

8.5.1 Data Conditioning

The first step in analyzing extracellular recordings is usually that of separating the LFP and high-frequency components using frequency filtering. In general,

---

2. The root mean square fluctuation in voltage is given by $V_{rms} = \sqrt{4kTR\Delta f}$.

the high-frequency component may contain action potentials from different neurons, and these have to be identified and clustered into groups corresponding to different neurons. This step is known as *spike sorting* and is discussed in the next chapter. A schematic representation of this separation of components for an extracellular recording is shown in figure 8.3. Occasionally, the clustering stage is abandoned and investigators simply use all action potentials without reference to the neuron from which they originate. Such signals are known as multiunit activity.

Having extracted the LFP and the spikes, the next step depends to some extent on the nature of the dataset. If the recording is from a few channels, the next step might be separate analysis of each of these channels beginning with noise and artifact removal. If many channels are involved, one might first use a dimensionality reduction method before going to next stage. These methods are illustrated in the chapters on EEG and optical imaging.

As mentioned in the previous section, one of the main sources of noise in extracellular measurements is electromagnetic interference, which is largely from the alternating current power supply which is ubiquitously present in

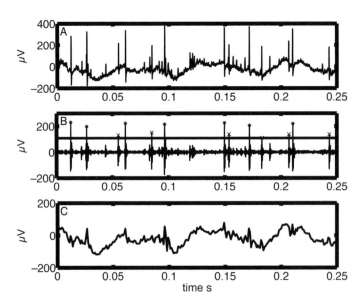

Figure 8.3: Separation of local field potential (LFP) and single unit activity from raw voltage recordings. (A) A segment of the raw voltage recording from a single channel of a tetrode. (B) The high-pass filtered signal is subjected to a spike extraction and clustering stage that aims to identify which of the spikes seen in the trace correspond to an individual neuron (points marked with * and x), a process known as spike sorting. (C) The low-pass filtered signal is the LFP. The typical low-pass frequency cutoff is at 200–300 Hz.

laboratories. Since the frequency at which this occurs[3] is in the frequency range of electrophysiological phenomena of interest, it is important to identify and suppress such "line" noise. A common practice is to use notch filters that remove all power in the signal in a narrow band around the signal. However, notch filters do not distinguish between signal and noise, and can cause spurious dips to appear in the signal spectrum. As mentioned in the chapter on time series analysis (chapter 7), a superior alternative is to use the harmonic F-test [219]. An example of line noise removal using this algorithm is given in chapter 10.

At the end of this series of preprocessing steps, raw data has been separated into two components: continuous valued time series representing the LFP and one or more point processes representing the spike times of the neurons. We now discuss the analysis of such data, beginning with classical characterizations of spiking activity based on the firing rate and then moving on to more complicated analyses. This is followed by a discussion of the LFP. We then discuss measures of association between two signals, both spikes and LFPs. Finally, we illustrate how response to periodic stimulation can be estimated. The discussion focuses on nonparametric techniques. Parametric models are discussed in a later section. This chapter ends with a brief discussion of methods to predict behavior from recorded neural activity.

An Example: Memory-Guided Saccade Task in the Macaque

As an example for detailed analysis, we consider a single spike train and a single LFP signal acquired from the same site in the lateral intraparietal area (LIP) of a macaque monkey. These data were recorded while the monkey performed a memory-guided saccade task [176], in which eye movements (saccades) must be made to remembered locations on a computer screen. At the start of each trial, the monkey fixated a light at the center of the screen. Then a peripheral target flashed 100 milliseconds at one of eight locations on a circle centered on the fixation point. After a variable delay of approximately one second, the fixation light was turned off, instructing the monkey to make a saccade to the location where the target stimulus had appeared. Note that this is a common task for studying short-term memory in primates. Eye movements were monitored, and the monkey was given a drop of juice for correct performance on a trial. If the monkey performed incorrectly (i.e., failed to make a saccade at the go signal to the target location), the trial was aborted and a new trial was initiated. Neural data was acquired continuously at a sampling frequency of 12 kHz. The aim in these experiments was to study the dependence of spiking and LFP activity on the target location (at the recording site).

---

3. A fundamental frequency of 50 Hz in Europe or 60 Hz in the United States.

Figure 8.4 displays three-second segments of spiking activity for a single neuron from the LIP dataset mentioned above. Each point represents a spike from one trial. The data were grouped by target direction and aligned with the onset of the memory period (shown by the vertical line at 1 sec.). The second vertical line (at approximately 2 sec.) indicates the mean saccade time. The saccades in correct trials followed the go signal at the end of the memory period. It can be seen from the figure that trials for which the target direction was $180°$ show the strongest modulation in firing rate (average number of spikes per second). In particular, the firing rate (1) increased rapidly at the onset of the memory period, (2) was sustained at an elevated level in the memory period, and (3) dropped shortly after the saccade. Such a sustained elevation of firing rate is often observed in tasks involving short-term memory and is thought to relate mechanistically to the memory or the motor plan.

8.5.2 Analysis of Spike Trains

Tuning Curves

The simplest characterization of the spiking activity of a neuron is in terms of its firing rate. When plotted against a parameter characterizing a stimulus or a behavioral state, the resulting plot is known as a firing rate tuning curve. In studies that were the first to attempt such characterization, Adrian and Zotterman [4, 6, 7] showed that the firing rate in fibers of the sternocutaneus

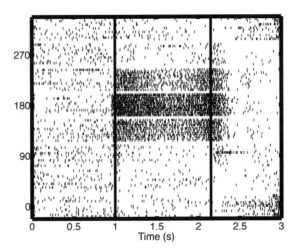

Figure 8.4:   Raster plot for a single neuron from area LIP during a memory-guided saccade task. See text for experimental details. The y-axis shows eight groups of target location, four of which are labeled (in degrees). The time interval between the two vertical bars corresponds to the memory period.

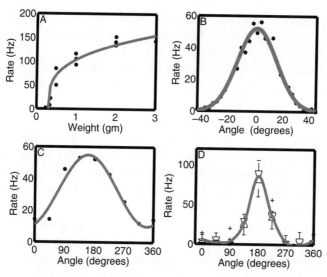

Figure 8.5: Tuning curves. (A) Firing rate as a function of load placed on the sternocutaneus muscle in frog. The solid curve is a guide to the eye (Adapted from [6].) (B) Firing rate of a neuron from cat V1 as a function of the orientation of bars of light moving at certain angles across the receptive field. The solid curve is a Gaussian tuning curve. (Adapted from [56] after [109]). (C) Firing rate of a neuron in M1 of monkey during two dimensional arm movements to one of eight directions arranged in a circle. The solid curve is a cosine tuning curve. (Adapted from [86].) (D) Boxplot of the firing rate from the LIP neuron shown in figure 8.4 in the 500-msec window during the middle of the memory period shows clear evidence of directional tuning. The solid curve is a local regression fit.

muscle (in the chest) of the frog varies with the load placed on it. Figure 8.5A shows the results one such experiment from [6]. As another example, figure 8.5B shows a neuron in the primary visual cortex (V1) of cat in response to bars of light moving at different angles across the visual field. Each point was obtained by averaging several trials, and the curve is a Gaussian fit to the average responses with mean $0°$, standard deviation $14.73°$ and amplitude $52.14\,\text{Hz}$ [56]. The data in figure 8C come from primary motor cortex (M1) in monkey. In these experiments the monkey made two dimensional arm movements to eight targets arranged in a circle and firing rate was measured during the whole of each trial. The solid curve is a fit to a cosine: $32.7 + 22.5\,cos(\theta - \theta_0)$ where $\theta_0 = 161°$.

Usage of Box Plots and Local Regression for Tuning Curves

The final panel (fig. 8D) shows the firing rate as a function of target location for the LIP neuron of figure 8.5 during a 500-millisec. interval from the middle of the memory period.[4] Because the monkey must remember a target location during this period, the plot can be thought of displaying the firing rate as a function of the memory or motor plan.

The uncertainty in the firing rate is quantified using the Tukey *box plot*, which is a useful way of summarizing variability in data. The horizontal lines in each box (from the bottom) displays the lower quartile, median and upper quartile. The notches denote a robust estimate of the uncertainty in the median. The limits of the "whiskers" (the vertical dashed lines on the top and bottom of the boxes) denote a robust estimate of the range, and outliers are denoted by isolated symbols (in the present case, black crosses). The fact that the notches for the preferred and antipreferred direction do not overlap means that the corresponding medians differ with 95% confidence. Thus, examination of box plots allows us to both generate and test the hypothesis of directional tuning in this neuron. The direction for which the firing rate is maximum is called the preferred direction, and the opposite direction, the antipreferred direction.

The fits in figures 8.5A and 8.5B were global in that a single function, a Gaussian in A and a cosine in B, were fit to the data from all angles. In contrast, the fit in figure 8.5D is a local regression fit. A brief discussion of local regression and likelihood is presented in chapter 13. Instead of attempting to fit a single parameterized function to the whole data, in local regression one fits a low-order polynomial to a local neighborhood of any point. Local regression provides a flexible method for smoothing and fitting functions to data without having to know a parametric functional form in advance.

Receptive Fields

The discussion on tuning curves tacitly assumes that dynamics does not play an important role. Either the stimulus input or behavioral output can be held steady, and the average firing rate measured during such a steady period; or alternatively, the stimulus or action is punctate, and the total number of spikes can be measured during the transient response. In each case, the activity of the neuron can be summarized in terms of a single number, which can then be used to define a tuning curve. However, more generally, the dynamics of the neuronal response has to be taken into account, which leads us to a discussion of temporal and spatiotemporal receptive fields.

In studies on the frog, Hartline [105, 106] showed that retinal ganglion cells respond most to illumination presented in specific regions of the retina and

---

4. We use the word *memory* in an operational sense to designate the delay period in the described task. There may be debate about whether this experiment is truly about short-term memory, attention, or motor plan. We do not wish to imply a particular position in this debate through the usage of the word "memory" in the text.

coined the term "receptive field" to describe these regions. Figure 8.6 shows the results of an experiment aimed at mapping the receptive field structure of a simple cell in the lateral geniculate nucleus (LGN) of cat.

In a static setting, the receptive field of a neuron is the region in space, such that stimuli placed in that region causes the neuron to have an altered firing rate (compared to baseline). More precisely, the spatial dependence of the neuronal response on the location of a punctate stimulus is known as the spatial receptive field. However, such a static description is inadequate, because neurons usually show larger responses to dynamic than to static stimuli. Transients in the neural response can be characterized by the spatiotemporal receptive field $R(\mathbf{x}, \tau)$, which could be defined as the response of a neuron at time τ due to a punctate stimulus presented briefly at $\mathbf{x}$ at time $t = 0$. The spatiotemporal receptive field can be determined by presenting stimuli with well-defined temporal and spatial frequencies. Alternatively, one can present a spatiotemporally white Gaussian noise stimulus $s(\mathbf{x}, t)$. It can be shown that $R(\mathbf{x}, \tau)$ is then given by the correlation between the spiking activity of the

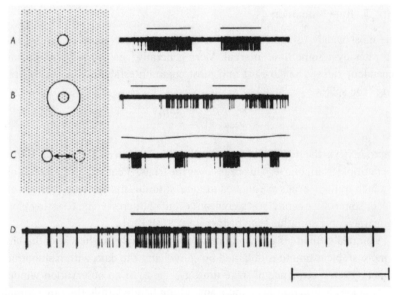

Figure 8.6:   The spiking activity of a single "on" cell in cat LGN. (A) A spot of light, $2°$ across, leads to high-spike discharge in this cell throughout the time of illumination. (B) When the annular illumination is presented concentric with the previous spot, the firing rate is almost zero during illumination. (C) Responses to the same spot as in A, moved back and forth. (D) Response to diffuse illumination while cat is asleep. In all panels, solid lines above the spike displays shows the time of illumination. The scale bar at the bottom is one second. Reproduced from Hubel, D. *J Physiol.* 150:91–104, 1968, with permission from Blackwell Publishing.

neuron at a given time t, $\rho(t) = \sum_i \delta(t - t_i)$, and the past history of the stimulus $s(\mathbf{x}, t - \tau)$,

$$R(\mathbf{x}, \tau) = \langle \rho(t)s(\mathbf{x}, t - \tau) \rangle \qquad (8.1)$$

Here, $\mathbf{x}$ denotes space, for visual stimuli, although more abstract stimulus spaces may also be considered (such as tone frequencies for auditory stimuli). Because the correlation is computed between the spiking activity and past values of the stimulus, the method is known as reverse correlation [31, 129, 130]. Note, however, that $R(\mathbf{x}, \tau)$ is also the correlation between the stimulus at a particular instant and the spiking activity at a later instant. A discussion of various types of receptive fields in the visual cortex can be found in Dayan and Abbott [56].

For the purposes of this book, the fact that the receptive field can be defined in terms of a cross-correlation function between white noise stimuli and neural responses is of note. This means that the measures such as cross-spectra and cross-coherency studied in the book, when applied the spike train and the stimulus, play the same role as temporal receptive fields.

Rate Estimation

The most widely used estimates of neural activity are based on average firing rates over some time interval. More generally, one is interested in time-dependent rates. The simplest and most common estimate is given by "binning" the spikes,

$$\lambda_{binning}(t) = \frac{\Delta N(t)}{\Delta t} \qquad (8.2)$$

where $\Delta N(t)$ is the number of spikes in the "bin" or interval $[t, t + \Delta t]$. If there are multiple trials, one also averages over the trials. A common situation is one in which multiple trials are aligned to some stimulus marker (e.g. the start of a trial or some other behavioral significant event of interest). The resulting plot is known as a peristimulus time histogram (PSTH; [90]).

A binned estimate is noisy and can depend strongly on the size of the bins. A more stable estimate is obtained by convolving the data with a smoothing kernel. Given a sequence of spike times $t_1, \ldots, t_N$ in an observation window $[0, T]$, a kernel function $K(x)$ and a smoothing bandwidth h, the rate estimate in this procedure is given by

$$\hat{\lambda}(t) = \frac{1}{h} \sum_{i=1}^{N} K\left(\frac{t - t_i}{h}\right) \qquad (8.3)$$

A kernel that is commonly used is the Gaussian. As before, the estimate can be averaged over multiple trials. However, estimates with a fixed bandwidth treat regions with relatively few spikes in the same way as regions with high spike density. A small bandwidth appropriate for regions of high spike rate may not give sufficient smoothing in regions with low spike rate. An estimate that is adaptive, so that regions of high density have shorter bandwidth, and regions of low density have larger bandwidths, would be preferable.

As illustrated by the tuning curve example presented earlier, local regression provides a flexible method for fitting nonparametric regression curves to data. Similar flexibility for the rate estimation problem is offered by local likelihood methods, discussed in chapter 13. Figure 8.7 shows the PSTH for the preferred direction for the spike train example displayed in figure 8.4. Superposed on the PSTH is a local-likelihood based estimate. The estimate was obtained by fitting a Poisson likelihood locally to the data. What this means is that at any given time point, the rate function in a neighborhood of that point is assumed to be an inhomogeneous Poisson process, with a time-varying rate given by a low-order polynomial. In the present example, the rate function within each window was taken to be a cubic polynomial, and the widths of the windows were chosen to include 35% of the data around any given time point. This is a simple method of adaptive bandwidth selection (see chapter 13 for other adaptive methods). Also shown are 95% local confidence intervals. Although the analysis here has involved multiple trials, local regression and likelihood methods can be usefully applied to single trials.

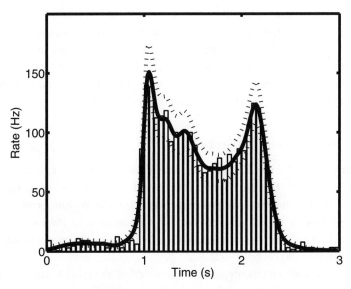

Figure 8.7: Smooth estimate of the rate of the LIP data for trials to the preferred direction using a local likelihood method. Also shown are 95% confidence intervals on the estimate.

Splines provide an alternative method for nonparametric function estimation. Adaptive techniques based on splines have also been applied to the estimation of spike rate functions [21, 59]. These techniques appear to be more computationally intensive than the local regression method. Both these approaches provide techniques for bandwidth selection and estimation of confidence intervals.

Fano Factor

Only for Poisson processes do rates provide a complete description of the process. As discussed in chapter 5, for a Poisson process the variance $V[N(T)]$ of the counts in an interval T is equal to the mean count $E[N(T)]$. The ratio of these quantities, $F(T) = V[N(T)]/E[N(T)]$ is known as the Fano factor [69] in the neuroscience literature, and has been measured to provide evidence for or against a Poisson process model [89, 100, 134, 173, 202, 209, 222, 253].

Figure 8.8 illustrates the relationship between the time-dependent Fano factor and the spike spectrum (equation 5.238), using trials in the preferred direction from the LIP data example. Because the spike rate shows strong time dependence, as seen in figure 8.7, the spectrum was computed on a data window taken from the memory period. The approximate constancy of spike rate in this window can be taken as a rough indicator of stationarity. Note the dependence of the Fano factor on the window length. As $T \to 0$, $F(T) \to 1$. The Fano factor is not identically one, indicating the non-Poisson nature of the process.

The long time limit of the Fano factor in figure 8.8 is less than 1, corresponding to the spectrum at zero frequency being different from the spectrum at high frequencies. The spike spectrum measures correlations in the spike train, and as equation 5.238 shows, the time-dependent Fano factor can be computed from the spike spectrum through an integral transform. The spike spectrum is therefore a direct measure of neuronal variability.

Interspike Interval Distribution

The distribution of time intervals between successive spikes is known as the inter-spike interval (ISI) distribution [90]. One reason for interest in ISI distributions [91] is that renewal processes (including the Poisson process) are defined entirely by the ISI distribution. For a homogeneous Poisson process with rate λ, successive ISIs are independent with an exponential probability density function, $P(\tau) = \lambda exp(-\lambda\tau)$.

For a process with a time-dependent rate function, the ISI distribution is not well defined because the probability of observing an ISI of a particular duration varies in time. However, the transformation

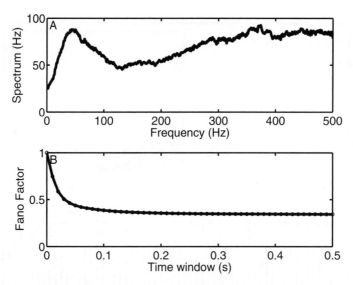

Figure 8.8: Illustration of the relationship between the Fano factor and the spectrum, discussed in chapter 6. (A) Spectrum computed from trials in the preferred direction, using data from the middle of the delay period. (B) Fano factor computed according to equation 5.238.

$$z_i = \int_0^{t_i} \lambda(t)dt \qquad (8.4)$$

where t_i are the spike times and $\lambda(t)$ the rate leads to new spike "times" that are realizations of a unit rate process. Note the difference between this rescaling, with respect to a fixed rate function, from that carried out in the time rescaling theorem, based on the conditional intensity process (discussed in chapter 5). In the latter case, the rescaling function depends on the particular realization of the process, and the rescaled times follow a Poisson process. In the former case, the rescaling function is independent of the realization. The rate function used in equation 8.4 is the first moment of the process, which can be estimated using one of the nonparametric methods indicated above.

Figure 8.9 shows a histogram and a local likelihood fit for the rescaled spike times, for the data example under consideration. The local likelihood rate estimate of figure 8.7 was used to rescale the times. The inset shows the distribution of the rescaled interspike intervals $\tau_i = z_{i+1} - z_i$. The dip in the ISI distribution close to zero occurs because of the relative refractory period. More salient is the bump between 1 and 2. It shows that the spike train is not simply a Poisson process with a time-varying rate. If that were the case, the rescaled ISI distribution would be exponential.

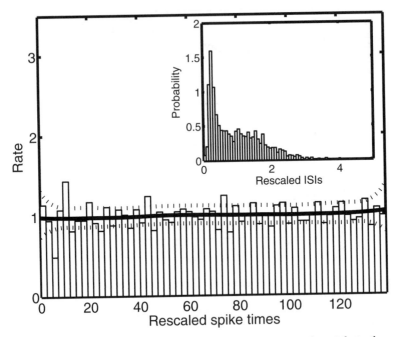

Figure 8.9: The spike rate in rescaled time. The spike times for trials to the preferred direction were rescaled according to equation 8.4. Note that the rescaled
rate is 1. The inset shows the distribution of rescaled interspike intervals (ISIs).

Interval Spectrum

Let the ISIs of a point process sample path be given by $\Delta t_1 = t_2 - t_1$, $\Delta t_2 = t_3 - t_2, \ldots$. The interval spectrum is defined as the spectrum of the discrete time stochastic process x_i defined by the sequence of ISIs, $x_i = \Delta t_i$. The interval spectrum is of interest both as a measure of correlations in a spike train, and as a diagnostic tool for renewal processes. Because the ISIs of a renewal process are independently and identically distributed random variables, the interval spectrum for a renewal process is white (constant as a function of frequency). Figure 8.10 shows the ISI spectrum of the rescaled process z_i, along with 95% jackknife and χ^2 confidence intervals. The spectrum deviates significantly from a constant, implying that the spike train cannot be described by a renewal process.

It should be noted that the number of ISIs (and hence length of the ISI series) is in general different across trials. To estimate an average spectrum for un-equal length trials, one procedure is to compute a different set of tapers for each trial, keeping the actual bandwidth $2W$ constant. Each trial is then multiplied by the corresponding tapers, and all trials are padded with zeros so as to have

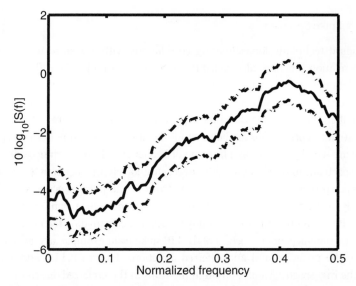

Figure 8.10: The interspike interval (ISI) spectrum of the rescaled process z_i shown in Figure 8.9. For a renewal process, the ISI spectrum should be constant. Confidence intervals based on the χ^2 distribution with an appropriate number of degrees of freedom (dashed lines), as well as jackknife based 95% confidence bands (dotted lines) are shown on a multitaper estimate of the ISI spectrum with estimation bandwidth 0.05. Note that the difference between the two sets of confidence bands is not noticeable except at low frequencies. At low frequencies, the jackknifed confidence bands are somewhat broader: as pointed out in chapter 7, the jackknife provides conservative confidence bands for the spectrum estimate.

equal length. Finally, the padded data are Fourier transformed and the multitaper spectrum estimate is computed as usual by squaring and averaging the fast Fourier transforms of all tapered and padded series. This procedure is computationally intensive but ensures a constant bandwidth across trials. Alternatively, a fixed time bandwidth product $2WT$ may be used, which ensures the same number of degrees of freedom per trial, but in this case the effective bandwidth depends on the distribution of the lengths of the ISI series.

The interval spectrum being flat as a function of frequency is a necessary, but not sufficient condition for the point process to be a renewal process. It is necessary to verify the other property of renewal processes, including the independence of all ISIs (not just the lack of correlation of nearest neighboring ISIs, as evaluated by the ISI spectrum). Further discussion of this issue can be found in Tuckwell [224]. However, it is unlikely that a nonrenewal process encountered in practice will have a flat ISI spectrum, because this would require fine-tuning of the structure of the process.

Spike Spectrum

A standard technique for estimating correlations within a spike train is the autocorrelation function, also called the autocorrelogram [175]. Although autocorrelation functions capture sharply peaked correlations well, direct time domain estimation of autocorrelation functions that are less localized in time from limited data presents difficulties (see the examples in figure 8.16, 8.19). Such extended correlations are better studied using the spectrum. Because spike spectra are usually smooth as a function of frequency, a lower variance estimate of the spectrum may be obtained by averaging locally in frequency (as in the multitaper procedure). Although the spectrum of the point process is mathematically related to the autocorrelation function through a Fourier transformation, it is better to estimate and study the spike spectrum directly. Figure 8.11 shows the time-dependent spectra of the LIP spike train example, averaged over trials to the preferred and antipreferred directions. Figures 8.11A and 8.11B show the raw spectrograms. Although the trials in the preferred direction show a change in spectral shape during the memory period, this is conflated with the change in the asymptotic value of the spectra at large frequencies due to spike rate variations. This can be rectified by displaying the spectrogram normalized by the time-dependent rate (recall that $\lim_{f \to \infty} S(f, t) = R(t)$):[5]

$$S_n(f,t) = \frac{S(f,t)}{R(t)} \tag{8.5}$$

The spectrograms normalized by the instantaneous firing rate are shown in figures 8.11C and 8.11D, making the enhancement of gamma band power in the memory period more apparent. In addition, there is evidence of a suppression of low frequency power (< 30 Hz). One could attempt to fit such a spectrum with the spectrum of a renewal process with an appropriate ISI distribution. This sort of fit could be used to argue that the spectral shape is explained by a particular form of the ISI distribution. Such an explanation presupposes that the spike train can indeed be described using a renewal process. In the current example, the ISI spectrum has been shown to be colored rather than white, so that a renewal process explanation is not tenable.

Figure 8.12 shows the spike spectra in a 500-millisec. window during the memory period for the two conditions. Jackknife-based 95% local confidence bands are displayed on the figure. For the preferred direction, in addition to the

---

5. Alternatively, one could first transform to rescaled times z_i based on the average rate $R(t)$. Note, however, that it is not very useful to carry out a spectrogram estimate after *trial-dependent* rescaling using an estimated conditional intensity process. With enough parameters in the estimate, such a procedure is more or less guaranteed to produce a constant spectrogram. This is not too surprising, because in general a different rescaling function is then used for each trial. The more restricted rescaling by the average rate is meant to remove *nonstationarity*, whereas modeling using a conditional intensity process will remove correlations from a *stationary* process.

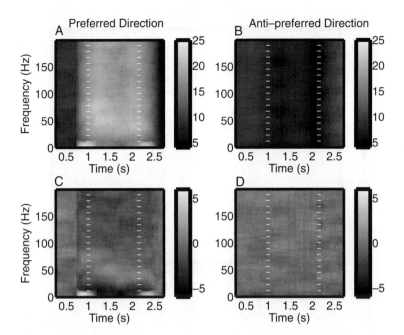

Figure 8.11: Spike spectrograms. (A, B) Spectrograms of the spike train from the LIP dataset, for the preferred and antipreferred directions. (C, D) The same spectrograms normalized by the instantaneous firing rates. The spectrogram was estimated using a sliding window with 500-millisec. duration and step size of 50-millisec. The multitaper spectral estimate was computed with a bandwidth $2W = 20\,\mathrm{Hz}$. The vertical lines dilineate the memory period.

clear suppression in the power at low frequencies, there is a small but significant increase in power at around 50 Hz and significant decrease at high frequencies. This contrasts with the relatively flat spike spectrum for the antipreferred direction.

The ISI distribution of spike trains that are Poisson apart for a "relative refractory period"[6] is sometimes modeled using a renewal process with a gamma distribution for the ISIs [43, 224]. For such processes, the spectrum has a dip at low frequencies [125]. A renewal process description would, however, not fit the present data example as pointed out earlier.

8.5.3 Local Field Potentials

The first moment for local field potential (LFP) activity ("evoked LFP"), analogous to the spike rate function, is given by the trial-averaged LFP for a given

---

6. This means that short ISIs are suppressed.

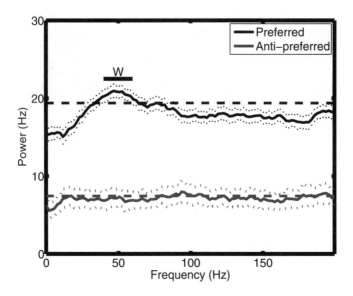

Figure 8.12: Spectra of the spike trains in the middle of the memory period for the preferred and antipreferred directions. All spectra were computed using 500 millisec. of data and a bandwidth $2W = 10\,\text{Hz}$. The horizontal lines indicate the firing rate for the preferred and antipreferred directions.

experimental condition. An example is shown in figure 8.13 for the data set under discussion. Sensory and motor events are visible in the evoked LFP. The estimate presented in the figure is a simple arithmetic average over trials. A smoother and more robust estimate may be obtained using local regression methods. We discuss this in the context of EEG data in the next chapter.

Figure 8.14 shows the spectrograms for the LFP for trials to the preferred and antipreferred directions. The appropriate evoked LFP is removed from each trial before spectrogram computations. The gamma band power in the LFP can be seen to be enhanced, during the memory period, for trials in the preferred direction. To check whether the observed elevation in gamma band power is statistically significant, a tuning curve based on total LFP spectral power in the range 30–80 Hz is shown in figure 8.15. The power was computed in a 500-millisec. window during the middle of the memory period and is displayed as function of target angle. Note the similarity between this tuning curve and the rate tuning curve from figure 8.5D. There are large differences in the power between the preferred and antipreferred directions. There are also significant differences between the preferred direction and the neighboring directions and between the neighboring directions and the anti-preferred direction.

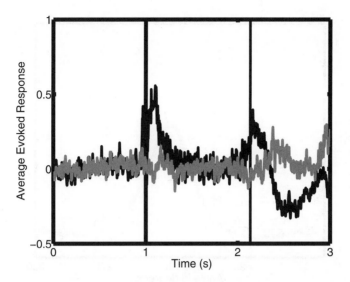

Figure 8.13: Evoked local field potentials for trials to the preferred direction (black) and antipreferred directions (gray). The vertical lines demarcate the memory period.

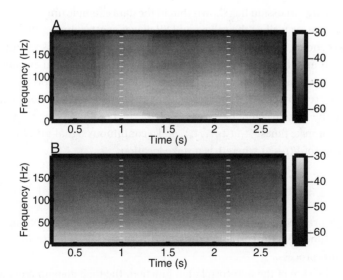

Figure 8.14: The local field potential spectrograms for trials corresponding to preferred direction (top) and antipreferred directions (bottom).

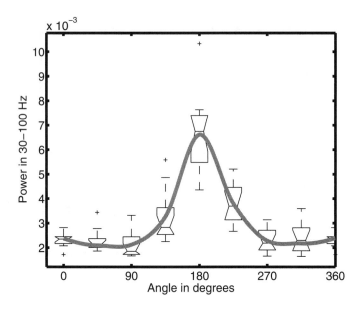

Figure 8.15:   Tuning curve based on the integrated local field potential power in the 30–100 Hz range from a window during the memory period. The solid curve is a local regression-based fit.

8.5.4   Measures of Association

Spike-Triggered Average

The preceding discussion has shown that in the data example under discussion, the spike rate, as well as the spike and LFP power spectra during the memory period depend on the target direction. It is therefore natural to ask whether the spike trains and the LFP are correlated with each other. This is an example of a *hybrid* correlation between a point process and a continuous process. A standard measure of association between spiking activity and a continuous signal is given by the spike-triggered average (STA) of the continuous signal. Given a sequence of spike times, $\{t_1, t_2, \ldots, t_n\}$, and a continuous signal $V(t)$, the STA is the average of $V(t - t_i)$ where t_i is a spike location

$$C(t) = \left\langle \frac{1}{n} \sum_{i=1}^{N} V(t - t_i) \right\rangle \qquad (8.6)$$

The angle brackets denote an average over trials. Clearly, this is nothing other than the time domain correlation function between the spike train and the continuous process.

As in the case of the autocorrelation function, the time domain cross correlation captures sharply peaked temporal correlations but has difficulties with

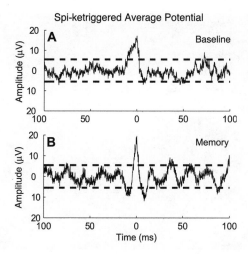

Spi-ketriggered Average Potential

Figure 8.16: Spike-triggered average of the local field potential (LFP) for the pre-ferred and antipreferred directions. The dashed horizontal lines show 95% confidence bands. Note that while oscillations can be seen, they fall within the confidence band computed locally in the time domain. In this case, the raw LFP signal was used, hence high frequency fluctuations visible in the data. (Adapted from [176].)

more extended correlations. Figure 8.16 shows an example of this difficulty in the spike triggered average of the LFP for the example data. Though there are clear oscillations in the preferred direction trials visible to eye, they fall within the confidence bands estimated locally in time. The difficulty arises from the fact that these confidence intervals are computed with the untenable assumption that successive time bins are independent. In contrast, estimates of the *cross-coherence* of a stationary process are approximately uncorrelated at frequencies separated by more that the estimation bandwidth. Moreover, the coherence is a normalized quantity; it is not clear how to properly normalize the STA.

Cross-Coherence Between Spikes and Local Field Potential

Figure 8.17 shows the coherence (the magnitude of the complex coherency) between a spike train and LFP from the example data set. The coherence is only displayed at points in the time-frequency plane for which it was significantly different from zero. To assess significance, the 95% points of the null distribution of the estimator (for zero true coherence) were computed from equation 7.82. Values of the coherence higher than this would be observed at approximately

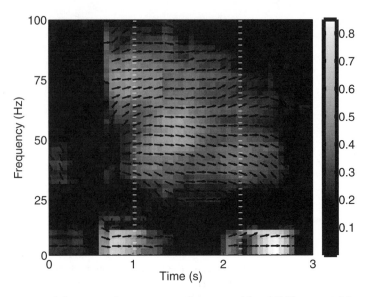

Figure 8.17: Coherogram between a single unit and local field potential from the data example. The gray scale indicates the amplitude and the arrows denote the phase of the complex coherency. Coherence is only displayed where it crosses the 95% level for the null distribution of the estimator.

5% of the points in the time-frequency plane. The estimated coherence crosses this threshold in a large region in the time-frequency plane, during the memory period, but not during baseline. The phase of the coherence, ϕ, is displayed as an arrow in the direction $(cos(\phi), sin(\phi))$. The displayed phases are close to zero.

Joint Peristimulus Time Histogram

When two spike trains are recorded simultaneously, it is desirable to estimate the degree of association between them. A popular measure of this relationship is the joint peristimulus time histogram (JPSTH) [93], corresponding to the second moment between the pair. Given simultaneously measured spike trains $x_1(t) = \sum_i \delta(t - t_i^1)$ and $x_2(t) = \sum_i \delta(t - t_i^2)$ of two neurons, the JPSTH or estimated cross moment, is given by

$$JPSTH(t, t') = \left\langle \frac{\Delta N_1(t)}{\Delta t} \frac{\Delta N_2(t)}{\Delta t} \right\rangle \tag{8.7}$$

where the angle bracket denote an average over trials. The JPSTH is an estimate of the cross moment $\mu_{12}(t, t') = E[x_1(t)x_2(t')]$. As with the PSTH, the spike trains are assumed to be aligned to some stimulus marker. For $t' = t$, the JPSTH represents the rate at which the two neurons fire simultaneously. When the

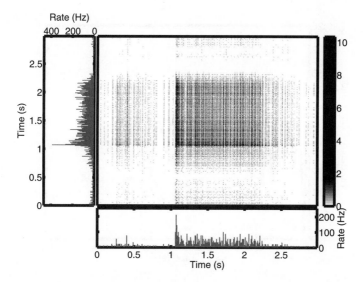

Figure 8.18: Joint peristimulus time histogram for two neurons recorded from area LIP of a macaque performing a task similar to the memory guided saccade task described in the data example.

binwidths are small enough that $\Delta N_1(t)$ and $\Delta N_2(t)$ can only take the values 0 and 1, the resulting plot is sometimes referred to as the JPST scatter plot [92].

Figure 8.18 shows an example JPSTH. The data here consists of two single units acquired from the area LIP of a monkey performing a coordinated reach and saccade task, similar to the one in example discussed above.[7]

The JPSTH corresponds to the second moment. In order to obtain the cross-correlation function, it is necessary to remove the product of the first moments $\rho_1(t) = E[x_1(t)]$ and $\rho_2(t) = E[x_2(t)]$:

$$C_{12}(t, t') = \mu_{12}(t, t') - \rho_1(t)\rho_2(t') \qquad (8.8)$$

The shift (or shuffle) correction [92, 93, 175] commonly used in the neuroscience literature is an equivalent procedure for performing this subtraction. The shuffle-corrected JPSTH is sometimes normalized by the product of the standard deviations of the spike counts (across trials) to give $JPSTH_{norm}(t, t')$. Figure 8.19 shows the corresponding normalized cross-correlation measure in a 500-millisec. window during the middle of the memory period. Apart from zero time lag, the estimated correlations in this data example are noisy and difficult to interpret.

7. The authors gratefully acknowledge the permission to use this data set, acquired by B. Pesaran.

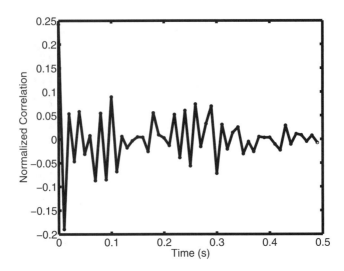

Figure 8.19: Normalized cross-correlation function during a 500-millisec. window in the middle of the memory period for the neurons shown in the preceding figure.

Coherence Between Spike Trains

Figure 8.20 shows the coherogram corresponding to the data shown in figure 8.19. The contrast between this figure and the previous one is striking. The estimate uses a sliding window of 500-millisec. duration, with 50-millisec. time steps. The coherence is shown only for points in the time-frequency plane where it is significantly above chance (see discussion for the figure on spike-LFP coherence). The black arrows indicate the phase angle. Note the strong coherence in the gamma band through out the memory period.

8.5.5. Periodic Stimulation

Periodic stimuli are commonly used in neuroscience experiments. This section illustrates the use of spectral measures to quantify neural responses to periodic stimuli.

The first example is from LFP recordings from the primary sensory (S1) cortex of rat, with periodic stimulation delivered to the vibrissae (whiskers) [10]. Figure 8.21 shows LFP spectra at a site in S1. In the absence of stimulation, intrinsic broadband oscillations were seen with fundamental $f_i = 5.5$ Hz and at harmonics ($2f_i$, $3f_i$, figure 8.21A). When the whisker was stimulated at $f_s = 8$ Hz, the spectrum showed additional peaks at $f_s = 8$ Hz and its higher harmonics ($2f_s$, $3f_s$, figure 8.21B). Interestingly, the spectrum also showed significant peaks at sum and difference frequencies $f_s - f_i$ and $f_s + f_i$, as well as peaks at $2f_s + f_i$ (figure 8.21B). Other experiments at different sites and for

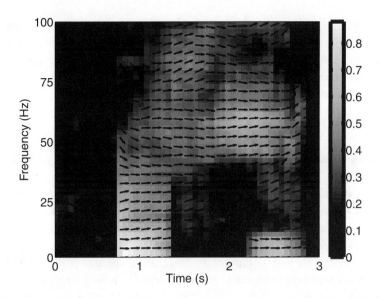

Figure 8.20: Coherogram between two simultaneously measured spike trains described in the text. The gray scale denotes the amplitude and the arrows denote the phase of the coherence.

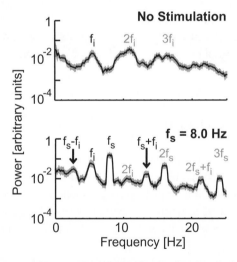

Figure 8.21: Comparison of local field potential spectra in the absence of stimulation (A, above) and in the presence of whisker stimulation (B, below) at $f_s = 8$ Hz. Note that the spectrum in the unstimulated condition contains peaks at $f_i = 5.5$ Hz and its harmonics. Stimulation at $f_s = 8$ Hz leads to the appearance of peaks in the spectrum at multiples of this frequency. In addition, there are peaks at sums and differences of the intrinsic and stimulation frequencies, and additional peaks at other combinations of f_i and f_s. Adapted from Ahrens, Levine, Suhl, Kleinfeld, [10]. Proc Natl Acad Sci, USA. 99:15176–15181, 2002. © National Academy of Sciences, 2002.

different animals also showed these patterns. These observations are of interest because a linear superposition of the spontaneous and the stimulus-driven activity cannot reproduce these results. A minimal model that produces the sum and difference frequencies from two periodic signals requires a product of the two signals. For example,

$$cos(2\pi f_i t)cos(2\pi f_s t) = \frac{1}{2}cos[2\pi(f_i+f_s)t] + \frac{1}{2}cos[2\pi(f_i-f_s)t] \qquad (8.9)$$

Thus, the presence of the these peaks is evidence for nonlinearity of the response [10].

The second example is from recordings in the primary sensory (S1) and primary motor cortices (M1) of a rat obtained with 5 Hz stimulation presented to the vibrissae [136]. Figure 8.22A shows the spectrum of an S1 neuron and panel C shows the spectrum of the M1 neuron. The S1 spectrum shows multiple peaks at 5 Hz and its harmonics. In contrast, spectral peaks in the M1 neuron are somewhat indistinct. This observation can be quantified through harmonic analysis of the spike train [125], using the Thomson F-test described in the chapter on time series analysis. Figure 8.22B shows the fitted amplitudes of the sinusoidal components for the S1 neuron, displayed at frequencies where the F-test was significant. The results of the same calculation for an M1 neuron are in panel D. The F-statistic for the S1 spike train is significant at 5 Hz and its harmonics, indicating that the S1 neuron has a periodic response at these frequencies. In contrast, the F-statistic for the M1 spike train is significant only at 5 Hz and is not significant at the harmonic frequencies, 10, 15 Hz, and so on.

8.6 Parametric Methods

In this section we present a brief discussion of parametric methods to model spiking activity based on likelihood functions. Likelihood models for point processes have been used to fit biophysical models [39], as well as to infer network connectivities in small networks of neurons [37, 38]. In most of this work the point process likelihood is expressed in terms of the conditional intensity process.

The reader may want to recall the discussion on conditional intensities from the theory of point processes in chapter 5. Given a sequence of points from a sample path $t_1, \ldots, t_n$ in an interval of time $[0, T]$, and the conditional intensity process $h(t|H(t))$ associated with the underlying point process, the joint occurrence density is given by (equation 5.209)

$$p(t_1, t_2, \ldots, t_n) = \exp\left[\sum_{i=1}^{n} \log\left[h(t_i|H(t_i))\right] - \int_0^T h(t|H(t))dt\right] \qquad (8.10)$$

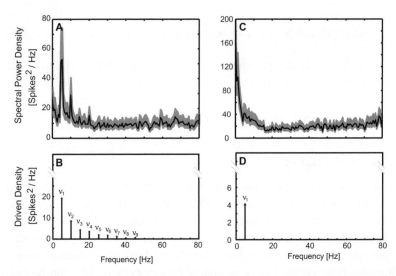

Figure 8.22: Comparison of response of two neurons, one in the sensory cortex and one in the motor cortex of rat in response to periodic stimulation. (A) Spectrum of sensory neuron to a 5-Hz stimulation. (B) The amplitude of the sinusoidal fit to the spiking activity of the sensory neuron at 5 Hz and its higher harmonics. (C) Spectrum of motor cortex neuron. (D) The amplitude of the sinusoidal fit to the spiking activity of the motor cortex neuron at 5 Hz and its higher harmonics. The data was 100 s long. Adapted from Kleinfeld, Sachdev, Merchant, Jarvis, Ebner [136]. Adaptive filtering of vibrissa input in motor cortex of rat. *Neuron* 34:1021–1034, 2002.

The conditional intensity process is defined in terms of the survival process $S(t|H(t)$, $S(t|H(t)) = \int_t^\infty p(u|H(u))du$

$$h(t|H(t)) = \frac{p(t|H(t))}{S(t|H(t))} \tag{8.11}$$

This description has served as the starting point for much of the work on the parametric modeling of spike trains. As emphasized in the tutorial section, the conditional intensity process is in general a stochastic process depending on the sample path, and should not be confused with the analogous rate function or first moment of the process. The latter is a fixed function of time that does not depend on the sample path. Only in the case of the inhomogeneous Poisson process do these quantities coincide.

The intensity process may also be conditioned on other variables or stochastic processes. In analysis of recordings of hippocampal place cells of a rat foraging in a disc-shaped arena [43], log $[h(t|H(t))]$ was modeled as a quadratic in the instantaneous position of the rat, $\mathbf{x}(t) = [x(t)y(t)]$ and periodic in the phase of the theta rhythm.

$$\log \left[h(t|\mathbf{x}(t), \phi(t)) \right] = \alpha - \frac{1}{2}\mathbf{x}(t)W\mathbf{x}^{\dagger}(t) + \beta \cos(\phi(t) - \phi_0), \qquad (8.12)$$

where α, β, and W are parameters to be determined. Substituting equation 8.12 in equation 8.10 gives a parametric form for the likelihood of the observed sequence of spike times. The parameters may be determined using a maximum likelihood procedure.

8.6.1 Goodness of Fit

Goodness of fit testing is carried out using the time-rescaling procedure [44], using the compensator process described in the section on conditional intensities. Each spike time is replaced by a rescaled time $\tau_i = \int_0^{t_i} h(t|H(t))dt$. If the conditional intensity process has been correctly estimated, τ_i should constitute a unit rate Poisson process. In particular, the ISI distribution obtained from the difference between successive τ_is should be exponential. This can be tested using the probability transformation on the ISIs, $z_i = 1 - \exp(\tau_i - \tau_{i+1})$. The z_i should be uniformly distributed between 0 and 1, which can be tested using parametric procedures or using nonparametric tests such as the Kolmogorov-Smirnov test described in chapter 6.

Other tests for Poisson processes may be employed on the rescaled sequence of times. A comprehensive review of this approach is contained in [41]. Note that the conditional intensity process used in the time rescaling is itself a stochastic process that is in general sample dependent (in contrast with the earlier discussion on rescaling using the rate function, which is not sample dependent).

8.6.2 Example

As an example, we consider a neuron recorded from the hippocampus of a rat foraging for food in a circular arena.[8] The trajectory of the rat and the positions at which it fired a spike are shown in figure 8.23.

Because the firing of the neuron occurred largely in a localized region of the disc, a Gaussian parametric form was used for the intensity process $h(t|x(t), y(t))$,

$$\log h(t|x(t), y(t)) = \beta_1 + \frac{1}{2}\left[\beta_2 x + \beta_3 y + \beta_4 x^2 + \beta_5 y^2 + \beta_6 xy\right] \qquad (8.13)$$

where the β_1 term represents background firing and the remaining terms represent the modulation of the firing rate due to the position of the rat in the arena. This model is a doubly stochastic Poisson process with a position-dependent rate. By discretizing time, this model may be treated as a general

---

8. We thank Emery Brown and Uri Eden for supplying the data and the code for this example.

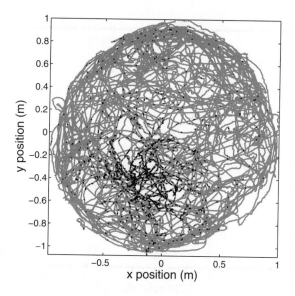

Figure 8.23:   Trajectory of a rat foraging in a disc-shaped arena. The positions at which the recorded neuron fired a spike are shown as black symbols. Note the as concentration of spikes in a small region of the arena.

linear model (GLM) discussed in chapter 6. Figure 8.24 shows the amplitudes of the GLM coefficients obtained using the maximum likelihood procedure.

Figure 8.25 shows a comparison between the model discussed above and one that is linear in the positions. Such a model cannot provide a localized firing pattern. As can be expected, the quadratic model provides a better fit. Note that although both models would be rejected by a hypothesis test, the idea behind these methods is to choose the best among a class of models. At this stage there are a number of possible extensions that could improve the model performance. These extensions could take two forms. First, one may add more covariates to the Poisson likelihood, for example, the phase of the θ rhythm or the velocity of the rat in the arena. Alternately, one might attempt a different form of the likelihood. More detailed discussion of these issues may be found in Barbieri et al [16].

8.7   Predicting Behavior From Neural Activity

In recent years, motivated in part by the desire to build neural prosthetic devices, the problem of predicting stimulus and behavioral characteristics from observations of neural activity in single trials has attracted increasing attention.

These problems are addressed in the framework of regression or supervized learning. First, neural responses to stimuli, or in behavioral or cognitive states

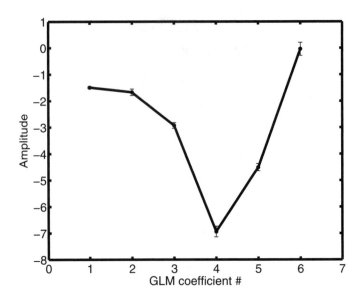

Figure 8.24: Amplitudes of the general linear model (GLM) coefficients β_i, $i = 1, \ldots, 6$ of equation 8.13. The last term is not statistically significant.

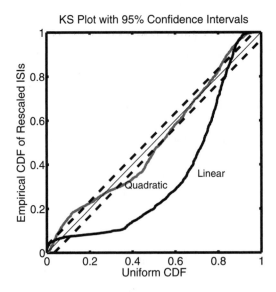

Figure 8.25: Comparison of two models for the intensity process conditioned on the position. Note that the quadratic model (gray), which corresponds to a Gaussian localization in space, is better than the model that is linear in the positions (black), which cannot produce localization in the middle of the arena. CDF, cumulative distribution function; ISI, interspike interval.

of interest, are quantified. This is the model estimation stage. Then, this relationship is reversed, in the prediction or "decoding" stage. A caveat to this description is in order. Separation between training and prediction applies in what are known as "open-loop" experiments where the subject cannot adapt to the outcomes of the prediction algorithm. Situations where the subject can learn from and adapt to the prediction algorithm raise their own unique questions that we will not discuss here, but see [45, 216, 241].

8.7.1 Selecting Feature Vectors

There are two aspects to a classification or prediction problem: choice of the feature vector and the choice of a learning algorithm. Most attempts to predict behavior from neural activity have used firing rates of one or more neurons as a summary of the signal. Recently, attention has also been directed to the use of LFP signals as the basis for prediction of motor activity and cognitive states [33, 152, 172, 176, 198].

There are many measures one can use to summarize the information carried by neural signals. For example, spectral power in specific frequency bands can be used as the features [172, 176, 198]. In particular, in [176] power in a single frequency band is used, whereas in [172, 198] the power in multiple frequency bands is used to construct feature vectors. In contrast, in [152] evoked responses in the time domain are used as the basis for constructing feature vectors.

We will discuss one particular feature vector in detail, because it is of interest in the light of time-frequency spectral analysis. The two-dimensional cepstrum may be defined as the two-dimensional Fourier transform of the logarithm of the spectrogram (over a chosen time and frequency range). If the time range is chosen to be $[0, T]$ and the frequency range $[0, f_{max}]$, then the two-dimensional cepstrum is given by

$$C_{2D}(\phi, \tau) = \int_0^T dt \int_0^{f_{max}} df \, \log \, [S(t, f)] e^{-2\pi i (f\tau + t\phi)} \qquad (8.14)$$

This quantity has been used for prediction of saccades from LFP recordings in LIP [33]. The advantage of using the two-dimensional cepstrum is that it provides a compressed representation of dynamics of the spectrum without making specific assumptions. In figure 8.26 the spectrograms and corresponding two-dimensional cepstra are displayed for two sets of trials from the LIP dataset discussed earlier in this chapter. Note that although the spectrograms are quite broad in frequency, the two-dimensional cepstra are well localized, with only a few leading values being significant. Thus, the two-dimensional cepstra compress the information present in the dynamic spectrum and may be used as a feature vector in prediction algorithms for both continuous and point processes. The two-dimensional cepstrum is related to high-order correlations

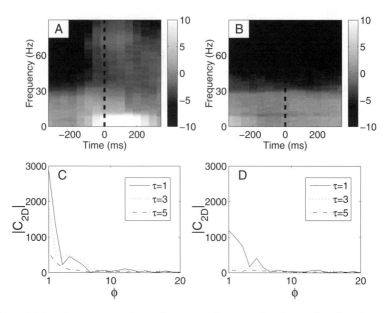

Figure 8.26: Comparison of two-dimensional cepstra for the preferred and anti-preferred directions in the LIP data example discussed earlier in this chapter. (A) Spectrogram for trials to the preferred direction. (B) Spectrogram for trials to the antipreferred direction. (C) Two-dimensional cepstrum corresponding to A. (D) Two-dimensional cepstrum corresponding to B. (Adapted from [33].)

in the time series. This connection is further discussed in the following chapter. In addition to the dynamic spectrum of individual neural signals, it has recently been shown that the coherence between two processes can also be used as a predictor on a single trial basis [250].

8.7.2   Discrete Categories

In certain situations, the stimulus states are discrete, data is given in trialized form, and one obtains a discrete pattern classification problem. This is an old problem in statistics and a number of algorithms have been developed [63, 107]. Many of these have been applied in neuroscience in the past few years. The simplest approaches include the usage of Fisher discriminants [176] and Gaussian mixture–based classifiers [198].

For the discrete classification problem, a standard way of assessing performance is given by the confusion matrix. Given a set of categories n categories and a classifier, the confusion matrix is an $n \times n$ matrix whose $(i, j)^{th}$ entry is the fraction of times the classifier predicts category i when the true category is j. A single number summary of the confusion matrix of a classifier is given by the mutual information between the true and predicted categories.

Classification of events into discrete classes in trial-based data is not the same as predicting the occurrence of these events without knowledge of trial markers. The former is a straightforward classification problem. The latter is a problem of detecting rare events in time, and is generally more difficult, except in cases where the events are associated with stereotyped signals that are well above the noise.[9] Further discussion of this issue and a framework for predicting discrete events from LFP signals may be found in [33].

8.7.3 Continuous Movements

Several studies have focused on prediction of continuous arm movement trajectories from recordings made in the motor cortex. For reviews, see [61, 164–166]. Similar work has also looked at continuous prediction of position using recordings from rodent hippocampus [40]. Two of the basic algorithms are discussed below.

Population Vectors

One of the earliest and simplest decoding methods is given by the population vector algorithm [86, 87]. Suppose there are n neurons in the population and $\mu(s)$ is an $n \times 1$ dimensional vector of the average firing rates of these neurons to presentation of stimulus s.[10] Given an observed $n \times 1$ dimensional vector of instantaneous firing rates $\lambda(t)$, the predicted value of the stimulus at time t is obtained by maximizing the normalized scalar product of $\lambda(t)$ with $\mu(s)$,

$$\hat{s}(t) = argmax_s \lambda(t) \cdot \mu(s) \tag{8.15}$$

Because $||\lambda(t) - \mu(s)||^2 = ||\lambda(t)||^2 + ||\mu(s)||^2 - 2\lambda(t) \cdot \mu(s)$, maximizing this dot product is equivalent to minimizing the residual sum of squares between the observed firing rate and the average firing rate. Therefore, the population vector algorithm is the well known nearest neighbor classification algorithm.

The population vector algorithm is normally described somewhat differently in work on prediction of arm movement velocities using multiple neurons recorded in motor cortex. If $\mathbf{n_i}$ denotes a unit vector in the direction of the *preferred* velocity of cell i, then the predicted velocity after some lag τ is given by the expression

$$\mathbf{v(t+\tau)} = \sum_{i=1}^{N} \lambda_i(t)\mathbf{n_i} \tag{8.16}$$

Although this description appears to be different from the preceding one, they can be seen to be equivalent if one assumes a linear transformation between

---

9. Spike sorting, discussed in the next chapter is an example.
10. For a scalar valued stimulus, this is a tuning curve.

the firing rates and the velocities. Then, minimizing differences in the n dimensional space of rates also minimizes differences in the space of velocities.

Linear Prediction

Reverse correlation was discussed earlier as a method that can be used to map receptive fields of neurons from examples of stimulus-response pairs. Equation 8.1 may also be used to predict the stimulus from the firing rates. To be more explicit, assume a linear model describing the relationship between the stimulus and the response

$$s = \lambda L \qquad (8.17)$$

where s is an $n \times 1$ dimensional vector of stimuli, λ is a $n \times p$ dimensional matrix whose i^{th} row is the time series of neural responses to the ith stimulus, and L is a kernel of dimension $p \times 1$. This is precisely the linear model discussed in the chapter on statistics (the notation used there was $y = x\beta$; the unfamiliar reader should revisit the discussion of the linear model at this point). The optimal linear kernel is given in the same form as the estimator for the parameters β for the linear model,

$$\hat{L} = (\lambda^\dagger \lambda)^{-1} \lambda^\dagger s \qquad (8.18)$$

Given a new vector of responses λ_{new}, one can predict the stimulus to be

$$s_{pred} = \lambda_{new} \hat{L} \qquad (8.19)$$

In the reverse correlation method to map receptive fields, the firing rate at a given point in time was related to the past history of the stimulus. In the prediction problem, these roles are reversed: the stimulus at a given point in time is related to the past history of the firing rates. This method was used in [240] and has since been used in [200, 201] to predict continuous arm movements in real time. It is to be emphasized that the methodology is identical to the classical statistical methods developed for the treatment of linear models.

9

Spike Sorting

9.1 Introduction

The point process component of an extracellular recording results from the spiking activity of neurons in a background of physical and biological noise (section 8.5.1). When a recording electrode measures action potentials from multiple cells, these contributions must be disentangled from the background noise and from each other before the activity of individual neurons can be analyzed. This procedure of estimating one or more single cell point processes from a noisy time series is known as *spike sorting*. When it succeeds, it can transform a weakness of extracellular recording, namely the inability to isolate changes in the firing rate of single neurons into one of its strengths—simultaneous measurement from multiple cells [43, 44].

A range of different approaches has been used to address this problem, from manual pattern recognition to more automated, algorithmic solutions (e.g., [1, 72, 143, 162, 179, 187]). The algorithmic approaches vary in their assumptions about noise statistics, incorporation of domain knowledge specific to the recording area, and the criteria for identifying single cells. Nevertheless, most of the algorithms can be viewed as different implementations of a common series of steps. This chapter develops a framework for these steps and proceeds to discuss the practical considerations of each level without reference to a specific computational approach. Throughout, the transformations of the data are illustrated by an idealized example modeled on recordings taken from the mammalian retina [226].

9.2   General Framework

In the general case, spike sorting takes a voltage trace containing action potentials from multiple cells and attempts to produce one or more collections of spike times, each corresponding to a putative single cell present in the raw trace. This transformation is accomplished through the following sequence:

1. Acquire raw signal containing extracellular action potentials.
2. Detect candidate neuronal waveforms.
3. Align waveforms to reduce temporal jitter.
4. Calculate shape parameters to simplify spike waveforms, if needed.
5. Identify waveforms with similar shape and segregate them into groups.
6. Judge the quality of these groups.

This transformation from raw signal to collections of similar waveforms can be given a quantitative interpretation as follows. If one considers the signal values in the neighborhood of a data sample, one can define a voltage waveform centered on each time point. One may choose to work directly with the voltage values of these waveforms or one may calculate a reduced set of shape parameters from them to ease visualization or computation. In either case, the waveforms are each associated with a numerical vector and they can be treated as a cloud of points in a high-dimensional space (section 5.2.1).

The detection of candidate waveforms is equivalent to the segregation of this cloud into points generated from background noise and points that appear to come from action potentials. If the variability in the action potentials recorded for a single cell is smaller than the differences in spike shape from different cells, the cloud of spike points will form distinct clusters. The basic goal of spike sorting is to identify these clusters of like points in the space of waveforms and use validation measures to judge whether each cluster is likely to have come from an individual neuron.

9.2.1   Manual Sorting

Before discussing automated algorithms it is useful to briefly consider manual sorting. A common, and labor-intensive approach is to reduce each waveform vector to two shape parameters, plot these parameters against one another, and manually identify clusters by visual inspection. This approach has the advantage that the experimenter can readily apply knowledge specific to the cell population under study. The waveforms, receptive fields, or firing patterns of putative single units can be compared to their known or expected characteristics. A researcher uses this knowledge to refine inclusion criteria and develop confidence that resulting analyses are based on the activity of a single cell.

Manual procedures are, however, of limited utility because (1) shape parameters designed for human inspection are inefficient at representing complex waveforms, (2) the labor-intensive process scales poorly to experiments performed with large numbers of electrodes, and (3) a subjective approach makes it difficult to design reproducible and reportable quality metrics. For these reasons, an algorithmic approach is desirable, and in fact, computational solutions with limited human monitoring have been shown to generally outperform manual sorting [104].

9.3 Data Acquisition

The first step in any spike sorting algorithm involves the acquisition of extracellular data in a form amenable to the detection of neuronal spikes.

9.3.1 Multiple Electrodes

An extracellular recording from a local group of neurons begins as an analog voltage signal on each of C electrodes, where C is defined as the number of electrodes in close enough proximity that a single neuron's activity could be recorded simultaneously on each (section 8.4.2). For example, consider an experiment with two tetrodes placed 2 mm apart, where each tetrode is a four-wire electrode bundle with an internal spacing of 50 μm. A spike from a single neuron is unlikely to appear simultaneously on the two bundles due to the large separation between them but may register on multiple wires within a given tetrode. For purposes of spike sorting, there is no advantage in considering all eight wires as a single source of intermixed spikes, and the signals from each tetrode should be sorted separately. In this case, C would be defined as 4.

Multichannel electrodes, often stereotrodes ($C = 2$) or tetrodes ($C = 4$), are used to gain an advantage in disambiguating waveforms [96, 151]. If two neurons with similarly shaped action potentials are equidistant from a single recording electrode, the resulting waveforms will appear indistinguishable. A larger number of recording sites makes it less likely that two neurons will be equally distant from all electrodes. Empirical studies confirm an increase in waveform discriminability obtained by using multiple electrodes [104].

9.3.2 Sampling

In general, the analysis of action potential waveforms requires the analog data to be filtered, sampled and digitized. The data acquisition process, although not specific to spike sorting, introduces several parameters that should be chosen with the sorting process in mind.

The fundamental parameter for acquisition is the sampling rate, F_s, measured in Hz. F_s must be large enough to ensure that multiple samples are recorded during the most rapid voltage swing of the extracellular spike. A rough estimate for a lower bound on F_s can be obtained as follows. The steepest voltage change in an intracellular sodium action potential occurs during depolarization, which lasts approximately 200 μsec at physiological temperature. Due to capacitive coupling, the extracellular action potential appears as a time derivative of the intracellular spike [101], so the signal will rise and fall in this interval. This suggests 5 kHz as a lower bound on the highest frequencies present in a recorded spike. Empirically, measured extracellular waveforms show significant frequency content at values up to about 8 kHz [71], and the sampling theorem (section 5.3.5) prescribes a minimum F_s of 16 kHz. Values of 20 kHz to 30 kHz are typically used in practice, exceeding the minimum somewhat to obtain smoother waveforms.

Before sampling, the analog signal must be low-pass filtered with a cutoff frequency below the Nyquist frequency of $F_s/2$ to avoid aliasing (section 5.3.5). The details of filter selection are beyond the scope of this discussion, but the general requirement is for a multipole filter with a cutoff set below $F_s/2$ to account for the roll off characteristics of real filters. The value used does not directly affect the spike sorting process but should be noted because it determines the correlation length of the sampled data. For example, data recorded with F_s equal to 30 kHz and low-pass filtered at 5 kHz will exhibit greater correlation in neighboring samples than if the recording used a low-pass cutoff at 10 kHz. The number of samples over which correlation is significant can be seen in the covariance matrix of the spike waveforms and determines the effective number of degrees of freedom in an N sample waveform.

As an aside, filters with a nonlinear phase response should be avoided because of the resulting distortion of the spike waveforms. Although this distortion may not interfere with spike sorting, the resulting spike shapes depend on the filter details and will therefore be difficult to compare to data taken with different equipment. Linear phase filters minimize this problem.

9.3.3   Data Windows

After acquisition, a high-pass filter is generally needed to isolate action potentials so they can be compared without regard to remaining differences in low-frequency baseline. The guiding factor is the expected duration of a spike. For example, to ensure that a waveform of duration 1.0 millisec will not show a baseline offset due to underlying low frequency activity, frequencies below 1 kHz must be removed from the raw recording.

The number of samples N taken as the duration of a spike also determines the length of the window used to define spike waveforms in the time series obtained from sampling. This window must be chosen so that successive appearances of action potentials from the same cell are as similar as possible from instance to instance. This requires that N be sufficient to span the interval over which spikes tend to be significantly different from background noise.

However, setting N too large increases the probability that action potentials from two different cells will occur in the same window, increasing variability. A value of 1.0–1.2 millisec is a reasonable compromise for mammalian cortical neurons at physiological temperature.

These data windows associate a vector describing a possible action potential with each time sample t_i as follows. The voltage values in a length N window centered at t_i are extracted from each of the C channels, and these values are collected to obtain a sequence of numbers that can be interpreted as vector with $N \times C$ dimensions. Vectors containing only low-amplitude background noise appear in a high-density cloud centered at the origin, and artifact events without a repeatable shape appear in regions of low density. Spike waveforms

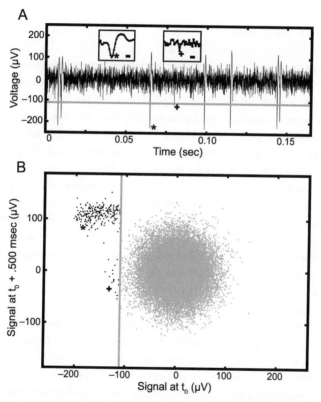

Figure 9.1:   Spike and noise events from a simulated data set based on primate retinal ganglion cells. (A) Segment of raw voltage time series. The horizontal gray line is the threshold used for spike detection; (*) and (+) mark example spike and noise events, respectively, that crossed threshold. The insets are expanded views of these events. Inset scale bar is 200 μsec. (B) Projection of selected windows of length N. Axes indicate voltage values at two times relative to the center of a data window, denoted t_0. The vertical line is the threshold for spike detection; (*) and (+) indicate the events marked in A.

should cluster together and show a clear separation from the central noise cloud.

This perspective is illustrated in figure 9.1. The raw data show several action potentials superimposed on background noise, with example data windows of $N = 32$ samples at $F_s = 20\,\text{kHz}$. The gray line defines a voltage threshold chosen to highlight candidate spikes (but see the next section). If we consider only those data windows that are below this threshold and describe each with two simple features, the result is a large central cloud (figure 9.1B) representing background noise. Of the data windows that cross threshold, we focus on those where the crossing occurs at the center of the window to avoid considering the same waveform at different offsets. These points comprise a smaller, distinct cluster (figure 9.1B).

9.4   Spike Detection

The extraction of spike waveforms for sorting thus requires separation of data windows associated with neuronal activity from those associated with noise. In this process, a detection function is applied to each data window. The function acts as a possibly nonlinear and time-varying filter that takes a length $N \times C$ input vector and reports the evidence for a spike at each time point. Output values above a chosen threshold are taken to be the location of spikes.

When the amplitude of a spike waveform is sufficiently large relative to the thermal and biological background noise, spike detection can be trivial. The detection function might simply reproduce the input signal, and a voltage threshold would be identified to detect large excursions from baseline. However, as the amplitude of spike events approaches the level of noise, a simple threshold includes an increasing number of noise events among the detected spikes. In this case, the statistics of noise and spike waveforms can guide the design of a filter that achieves better separability. For example, figure 9.1B demonstrates that spike waveforms that are not well separated from noise using a simple threshold may be easily separable in a higher dimension.

A model of background noise can be developed directly from the recorded data [60, 180]. Epochs of time known to be free from spiking activity can be used to estimate the parameters of a noise model. For example, if noise is assumed to arise from a Gaussian distribution, the necessary parameters are the mean and covariance. A data window that has a low probability under such a noise model would be considered an action potential. Because biological noise sources are typically nonstationary, the parameters may need to be locally re-estimated throughout the data.

The most direct way to develop a signal model is from a library of prototype spike waveforms. In the presence of white noise, the optimal linear filter for spike detection is a matching filter that convolves the data with the expected waveform shape. If spike sorting is performed in an iterative fashion, the mean waveforms of clusters determined from one round of spike sorting can be used as the matching filters for the next iteration.

When an explicit model of noise or waveform shape is unavailable, a more ad hoc approach is necessary. Heuristic approaches are typically based on two observations. First, background noise has zero mean and short autocorrelation. Second, spike events consist of abrupt increases in absolute voltage levels. From these observations, several methods have been developed to detect significant voltage excursions (for a comparison see [169]). Although these techniques may not require the estimation of model parameters, they do not have the optimal properties of explicit models.

In all of these methods, the choice of threshold for detection of a spike event is a trade-off between avoiding false positives (i.e., type I errors) and false negatives (i.e., type II errors). A low threshold will capture the most spike events but will erroneously admit many noise events. A high threshold rejects the most noise but also misses the most spikes. When a statistical model of noise is used, the threshold can be calibrated to a desired ratio of type I to type II errors. In most cases, a more permissive threshold is desirable because windows of noise can be removed in later stages of processing.

9.4.1 Alignment

Once spike events are detected, the waveform of each action potential is extracted from the data. As discussed previously, a data window is taken from around the time of each spike event. In the case where $C > 1$, this window includes the waveforms from each electrode.

Before the waveforms are clustered, it is important that they are correctly registered with one another. The comparison of voltage values for different instances of an action potential from the same cell is sensitive to the temporal alignment of the two waveforms. It is common to align spike events on the threshold crossing found in spike detection, but this is often inappropriate.

The precise moment at which an analog voltage trace crosses threshold will in general occur between two consecutive samples. The first sample recorded above threshold then lags the actual crossing by a duration between 0 and $1/F_s$ sec, and the extracted samples for the entire waveform are equally shifted in time. This process causes two identical waveforms to appear different even in the absence of noise. Background noise compounds this effect by randomly advancing or delaying the actual threshold crossing for each event, possibly by multiple samples.

One solution to misalignment is to digitally resample the data at a higher frequency. When electrophysiological signals are sampled at more than twice the Nyquist frequency, the sampled waveform contains the information needed to reconstruct the continuous analog signal. Interpolation of values between samples increases the effective F_s and yields an alignment with a higher temporal resolution. If the new alignment is based on a single sample, such as a threshold crossing, it will still be sensitive to noise. A more robust alignment point would be a function of the entire waveform, such as its center of mass. After an improved alignment is found, the data can be downsampled to retain the original dimensionality of the spike waveforms. Figures 9.2A and 9.2B show a sample data set before and after alignment, demonstrating the reduction in temporal variability.

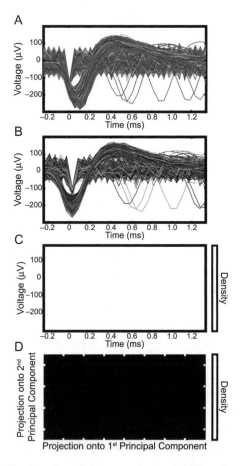

Figure 9.2: Visualization of candidate waveforms. (A) Waveforms of all events, before alignment. (B) Waveforms of all events, aligned on their peaks. (C) Voltage versus time histogram corresponding to B. (D) Two-dimensional histogram of waveforms from B projected onto the first two principal components of the data set.

9.4.2　Outlier Removal

The detection step produces a set of waveforms that may include outliers, defined here as spike events that are dissimilar to all other waveforms. Outliers may arise from unusual noise events, neurons with very low firing rates, and overlapping waveforms from simultaneously firing neurons. These events are problematic for spike sorting algorithms because they will not appear as dense clusters. Further, many clustering algorithms are not robust to outliers and will distort true clusters in an attempt to account for them. When this is a concern, spikes in low-density regions of the waveform space can be set aside as outliers. This can be accomplished, for example, by partially sorting spikes and removing those waveforms that are not well captured by any cluster.

9.4.3　Data Visualization

Even in automated algorithms, it is useful to visually examine the data to confirm that the results capture the gross structure of the data. This allows the experimenter to understand the degree of separation between signal and noise, the nature of any outliers, and to make corrections to the clustering if necessary.

For example, Figure 9.2B, 9.2C, and 9.2D show three different views of the spikes detected from the data in figure 9.1 after they have been aligned on their peaks. Apparent in the plot of superimposed waveforms are noise waveforms, such as the one marked by a+ in figure 9.1A, that crossed the detection threshold by a chance fluctuation. Also clear is a group of waveforms that have the expected shape for an action potential, with the variability between waveforms clearly smaller than the separation from noise. A small number of gross outliers can be seen with large secondary peaks.

The superimposed waveforms portray the range of data but can misrepresent the frequency of different events. Figure 9.2C emphasizes common events in a voltage versus time histogram, where each column corresponds to a histogram of voltage values at a given time point. The background noise vanishes here, except for a small peak visible at $t = 0$, because the noise waveforms are highly variable. Similarly, the outliers are not visible because of their low relative frequency. The putative spikes, by contrast, have a highly stereotypical waveform. The maximum variability in these waveforms, judged from the voltage spread at each time point, occurs in the samples near the peak of the spike at $t = 0$.

A final perspective on the data comes from treating the waveforms as high-dimensional points, as discussed previously, and projecting them into a two-dimensional subspace (section 5.2.4). A convenient, although potentially suboptimal, choice of subspace comes from a principal components analysis (chapter 5) on the set of spike waveforms. A projection of the data points onto the first two principal components preserves as much of the variation as is possible in an orthogonal two-dimensional representation. When the separation between clusters is significantly larger than the noise within clusters, this maximum variance subspace also approximates the subspace that best preserves cluster separation. Such a projection is shown in figure 9.2D, plotted as a two-dimensional histogram to highlight regions of high density. The cloud of noise points corresponds to the low-density region on the left, and the spike waveforms yield the brighter regions to the right. In particular, this projection suggests that the action potentials are divided into two similar but distinct clusters.

These plots thus demonstrate at a glance what the sorting algorithm should find: two very similar stereotypical waveforms, a background noise cluster, and a small number of outliers.

9.5 Clustering

All complete spike-sorting algorithms include a definition, either explicit or implicit, of what is to be considered a cluster of points, and divide up the data space in a way that best fits that definition. For example, an isotropic Gaussian noise model defines a cluster as a compact set of points and an associated mean vector such that points within the cluster are closer in Euclidean distance to their mean than to the mean of any other cluster. The solution, for a given number of neuronal sources K, finds the K mean vectors that minimize the average distance from any point to its cluster mean.

Because many physical sources of noise follow a Gaussian distribution, models that assume Gaussian noise are often reasonable and have well-defined solutions. The case in which the noise added to each of K prototypical neuronal waveform is assumed to be from an anisotropic Gaussian distribution is of particular interest because this model has a known optimal solution. As in the previous example, the a cluster is defined such that members $\mathbf{x}$ are closest to their corresponding means μ, with the metric given by the Mahalanobis distance $(\mathbf{x} - \mu)^{\dagger}\Sigma^{-1}(\mathbf{x} - \mu)$, which involves the inverse of the covariance matrix Σ. The anisotropic Gaussian mixture model allows for noise that varies unequally over a waveform. This could occur if, for example, the amplitude of the spike peak was less variable than the spike trough due to variability in after-hyperpolarization currents.

The full definition of a Gaussian mixture model requires a mean and a covariance matrix for each of K clusters, as well as mixing parameters describing the relative frequency of the different clusters. Such models are usually solved using an iterative expectation-maximization procedure to estimate maximum likelihood model parameters [63]. In practice, the main difficulty encountered in this approach lies in determining the number of clusters. Model selection criteria, such as the Akaike information criterion, can find a compromise between goodness of fit and model order by effectively comparing solutions obtained with different numbers of clusters. This approach has been evaluated in an experiment in which simultaneous intracellular and extracellular recordings allowed the results to be validated, and it appears to perform well in many situations [104, 110].

If noise is not Gaussian, for example due to electrode drift or variation in action potential shape during bursting, then more general definitions of a cluster are needed. Several definitions and techniques are available from the larger literature on clustering (e.g., [63, 213]). One particular notion of a cluster that may be applicable in the non-Gaussian case is the idea of a contiguous set of points with no dips in local density larger than some threshold. This idea is appealing because the threshold allows a hierarchy of clusters, where the predicted number of clusters depends on the amount of discontinuity the experimenter is willing to tolerate. Algorithms such as those designed by [72] and [187] have been applied to spike sorting are effectively nonparametric density-based approaches. When the shape of an action potential varies relatively smoothly, as in the slow change of amplitude with electrode drift, these approaches can capture structure missed by Gaussian models.

An example applying the algorithm proposed by [72] to the data from figure 9.2 is shown in figure 9.3. The voltage vs. time histograms for the five resulting

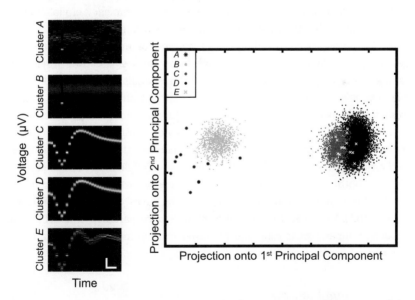

Figure 9.3: Results of spike clustering. Left: voltage versus time histogram of the waveforms of each identified cluster. Scale bar is $100\,\mu V$ by $200\,\mu sec$. Right: waveforms of each cluster projected onto the first two principal components.

clusters are shown on the left and the projection onto the first two principal components is on the right. As predicted, these clusters include noise (cluster B), two similar neuronal waveforms (clusters C and D), and two groups of outliers (clusters A and E).

9.6 Quality Metrics

The clusters returned by a sorting algorithm must be evaluated to determine whether they truly represent the output of single cells. Quantitative measures of confidence are necessary to identify clusters suited for single unit analysis. For example, an analysis showing a 5% increase in firing rate should only be performed on units with an estimated false positive rate of less than 5%.

A common measure of quality is whether the point process associated with a given cluster shows interspike intervals (ISIs; section 8.5.2) of less than a typical refractory period. Because neurons cannot produce action potentials closer together than a few milliseconds, with the details depending on cell type, a single unit cluster will not have ISIs in this range. Conversely, a multiunit collection of spikes with no biophysical refractory period will have a frequency of short ISIs that is predictable from the mean firing rate of the cluster spikes. The frequency of these refractory period violations, characterized by an ISI histogram or autocorrelation function, will increase as the false-positive (type I) error rate of a cluster goes up. When the mean firing rate is large enough that a significant number of violations are expected by chance, a low frequency of violations is strong evidence that the cluster was generated by a single cell.

While the refractory period provides a measure of multiunit contamination based on spike times at sufficiently high firing rates, it does not provide an estimate of type II or false-negative errors, corresponding to missed spikes. For example, it is possible to generate clusters without any short ISIs by simply excluding the offending spike. A complementary metric is therefore needed to describe how often similarly shaped spikes are not counted in the same cluster. Although no such metric is currently in common use, the proximity of clusters in the waveform space relative to their internal variability is a natural place to estimate both type I and type II errors. An explicit estimate is theoretically possible for parametric models by computing the Bayes' error integral of cluster overlap [63]. In models that do not form an explicit parametric model for the clusters, nonparametric estimates of cluster overlap may still be valuable for purposes of comparison.

9.6.1 Manual Review

In addition to the quantitative calculation of error estimates, human inspection of the results of a sorting algorithm is needed to confirm the quality of the sorting and to deal with cases in which an algorithm fails. The most common problem arises when an algorithm poorly estimates the number of clusters present in the data, either inappropriately lumping clusters that should be kept distinct or splitting apart collections that seem to be from a single cell.

As an example, figure 9.4 shows plots used to judge the quality of the clusters from Figure 9.3. Figure 9.4A shows autocorrelation functions indicating that the spikes from clusters C and D both demonstrate refractory periods, because the number of events goes to zero for very short latencies. The noise spikes in cluster B do not show a clear absence of events at these short latencies, although the low frequency of the noise events makes it difficult to accumulate statistics.

In contrast to the variance-maximizing principal components analysis, once the data has been divided into clusters it is possible to explicitly find the subspace that maximizes the separation between clusters. In particular, given any two clusters, the Fisher linear discriminant [63] defines the one-dimensional projection with the least cluster overlap. Thus figure 9.4B demonstrates that the action potential cluster B has no overlap with noise cluster D. Figure 9.4C uses the same principle to show that the waveform clusters C and D are in fact separated by a region of low density, despite the high degree of apparent overlap

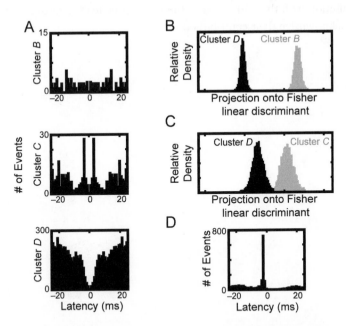

Figure 9.4: Quality metrics applied to spike sorting. (A) Spike train autocorrelation for selected clusters. (B) Histogram of spike waveforms in cluster B and cluster D when projected onto the Fisher linear discriminant between them. (C) Linear discriminant analysis applied to cluster C and cluster D. (D) Cross-correlation of spike trains from cluster C and cluster D.

in the principal components projection visible in figure 9.3. It is therefore tempting to conclude that these are two different cells with similar waveforms.

However, figure 9.4D shows the cross-correlation of the spike trains for clusters C and D and indicates that spikes from cluster B are very often preceded by spikes from cluster A. This is apparent in the original signal shown in figure 9.1A, where two short spikes are seen preceded by taller spikes. In this case, knowledge of the recording site is required to understand the cause of this correlation. The cells often fire doublet spikes, suggesting that cluster B represents a second, smaller spike from the same cell in cluster A. It is also possible that the two waveforms represent two cells, one driving the other. This evaluation may require human judgment, because the range of factors needed to distinguish these unusual cases is often difficult to define algorithmically. In these cases, a general spike sorting algorithm should compute a best guess solution and present this solution in a way that allows rapid manual confirmation.

Acknowledgments

This chapter was prepared by Samar Mehta, David Kleinfeld, and Dan Hill, in consultation with the authors, who then further edited the results. We gratefully acknowledge their contribution.

10

Electro- and Magnetoencephalography

10.1   Introduction

Charge and current sources in the brain generated by electrical activity give rise to electric and magnetic fields. The study of these fields is the subject of electroencephalography and magnetoencephalography (EEG and MEG, respectively). These provide the most direct noninvasive methods for studying the dynamics of brain function. EEG is also the area of neuroscience that has traditionally had the closest contact with time series analysis techniques.

This chapter is organized as follows. We begin with a brief discussion of early references in the application of time series analysis techniques to the analysis of EEG data. We then discuss the physics of EEG and MEG signals, the measurement techniques, and noise sources. Following this, we discuss analysis of issues connected to denoising of these datasets. Finally, we extend the discussion of time series analysis methods from Chapter 8 using EEG and MEG data.

10.2   Analysis of Electroencepalographic Signals: Early Work

The first human EEG recordings were published by German physiologist Hans Berger (1873–1941) in 1929 [24]. Berger had begun his studies of the human EEG in 1920 and made the first recordings of human epileptic seizures. In his normal and clinical subjects he noted that alpha waves (8–13 Hz) appeared on the scalp when the subjects closed their eyes and were unoccupied with any task, and disappeared when the subjects opened their eyes or were otherwise occupied with a mental task. He also noted that the waves occurred with higher amplitudes over fissures in the skull and concluded that they had a cortical origin. However, Berger's work was not widely accepted until Adrian [5] performed a series of controls to rule out the possibility that the waves were produced by eye movements and muscle discharges. The α wave observed by Berger and Adrian is evident from visual inspection of the EEG signal. In fact, early work on EEG involved examining and detecting patterns by eye, essentially by counting the number of zero crossings [167].

Visual inspection of patterns was quickly augmented with quantitative methods, including frequency domain analyses. The first computation of the spectrum of EEG signals appears in a paper by a collaborator of Berger [58]. The first examples of EEG spectra from an English language publication are found in [95]. Norbert Wiener played an important role in the development of EEG analysis from the late 1940s to the early 1960s, an excellent early example of the use of quantitative spectral estimation for understanding EEG data is contained in his book [244]. Wiener estimated confidence intervals for an EEG spectrum with two closely spaced α peaks (at about 8.95 and 9 Hz), separated by a small dip, and concluded, based on these confidence bands, that the dip was a statistically significant phenomenon. Although this is a later addition to the original 1948 edition [243], this book and another one on time series analysis [245] were both quite influential [18] in the processing of neural signals. The first estimates of cross-correlations between electrodes seem to be in [36]. Some other important references up to the fifties are [19, 35, 36, 55, 123, 238, 239, 246].

Although the earliest work [95] used a special purpose analog machine for spectral analysis, subsequent studies [19, 238, 239] largely used special or general purpose computers. The development of the fast Fourier transform and general purpose computers led to an increase in the application of time series analysis techniques to the analysis of EEG data. Cross-correlation of EEG signals recorded at different locations over the hippocampus of cats performing maze navigation tasks showed consistent differences in phase patterns between correct and incorrect trials [2]. One of first extensive discussions of spectral methods in the context of EEG data may be found in [237]. Particularly notable in this reference is the emphasis on confidence intervals. Spectrograms and coherograms were apparently introduced into the EEG literature in [236]. The use of correlations to quantify responses induced by sinusoidally varying visual stimuli are found in [190, 191]. In [67], a χ^2 test is used to demonstrate that a mental task caused strong departures from Gaussian behavior in the EEG signal. Autoregressive spectral estimation techniques were introduced into EEG analysis in [88], and in [217] these methods were used to assess the focus of seizure in humans using autoregressive partial coherence estimates. A summary of the early developments, and particularly Wiener's role, can be found in [18]. A more general time-line of important developments in EEG is in [215].

The list of references in the previous paragraphs not meant to be exhaustive, but it should convey the idea that time series analysis techniques have been used in the analysis of EEG signals almost since the inception of the field. The power spectrum of the EEG signal is somewhat arbitrarily broken up into named frequency bands as δ (1–4 Hz), θ (4–8 Hz), α (8–13 Hz), β (13–30 Hz), and finally γ (>30 Hz). Although conventional, this procedure has caused much confusion because these bands do not necessarily correspond to well defined discrete peaks in the power spectrum. In addition to oscillatory behavior seen in the ongoing EEG, neural responses to specific tasks, known as event-related potentials (ERPs) are part of the basic EEG phenomenology. ERPs have also been observed to show stereotyped patterns. For reviews of EEG phenomenology, the reader can consult [148, 192]. The first chapter of [148] contains a brief discussion of evoked response potentials. In recent years, analysis of ERPs in single trials has attracted considerable attention, in part because of interest in prosthetic applications [249].

10.3 Physics of Encephalographic Signals

A comprehensive understanding of the relationship between the recorded EEG and MEG, and the underlying sources, remains an area of active research. It is thought, however, that the recorded fields are related to current dipoles produced in the cortex due to neural activity [13, 167]. Because the electromagnetic fields reflect the instantaneous distribution of currents in the brain, EEG and MEG signals theoretically have resolutions in the millisecond range.[1] The spatial resolution is poor, however. It is limited both by the number of sensors that can be used and by the ill-posed nature of the inverse problem that relates the sources to the fields. Multiple source distributions can give rise to the same measured EEG and MEG signals [13, 102, 153].

10.4 Measurement Techniques

EEG is measured by using metal electrodes that contact the scalp and draw current. The placement of electrodes is standardized, with the 21 positions of the 10/20 system [126] being the basis for more dense arrays. Clinical practitioners typically use the traditional 10/20 system. For basic research studies,

---

1. Because EEG and MEG power spectra typically decay away by about 100 Hz, in practice there is no measurable power in the signal at 1 kHz. Therefore, the time resolution is really closer to 10 millisec rather than 1 millisec, and statements that EEG/MEG have millisecond resolution are overly optimistic. Given a large enough signal-to-noise ratio, individual peaks can be localized with higher accuracy, as can be the time delay between signals. These should not, however, be conflated with the *time resolution* of the signal, which is strictly speaking set by the spectral bandwidth.

the number of electrodes is larger, and systems with 128 and even more electrodes, known as high-density EEG systems, are becoming increasingly more common. Besides recording from the scalp, EEG studies may sometimes use electrodes implanted on the surface of the cortex. Such recordings are known as intracranial EEG or electro corticograms. These methods offer substantially improved spatial resolution over conventional scalp EEG and suffer from relatively few of the artifacts seen in the latter. Their use is limited, however, to patients in neurosurgical care. In chapter 8, we mentioned that although the intracellular voltage spikes have amplitudes on the order of 100 mV, the extracellular potential is of the order of a millivolt or less. The EEG signal is smaller still, because it is measured on the scalp, typical values being in the tens of microvolt range.

An important issue in EEG recordings is the choice of the reference and much discussion can be found in the literature about the "proper" choice. Ideally, a reference electrode would be affected by extraneous noise in the same way as scalp electrodes and unaffected by the neural signals of interest so that subtracting the electrode potential from the reference potential leaves a clean signal. In reality, no reference is ideal. Common strategies include using electrodes on the mastoid process of the skull behind the ear or some other location on the head somewhat far away from the region of interest, referencing to the average of the potentials recorded at all electrodes, and finally, computing a surface Laplacian. The last method is a way of approximating the current in the region around the electrodes. A detailed discussion of these issues can be found in [167].

MEG is recorded using arrays of coils and measuring the current induced in them by the magnetic field. Magnetic fields generated by the brain are very small (in the pico Tesla range; in comparison, the earth's steady magnetic field is $10^{-4}T$). Similarly, other environmental magnetic fields, and fields generated by the heart, the skeletal muscles, and even the human eye, are larger than the brain's magnetic field [102]. For this reason measuring magnetic fields generated by the brain is difficult, and while the first EEG was recorded in human in the 1920s [24], MEG was first recorded only in 1968 [48] in a magnetically shielded room.

To shield the subject from the magnetic fields in the environment, a combination of three methods is used. Magnetically shielded rooms are built that exclude most external fluctuating fields [49]. The sensors themselves often consist of coils of different orientations placed close together in so-called gradiometer configurations.[2] Because distant fields are relatively uniform near the detector (compared to fields from the brain), use of gradiometers approximately cancels the contribution from the distant fields. Finally, MEG systems also use dedicated

---

2. Occasionally the sensors may consist of a single coil, in which case they are known as magnetometers.

reference channels placed further away from the head, to measure the environmental fluctuations in the magnetic field. The first MEG recordings [48] used sensors consisting of copper coils. However, for increased sensitivity these were replaced by superconducting quantum interference devices (SQUIDS; [47]).

Finally, as with microelectrode recordings, encephalographic studies are performed either to study spontaneous or evoked activity. However, one important difference between evoked responses seen in EEG and MEG and those seen in microelectrode recordings is that the magnitude of spontaneous activity in the former is often substantially larger than the evoked components. Thus, although the amplitude of spontaneous α activity in EEG is $10-100\,\mu V$, the event related signals are only of the order of $1\,\mu V$. This makes analysis of these signals considerably more difficult than for microelectrode recordings.

10.4.1   Noise

The dominant sources of noise in EEG and MEG are the electric and magnetic fields generated by other parts of the body. Thus, eye blinks and saccades, discharges of facial and cranial muscles, and cardiac signals are common contaminants in both EEG and MEG experiments. Partly for this reason, EEG and MEG recordings may be accompanied by electro-oculograms (measurements of the electric potentials due to eye movements, EOG), electromyograms (measurements of muscle potentials, EMG), and electrocardiograms (ECGs). Like in microelectrode recordings, instrumental noise takes the form of line noise at 50 or 60 Hz.

10.5   Analysis

The preceding discussion has highlighted that physiological artifacts substantially affect encephalographic recordings. These artifacts and the high dimensionality of EEG/MEG datasets necessitate an emphasis on denoising and dimensionality reductions methods in the analysis protocol. However, once such data reduction and denoising has been carried out, the techniques for analysis of EEG/MEG data are quite similar to those for local field potential recordings. Therefore, in this and the next two chapters, the aim is to elaborate on analysis techniques that were not covered in the chapter on microelectrode recordings.

10.5.1   Denoising and Dimensionality Reduction

Local Detrending and Line Noise Removal

EEG and MEG recordings often show low-frequency fluctuations due to eye movement, breathing, subject motion, and so on. Because such fluctuations can mask important experiment-related activity, they are commonly suppressed using high-pass filters. However, a high-pass filter can introduce spurious Gibbs ripples at the edges of the time series. A better procedure, that does not introduce such artifacts, is to model slow fluctuations using local regression on low-order polynomials. A procedure that is similar in spirit is to perform linear regression on overlapping data segments, and averaging the regression lines to obtain the desired fit. The fit is then subtracted from the data, a procedure which may be called local detrending (in contrast with global detrending, where a straight line fit to the entire data segment is removed).

Figure 10.1A shows approximately eight seconds of an MEG recording from human subjects [119]. Figure 10.1B shows the spectrum of this time trace computed using the multitaper method. Note the low-frequency peak, which corresponds to the slow variations seen in figure 10.1A. There is also a peak at 60 Hz, corresponding to line noise. This peak has a characteristic box shape, expected in the multitaper method from a sinusoidal oscillation. The width of the peak is the bandwidth of the estimate (≈ 1.3 Hz).

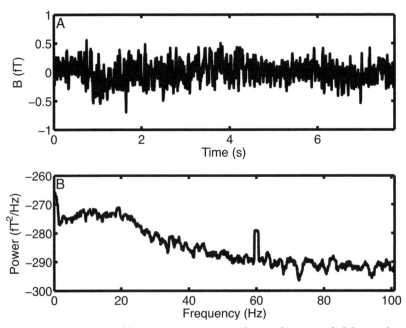

Figure 10.1: Segment of line noise contaminated MEG data recorded from a human subject. (A) Raw data. (B) Spectrum showing a peak at 60 Hz in the shape characteristic of line noise. The spectrum estimation was carried out with 5 data tapers, corresponding to a bandwidth $2W = 1.3$ Hz.

Figure 10.2 summarizes the result of applying the local detrending procedure and the harmonic analysis discussed in chapter 7 to this data. Because the data are roughly linear over a 1-sec period, the local detrending procedure used a 1-sec long-moving window, stepped through 0.5 sec. Figure 10.2A shows the F-statistic for this segment of data. Because the F-statistic is computed over a range of frequencies, a Bonferroni correction was used to assess significance: to compute the threshold at the level α, the $(1 - \alpha)/N\%$ point of the F distribution was used. This is shown by the dotted horizontal line ($\alpha = 0.05$). Figure 10.2B shows the spectrum of the data, with the slow variations as well as the fitted sinusoid at 60 Hz removed. In this example, a

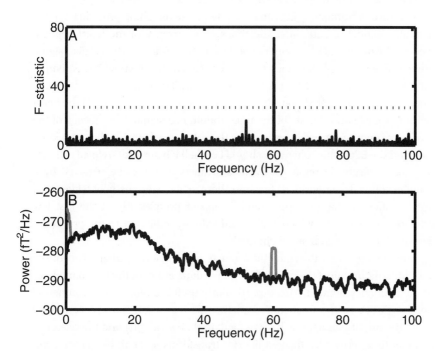

Figure 10.2: Line noise removal using the Thomson F-test. (A) F-statistic as a function of frequency. The threshold is a $(1 - 0.05/N)\%$ point of the cumulative F distribution with the appropriate number of degrees of freedom, and N is the number of independent frequency bins, given by the product of the data length and the digitization rate. The peak at 60 Hz is the only significant peak. The computation used five tapers. (B) Spectrum of the data with local detrending and the 60 Hz component removed. Also shown is the original spectrum. Note that the F-test removes just the 60-Hz sinusoid, leaving neighboring frequencies unchanged. Similarly, the local detrending method removes just the low-frequency peak.

constant amplitude sine wave was fitted to the entire data segment. In general, one may fit time-varying amplitudes using moving windows. An example can be found in [159].

Cardiac and Distant Sources

In MEGs, the use of gradiometers is the simplest method to cancel contributions to the signal from the heart and other environmental factors. In some MEG experiments, the sensors are arranged in a magnetometer configuration, but the reference channels may still be used for this purpose. Cardiac and EOG artifacts also appear in EEG, where it is more difficult to cancel these contributions through a subtraction procedure.

The simplest and most widely applied technique to remove cardiac artifacts is to acquire simultaneous ECG and use a template matching procedure. Given a single channel of data, $y(t)$, and times of occurrence of the heart beats, t_i (acquired from the ECG), segments of data $y_i(t)$ containing the cardiac signal are extracted around the times t_i. Because the cardiac component is temporally localized, this procedure is usually feasible. The extracted segments are smoothed and subtracted from the raw signal in the neighborhood of the heart beat to produce an estimate of the uncontaminated signal. The efficacy of the procedure may be verified by estimating the coherence between the cleaned-up data and the ECG. This coherence should be small if heart beat–related artifacts have been effectively removed. Cardiac artifacts may also be removed by a singular value decomposition. Because these artifacts are usually widespread on the different channels, they tend to appear prominently in the first few principal components, which can be individually subjected to the procedure described above for individual channels.

Another approach to removing artifacts is to perform a regression of the EEG/MEG data against the reference channel data, either in the time domain or in the frequency domain. This is particularly useful to remove environmental noise in MEG. In the frequency domain, this regression may be performed using the multitaper approach. Given a data time series $y(t)$ and the reference channel time series $x(t)$, tapered Fourier transforms $\tilde{y}_k(f)$ and $\tilde{x}_k(f)$ are computed. The K dimensional vector $\tilde{y}_k(f)$ can be regressed against $\tilde{x}_k(f)$ (K being the number of tapers) to obtain the transfer function between the two

$$T(f) = \frac{\frac{1}{K}\sum_k \tilde{y}_k(f)\tilde{x}_k^*(f)}{\sqrt{S_{MT}^x(f)S_{MT}^y(f)}} \qquad (10.1)$$

where $S_{MT}^{x,y}(f)$ are the multitaper estimates of the spectra of x and y. Note that in addition to using multiple tapers, one may also use multiple data segments. In this case, the sum in equation 10.1 additionally includes the different seg-

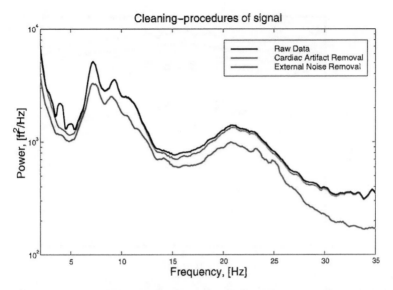

Figure 10.3: Removal of cardiac and distant source artifacts from MEG data. Cardiac sources were removed by combining a template matching procedure with an singular value decomposition. The distant sources were removed by frequency domain regression. (Adapted from [146].)

ments or trials. The results of such a procedure, in combination with the singular value decomposition, is shown in figure 10.3.

Eye Movement and Muscle Discharge Artifacts

Muscular discharges due to scalp and facial muscles, as well as eye movement potentials, are the largest sources of noise for EEG/MEG data and pose non-trivial challenges. A number of methods have been used in the literature to remove these artifacts, including filtering (high pass to remove ocular artifacts and low pass to remove muscle artifacts) [17, 94, 124], regression against the EOG signal in the time domain [186] and frequency domain [83, 84, 248], principal component analysis [140, 144, 145], and independent component analysis [131, 132, 234]. There is currently no consensus on the best method; reviews can be found in [51, 52, 70]. Also, visual inspection of data followed by removal of strongly noise contaminated signals remains a useful if laborious method for ensuring that these noise components do not dominate.

Singular Value Decomposition

MEG and EEG recordings typically involve many channels. Although examination of channels on an individual basis may be necessary and even required

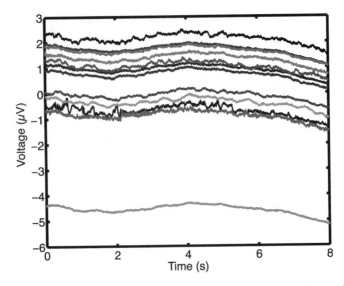

Figure 10.4: Example of intracranial EEG data showing one channel in each brain region. Note the slow variations seen in all channels.

in certain situations, analysis of multivariate data usually requires some form of dimensionality reduction. The most common method of reducing dimensionality of multivariate data is the SVD discussed in chapter 5. Besides providing a reduced representation of the data, such methods can also serve to help in the noise removal process. Here we show an example in which the SVD approximately segregates 60-Hz noise from the signal generated by the brain.

An intracranial EEG data set was acquired from a patient with intractable epilepsy.[3] The patient had 60 electrodes located on the surface of the scalp, under the dura: 24 electrodes in the frontal lobe, 12 in the parietal lobe, and 24 in the temporal lobe. In addition, 16 depth electrodes were located in the middle temporal lobe. The recordings were acquired for eight seconds while the patient performed a maze navigation task on a laptop. The sampling frequency was 500 Hz.

Figure 10.4 shows the voltage measured at one channel from each of the brain regions, and figure 10.5 shows the corresponding spectra. The slow variations seen in the figure occurred from movement of the patient in the hospital bed. Therefore, before computing the spectra, these slow fluctuations were suppressed using the methods discussed in the previous section 10.5.1.

3. We acknowledge Keith Purpura, Erik Kobylarz, Doug Labar, Ted Schwartz, and Dan Weisholtz for sharing these data with us.

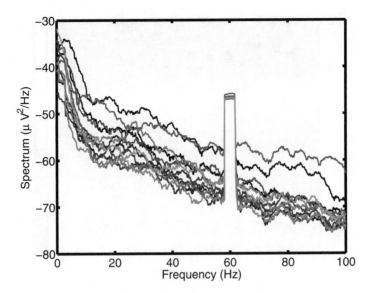

Figure 10.5: Spectra of channels shown in figure 10.4 showing the 60-Hz peak. Because the recordings are almost 8 sec long, these spectra were computed with a large time-bandwidth product, $2TW = 30$.

Given an $n \times m$ data matrix $M(t, x)$ (with $n > m$), where t denotes time and x denotes space, the SVD of the data matrix is usually written as

$$M = U\Lambda V^{\dagger} \qquad (10.2)$$

$$M(t, x) = \sum_{i=1}^{m} \lambda_i u_i(t) v_i(x),$$

where λ_i are the singular values (diagonal elements of the diagonal matrix S), $u_i(t)$ are the "temporal modes" and $v_i(x)$ the "spatial modes." The modes are ordered according to decreasing variance.

Restricting the computation to the frontal lobe channels, the SVD was computed on a 4000×24 matrix corresponding to 4000 time points and 24 channels. Figure 10.6 shows the spectrum of the resulting temporal modes (i.e. the spectra of the columns of U). The first mode shows an artifact at a very low frequency and contains most of the 60-Hz line noise. In contrast, the higher order modes contained a broad peak in the spectral power centered at around 25 Hz, likely to be of neural origin. Partially denoised data may be reconstructed by discarding some modes that are strongly contaminated. In the present case, this may be accomplished by discarding the first mode

$$M_{2-24}(t, x) = \sum_{i=2}^{24} \lambda_i u_i(t) v_i(x) \qquad (10.3)$$

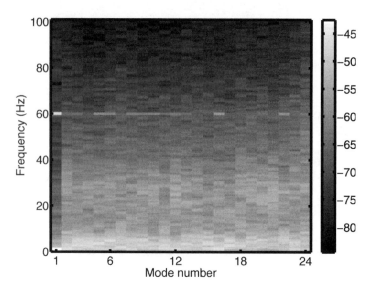

Figure 10.6:   Spectra of each temporal mode.

Figure 10.7 shows the mean spectrum of $u_1(t)$ and $u_{2-24}(t)$. It is seen that the low frequency component and the 60-Hz noise segregated largely with the first mode.

Notwithstanding the separation seen above, it should be emphasized that *individual* eigenmodes computed from the space-time SVD (as well as modes obtained using Independent Component Analysis or other matrix decomposition algorithms) do *not* necessarily have biological meaning. When modes can be identified with particular physiological sources, this sort of procedure is useful, especially in exploratory data analysis. Nevertheless, these are mathematical algorithms and there is no necessity that such segregation will occur. The SVD, for example, imposes the constraint that the individual modes must be orthogonal. However, there is no reason to assume that neurobiologically relevant modes are orthogonal to one another. For this reason, these decomposition algorithms have limited utility as methods for separating different noise and signal sources. Even in the example discussed here, there is some 60 Hz in the remaining modes, which needs to be removed separately. The best way for line noise removal is still the F-test used in the previous section, because this procedure uses the knowledge that this artifact is in the form of sharp spectral peak. The removal of the line noise may be aided by first using the SVD or some other procedure to first reduce the line effects to a few modes. In general, modes taken from an SVD procedure need to be considered in groups. Rather than consider individual components, it is better to consider

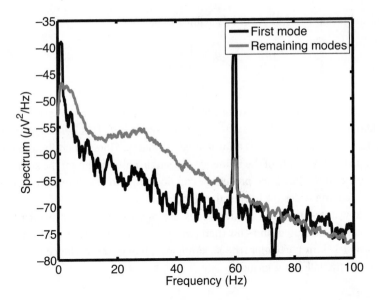

Figure 10.7: Mean spectrum of the data reconstructed from the first mode and the remaining modes. Note the peak at 25 Hz in the spectrum of the data reconstructed from the higher order modes. Note also that line noise and the low-frequency artifact are both suppressed in the higher modes.

entire subspaces consisting of groups of modes, which have a better chance of segregating noise or signal sources of interest.

10.5.2   Confirmatory Analysis

Single Group Jackknife

The jackknife procedure was introduced [184, 185] for reducing bias in estimates. Tukey is credited with popularizing this technique and proposing that it be used both to reduce bias and to estimate confidence intervals [155]. The technique is reviewed in [157], and extensive discussion of the jackknife and other resampling techniques may be found in [65, 66].

Let $x_1, \ldots, x_n$ denote samples drawn from a given probability distribution with an associated parameter θ. Let $\hat{\theta} \equiv \hat{\theta}(x_1, \ldots, x_n)$ denote an estimator of θ using all the samples, and $\hat{\theta}_i \equiv \hat{\theta}(x_1, \ldots, x_{i-1}, x_{i+1}, \ldots, x_n)$ denote the estimator obtained from all but the ith sample. So-called *pseudovalues* $\tilde{\theta}_i$ are defined as

$$\tilde{\theta}_i = n\hat{\theta} - (n-1)\hat{\theta}_i \tag{10.4}$$

and the jackknife estimate of θ is defined to be

$$\tilde{\theta}_J = \frac{1}{n} \sum_{i=1}^{n} \tilde{\theta}_i \qquad (10.5)$$

To gain an intuitive understanding of this procedure, consider the case where θ is the mean of the distribution, and $\hat{\theta} = \sum_{i=1}^{n} x_i/n$. Then, $\tilde{\theta}_i = x_i$, and the jackknife estimator $\tilde{\theta}_J$ is equal to original estimator $\hat{\theta}$. This is not surprising, because the sample mean is an unbiased estimator. More generally, the pseudovalue is an estimate of the influence of a single observation on the statistic of interest, and the jackknife procedure can be shown to asymptotically remove bias to leading order ($O(1/n)$ in the sample size n).

Tukey noted that the pseudovalues are approximately independent and identically distributed and can therefore be used to construct confidence intervals [157]. In particular, the jackknife estimate of the variance of θ, $\tilde{\sigma}_J^2$, is given by the following formula:

$$\tilde{\sigma}_J^2 = \frac{1}{n(n-1)} \sum_{i=1}^{n} (\tilde{\theta}_i - \tilde{\theta}_J)^2 \qquad (10.6)$$

It can be shown that

$$\frac{(\tilde{\theta}_J - \theta)}{\tilde{\sigma}_J} \qquad (10.7)$$

approximately follows a t-distribution with $n-1$ degrees of freedom. This formula may be used to estimate confidence intervals on θ.

The jackknife does not work well in certain situations (e.g., when θ is the median) [see 155 for this and other examples]. However, it has been shown to work well in many cases where the statistic is locally linear in the observations. In particular, it works for variances [156] and correlations [112]. We should also note that in addition to leaving out one sample in turn, one can also carry out the jackknife procedure by leaving out groups of samples in turn [157].

The jackknife procedure cannot in general be applied to time series data by leaving out individual time points, because successive time points are usually correlated. However, the jackknife procedure is well suited to multitaper spectral analysis, because the tapered Fourier transforms of the data are approximately uncorrelated for locally flat spectra and may be treated as samples that are subjected to the leave-one-out procedure [221]. This is a principle reason for our interest in the procedure.

Jackknife for Two Groups

The previous discussion on the single group jackknife can be extended to statistics involving two or more groups of observations drawn from different distributions. Let $x_1, \ldots, x_n$ and $y_1, \ldots, y_m$ be two groups of samples from distributions F and G. Let θ denote a parameter involving both distributions F and G, and let $\hat{\theta} \equiv \hat{\theta}(x_1, \ldots, x_n, y_1, \ldots, y_m)$ denote the estimate of θ obtained from all samples of both groups. Define $\hat{\theta}_{i0}$ as the estimate computed after dropping the ith sample of the first group and $\hat{\theta}_{0j}$ denote an estimate with the jth sample of the second group dropped. Then, defining pseudovalues

$$\tilde{\theta}_{i0} = n\hat{\theta} - (n-1)\hat{\theta}_{i0}$$
$$\tilde{\theta}_{0j} = m\hat{\theta} - (m-1)\hat{\theta}_{0j} \qquad (10.8)$$

the jackknife estimate of θ is given by

$$\tilde{\theta}_J = \frac{1}{n+m}\left[\sum_{i=1}^{n} \tilde{\theta}_{i0} + \sum_{j=1}^{m} \tilde{\theta}_{0j}\right] \qquad (10.9)$$

The jackknife estimate of the variance is given by

$$\tilde{\sigma}_J^2 = \frac{1}{n(n-1)}\sum_{i=1}^{n}\left[\tilde{\theta}_{i0} - \bar{\tilde{\theta}}_{i0}\right]^2 + \frac{1}{m(m-1)}\sum_{j=1}^{m}\left[\tilde{\theta}_{0j} - \bar{\tilde{\theta}}_{0j}\right]^2 \qquad (10.10)$$

As in the single group case, these estimators may be used to obtain approximate confidence intervals for θ.

The discussion here follows a procedure proposed in [11]. This is not the only possible procedure: alternate proposals have been put forth [9, 197]. However, for application of these methods to the problem of comparing spectra and coherences the method discussed here has proven to be adequate [32].

Confidence Intervals for Spectrum and Coherence Estimates

The multitaper method generates multiple degrees of freedom at a given frequency for all of the estimators of interest. In particular, for N trials and K tapers, there are NK degrees of freedom corresponding to individual tapers and trials. Therefore, one may drop individual taper-trial combinations in turn, to apply the jackknife procedure [221]. The jackknife is usually performed after variance stabilizing transformations: the logarithm for the spectrum ($\log(S(f))$) and the Fisher transform for the coherence ($\tanh^{-1}(C(f))$), discussed in chapter 7. The double-sided $1 - \alpha$ confidence interval for $S(f)$ is given by

$$\hat{S}(f)e^{-t_{n-1}(1-\alpha/2)\hat{\sigma}} < S \le \hat{S}(f)e^{t_{n-1}(1-\alpha/2)\hat{\sigma}} \qquad (10.11)$$

where $\hat{S}$ is the mean spectrum, $\hat{\sigma}$ is the jackknife estimate of the variance of $\log(S(f))$, and t_{n-1} is the t-distribution with $n-1$ degrees of freedom. The same procedure is applied to $\tanh^{-1}(C(f))$ to generate confidence intervals on the coherence. Note that orthogonality of the tapers ensures that the NK estimates are approximately independent and validates the use of the jackknife; further details may be found in [221].

Comparison of Spectra and Coherences

The problem of comparing measured quantities between two different experimental conditions is an important one in neuroscience. Confidence intervals around individual estimators may be used to assess such differences. A more direct procedure is to use the two-group jackknife to provide confidence intervals on the *difference* between the two quantities of interest. We consider the example of comparing the estimated coherence for two conditions.

Because coherence estimates have a bias that depends on the degrees of freedom (see equation 7.28), a simple difference between the estimates in the two conditions is not a suitable statistic. Even if true coherences are equal, their estimates can differ quite significantly due to estimation bias terms, if the number of degrees of freedom are different. Figure 10.8 illustrates this difficulty. The data consists of two pairs of simulated Gaussian processes, constructed to have equal coherence of 0.5. The first pair has fewer trials, however, and hence the expected value of the estimated coherence for this pair is higher than 0.5.

This difficulty can be solved by using a bias-corrected test statistic

$$\Delta y(f) = \frac{(y_1(f) - B_1) - (y_2(f) - B_2)}{\sqrt{V_1 + V_2}} \tag{10.12}$$

where $y_1(f)$ and $y_2(f)$ are the estimators (of the variance stabilized spectrum or coherence) in each group, B_1 and B_2 are the bias terms, and V_1 and V_2 are the corresponding variances. If the underlying processes in the two groups have the same distribution, then the expected value and variance of $\Delta y(f)$ are

$$E[\Delta y(f)] = 0 \tag{10.13}$$
$$V[\Delta y(f)] = 1 \tag{10.14}$$

The null hypothesis $\Delta y(f) = 0$ may be tested using the percentage points of the unit normal distribution, $N(0, 1)$.

The arguments presented in the previous paragraph are valid asymptotically for large degrees of freedom. For finite sample sizes a better procedure is to use the percentage points of $N(0, \tilde{\sigma}_j^2(f))$, where $\tilde{\sigma}_j^2$ is the *jackknife estimate* of the variance of $\Delta y(f)$. This has the added benefit of providing a test for non-Gaussian behavior in the original process. A large discrepancy between $\tilde{\sigma}_j^2(f)$ and the value of 1 valid for Gaussian processes is indicative of non-Gaussian behavior or heterogeneity in the experimental conditions that needs to be further investigated. Conversely, if the jackknife estimate of the variance is close to 1, the procedure is consistent and may be used to assess the difference between the two groups.

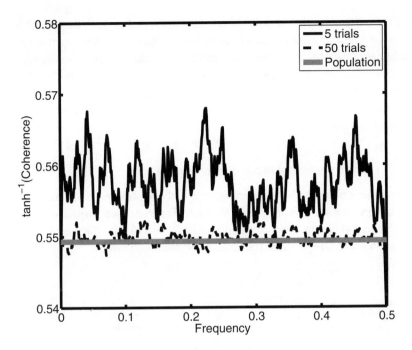

Figure 10.8: Coherence for two groups of simulated Gaussian processes, show-ing that the bias of a coherence estimate depends on the number of trials. Fewer trials lead to larger bias. The coherences were computed using the multitaper method with a time-bandwidth product $NW = 5$ and $K = 2NW - 1 = 9$ tapers. This first pair had 5 trials and the second pair had 50 trials (this corresponds to 90 and 900 degrees of freedom). (Adapted from [32].)

Because the test statistic $\Delta y(f)$ is a function of frequency, the null hy-pothesis $\Delta y(f) = 0$ will be rejected at a fraction α of the frequencies under consideration, by chance fluctuations. This is related to the so-called multiple comparisons problem. A general discussion of multiple comparisons is con-tained in the next chapter. However, if the excursions are over large and contiguous portions of the frequency range, then multiple comparisons are less likely to be an issue.

Figure 10.9 shows an application of the procedure detailed above, to assess the equality of coherence between an MEG time series and an EMG time series, obtained under two different experimental conditions.[4] The MEG-EMG coher-ence in these two conditions are shown in figure 10.9A. Figure 10.9C shows

4. The MEG and EMG signals were recorded simultaneously from a human subject. The subject periodically extended the right wrist for intermittent periods of eight seconds. The behavior was categorized into two conditions: (1) Relaxation condition, when the subject's wrist was relaxed, and (2) isometric contraction, when the subject's wrist was extended. Further details may be found in [32].

that the jackknife variance of the difference statistic is close to 1, showing that the procedure is reliable in this instance. Finally, figure 10.9B shows that the statistic is outside the 95% confidence band for a range of frequencies between 20–26 Hz and 28–45 Hz (figure 10.9B). Because the bandwidth of the spectral estimate is $W = 10$ Hz, the excursion of the test statistic out of the confidence bands for the 20–26 Hz range may be due to a chance fluctuation. More examples can be found in [32].

Global Confidence Bands: Permutation Tests

The two-group jackknife procedure described above provides *local* confidence bands. Permutation tests provide an alternative approach, and are particularly suitable in estimating *global* confidence bands. We illustrate the use of a permutation procedure to check the equality of two functions.

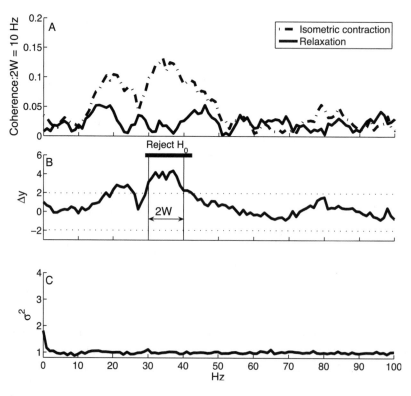

Figure 10.9:   MEG-EMG coherence for contraction and relaxation conditions. (A) Estimated coherences. (B) The test statistic Δy, the $p = 0.05$ confidence band (dashed lines) around zero based on $N(0, 1)$ and the frequencies at which the null hypothesis of equal coherence was locally rejected (thick horizontal line). Adapted from [32]. (C) The jackknifed variance is close to 1.

Let $F(t)$ and $G(t)$ be two functions estimated from data. These functions could be frequency-dependent spectra or coherences discussed in the previous section or other functions of interest. Define a statistic corresponding to the maximum absolute deviation between the two functions, $D_{max} = max_t \mid F(t) - G(t) \mid$. If $F(t)$ and $G(t)$ are significantly different from each other, the maximum deviation statistic D_{max} should be significantly different from zero. A permutation procedure may be applied to the pooled set of $n + m$ samples to generate a distribution of D_{max} under the null hypothesis that the groups are identical; the corresponding samples *exchangeable*.

As an illustration, consider the problem of comparing evoked responses to the two directions adjacent to the preferred direction, in the LIP dataset discussed in chapter 8. Applying the test as described above to the simple trial averaged evoked response does not produce usable results because the response is noisy (figure 8.13). Instead, the evoked responses were first smoothed using local regression, and the permutation test applied to the smoothed responses.

Figure 10.10A shows the two evoked responses for a 1-sec period, 0.5 sec before and 0.5 sec after the onset of the memory period. Figure 10.10B shows a

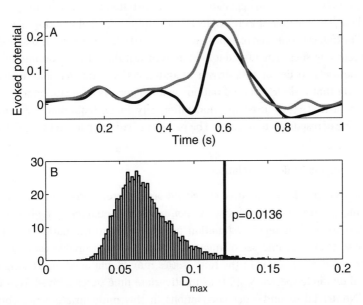

Figure 10.10: Assessing the equality of functions using the permutation procedure. (A) Evoked local field potential responses for trials corresponding to two conditions from the data example considered in chapter 8. (B) The empirical null distribution of the maximum absolute deviation obtained from the permutation procedure, and the value observed for D_{max}. Note that D_{max} falls at the $p = 0.0136$ point of the null distribution. It is therefore unlikely that the underlying responses are equal.

histogram of the maximum absolute deviations, resulting from an application of the permutation procedure to the pooled sample from the two groups. The maximum deviation of the estimated responses was 0.12; the probability that $D_{max} > 0.12$ estimated empirically from this histogram was $p = 0.0136$ (the shaded area). Thus, at a 5% level the null hypothesis of equality of the evoked responses would be rejected.

Nonstationarity

When estimating dynamic spectra or coherences, an important question is whether the estimated dynamics reflect real nonstationarities in the underlying stochastic process, or are sampling fluctuations in the estimator, with the data being actually drawn from a stationary stochastic process. If the experiment has a well defined "baseline" period, dynamics in the spectrogram or coherogram may be assessed relative to this period. However, when studying ongoing activity, there is no obvious baseline. Thus, it is useful to be able to directly assess the significance of observed power variations in the estimated spectrogram or coherogram. A statistic to assess non stationarity in the dynamic spectrum, was presented in chapter 7.

Figure 10.11 shows an application of the nonstationarity test to intracranial EEG data [188] acquired from subjects performing a verbal working memory task. The dataset consisted of approximately 200 trials per subject and a total of 247 recording sites. The high data volumes meant that visual examination of these datasets to detect task-driven modulations was not feasible. Instead, reasoning that task-driven modulations would appear as nonstationarity, the authors of that study used the nonstationarity index (equation 7.73) as a diagnostic of responses to the task. The results are summarized in figure 10.11.

Higher-Order Correlations

The discussion so far has focused on second-order correlations, estimated using dynamic spectra and coherences. As pointed out in chapter 7, higher-order correlations present severe estimation problems due to the curse of dimensionality. However, one set of measures that gives reasonable estimates of higher order correlations in the times series may be obtained by treating estimated dynamic spectra $S_{est}(f, t)$ as multivariate time series derived from the data. Nontrivial second-order correlations in this multivariate series correspond to nontrivial higher-order correlations in the original series. By nesting the evaluation of second-order statistics, the good statistical properties of these estimators may be maintained, thus providing a statistically sound route to the high-order correlations in time series data. An alternative procedure, which we will not discuss here, would be to use hidden Markov models or analogs, as used for speech signals.

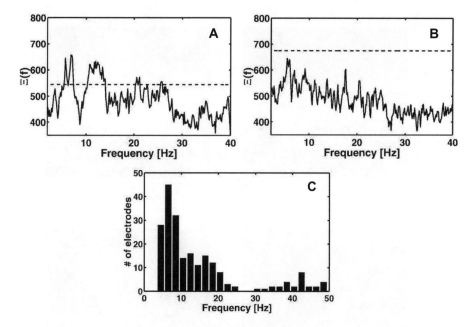

Figure 10.11: Intracranial EEG data recorded during a working memory task show significant task-related nonstationarity, predominantly in the theta frequency band. Nonstationarity index shown for two representative electrodes. (A) Subject 1. This electrode exhibits significant nonstationarity in the theta and beta bands, as well as some peaks in the 20–30 Hz range. (B) Subject 3. This shows an electrode that has no significant peaks. In both cases, the average power spectrum had peaks in the theta frequency range. (C) Summary plot of the number of electrodes which showed significant nonstationarity as a function of frequency. A given electrode could show nonstationarity at several different frequencies. (Reproduced from [188], © 2001 by the Society for Neuroscience).

One way to approach the second-order statistics of the estimated dynamic spectrum, is through the two-dimensional cepstrum introduced in chapter 8 as a method to build a compressed feature vector for prediction problems. First, compute the two-dimensional Fourier transform of the (mean subtracted) log spectrogram

$$C'_{2D}(\phi, \tau) = \int_0^T dt \int_0^{f_{max}} df\, \delta \log\left(S_{est}(t, f)\right) e^{2\pi i [t\phi + f\tau]} \qquad (10.15)$$

It is understood that this computation is done on a given time-frequency window; although the dependence on this window will not be explicitly denoted, the considerations below depend on the choice of the parameters defining the window. It is also important to note that $S_{est}(t, f)$ is the *estimator* of the dynamic spectrum and a function of the data, not the true underlying quantity in the

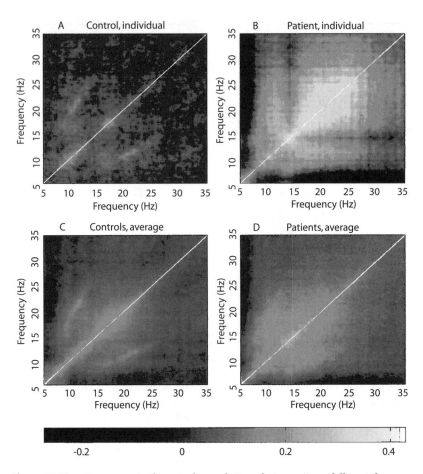

Figure 10.12: Assessment of spectral correlations between two different frequencies in magnetoencepalography data from human subjects. The experiments involved nine healthy control subjects and nine patients suffering from chronic neurological disorders. (Adapted from [146].)

probability distribution of the stochastic process. The absolute value squared of $C'_{2D}(\phi, \tau)$ is given by

$$|C'_{2D}(\phi, \tau)|^2 = \int dt\,df\,dt'\,df'\,\delta \log\left(S_{est}(t, f)\right)\delta \log\left(S_{est}(t', f')\right)e^{2\pi i[(t-t')\phi + (f-f')\tau]}$$

(10.16)

Now consider averaging this quantity using a moving time window. This provides an estimate of a higher order correlation of the process, which we will write in implicit form by taking an expectation value of the equation above:

$$\langle|C'_{2D}(\phi, \tau)|^2\rangle = \int dt\,df\,dt'\,df'\,C_4(t, t', f, f')e^{2\pi i[(t-t')\phi + (f-f')\tau]}$$

(10.17)

where C_4 was defined in equation 7.109. The quantity $\langle |C'_{2D}(\phi, \tau)|^2 \rangle$ is related closely to the so-called "modulation spectrum" [205]. The more general quantities C_4 and C_3 defined in chapter 7 may also be considered. Setting $t = t'$ in C_4, one obtains the instantaneous correlation between the spectral power at two different frequencies.

Figure 10.12 shows the instantaneous correlation coefficient between the log spectral power at two different frequencies, $\log[S(f, t)]$ and $\log[S(f', t)]$, in MEG data [146] acquired from a mixed population of healthy controls and patients with neurological disorders (equation 7.111). Although all subjects showed evidence of non-Gaussian fluctuations, the nature of those fluctuations were found to be different in the healthy subjects as compared with the patient population. In particular, spectral correlations between different frequencies were much broader for the patient population than they were for the controls. The bandwidth of the spectral estimate was $2W = 0.8$ Hz. The computation was carried out by segmenting the continuous data into nonoverlapping windows and using the different windows as independent samples in estimating the spectral correlation.

11

PET and fMRI

11.1 Introduction

The development of positron emission tomography (PET) and functional magnetic resonance imaging (fMRI) as noninvasive methods for measuring brain activity has given rise to a relatively new field of neuroscience research in recent decades. Electroencephalography (EEG) and magnetoencephalography (MEG) discussed in chapter 10 are direct measurements of neural activity. In contrast, the signals measured with PET and fMRI have an indirect relationship with the underlying neural dynamics, mediated by the response of the cerebral vasculature.

However, PET and fMRI have the important advantage of better spatial localization compared with EEG/MEG. In both cases, standard image reconstruction techniques exist that can create relatively high-resolution image volumes from the raw recordings, although better image reconstruction does still remain a topic of research. The problems faced by the functional neuroimaging community are ones of multidimensional signal processing and statistical inference.

In the remainder of this chapter we provide a brief overview of the biophysical bases of PET and fMRI, followed by a survey of experimental and analysis protocols. The analysis procedures discussed focus largely on fMRI rather than PET, since the former give rise to longer time series data sets to which the methods described in this book may be applied. More comprehensive coverage of the material is available in the literature [77].

11.2 Biophysics of PET and fMRI

Both PET and fMRI are based on the response of the cerebral vasculature and blood flow to neural activity. In fMRI, the source of contrast is intrinsic, whereas in PET an extrinsic contrast agent is used.

11.2.1 PET

PET uses tracers consisting of radioactive isotopes incorporated into biologically relevant molecules injected into the bloodstream of the subject or inhaled as a gas. Different types of tracers are used to measure different aspects of physiology (e.g., F^{18}-fluoro-deoxyglucose (FDG) to measure glucose metabolism, O^{15} water to measure cerebral blood flow, or C^{11}/O^{15} carbon monoxide to mea- to measure cerebral blood volume). Because the tracers are very similar to the corresponding naturally occurring compounds, they become concentrated in the same areas with high concentrations of the natural counterpart. When radioactive tracers decay (those used in PET have a half-life between a few minutes and a few hours), they emit *positrons* as they transform from an unstable isotope to a stable one. Emitted positrons collide with electrons within a few millimeters of their origin, converting the mass of both particles to energy in the form of two gamma rays traveling in opposite directions. These gamma rays leave the subject's body and are measured by detector arrays in the PET scanner instrumentation, which detect coincident arrivals of photons at two detectors, thereby forming a single line through physical space that determines the origin of the photons. The count of photons along a line is proportional to the sum of all activity concentrations along that ray. By measuring many such projections, it is then possible to reconstruct images using methods similar to x-ray computed tomography.

The spatial resolution of PET images is limited by the mean free path of emitted positrons prior to annihilation (a few millimeters), the finite number and size of detector arrays, and the point spread function of the underlying physiological cause of the signal (e.g., blood flow). The temporal resolution is also quite limited, with single measurements requiring tens of seconds to acquire (table 8.1).

11.2.2 fMRI

Magnetic resonance imaging (MRI) is based on the phenomenon of nuclear spin resonance. Nuclear spins placed in a magnetic field exhibit Larmor precession at a frequency proportional to the strength of the magnetic field and can resonantly absorb energy from an oscillating electromagnetic field. If a spatial gradient is superposed on the magnetic field, then the Larmor frequency becomes a function of space. This mapping between resonant frequency and spatial location is the basis of MRI.

Although in principle the imaging could be performed by scanning resonance frequencies, in practice time domain methods are used, where non-equilibrium configurations of the nuclear spins are created using short excitation pulses, and the relaxation back to equilibrium is measured in the presence of controlled gradients in the magnetic field. Notable for the purposes of this book, is that the measured raw signal corresponds to the *spatial Fourier transform* of the density of nuclear spins. In fMRI, the nuclear spin corresponds to water protons, although other nuclei are also used in some imaging studies.

Because the measurements are made during relaxation back to equilibrium, the relaxation rates of the proton magnetic moments determine the strength of the measured signal. These relaxation rates vary in space due to a variety of biophysical mechanisms, and are the source of contrast in the image. The longitudinal relaxation rate T_1 for the component parallel to the applied field depends on the local biochemical environment (e.g., it is different between white matter and gray matter). The transverse relaxation rate for a homogeneous applied field T_2 is similarly dependent on the biochemical environment. Inhomogeneities in the magnetic susceptibility of the material generate spatial fluctuations in the applied field, which cause the transverse relaxation rate to become shorter (denoted T_2^*). Deoxygenated hemoglobin is paramagnetic, whereas oxygenated hemoglobin is diamagnetic, providing a susceptibility contrast that can influence T_2^*. The oxygenation level of blood in the cerebral vasculature depends on neural activity, thus providing a connecting link between neural activity, and the NMR signal. This "Blood Oxygen Level Dependent" (BOLD) contrast mechanism discovered by Ogawa [171] was key to the development of functional MRI or fMRI. The relation between the blood oxygenation levels, blood volume and flow rates—and the NMR signal intensity— is now relatively clear. The precise nature of the coupling between neural activity and cerebrovascular activity remains the subject of active research.

11.2.3 Noise Sources

PET images are subject to noise in photon counts due to scattering and detection of false-positive (random) coincidences. Noise in PET images is highly dependent on the details of the reconstruction algorithm used. Shot noise, which takes the form of "streaks," is a common characteristic of images reconstructed with the filtered back projection method. Additional noise may be added by the system electronics and recorder systems, motion of the subject, or environmental noise. We focus here on fMRI time series rather than on PET because the higher sampling rate allows for additional types of analyses and also invites different forms of noise.

Functional MRI measurements are subject to noise from a number of disparate sources. Noise sources can be broadly grouped into two major categories: (1) biological and (2) nonbiological noise. Nonbiological noise sources include instrumentation noise such as scanner drift, thermal noise from the subject and scanner, 60-cycle electrical noise, and environmental noise. Finally, fMRI signals may contain noise in the form of susceptibility artifacts, which cause warping or local signal loss in the image and originate from inhomogeneities in the magnetic field. These can be introduced by the subject or by some foreign object. For example, such artifacts can occur during swallowing or speaking [26] or by a magnetic object being placed within the scanner field of view.

Biological "noise" arrives from physiological sources, including respiratory and cardiac cycles, vasomotor oscillations, fluctuations in brain metabolism and blood flow, and "background" neural activity unrelated to the stimulus. Respiratory, cardiac, and vasomotor effects can be quite regular, with energy primarily in the ~ 0.3, ~ 1, and ~ 0.1 Hz bands, respectively. If the sampling rate used is less than twice these frequencies, then such artifacts are aliased down to lower frequencies but may still remain localized in frequency. Additionally, subject motion, which is sometimes correlated with respiration, is an important source of noise, especially at low frequencies.

The physiological noise sources dominate over the instrumental noise sources in fMRI, resulting in a colored (i.e., nonflat) noise spectrum. Physiological noise exhibits a complex pattern of spatiotemporal correlations that must be taken into consideration when assessing functional imaging data sets [158, 182, 254]. Although not commonly practiced, it is useful when possible to make other physiological recordings simultaneous with Magnetic Resonance (MR) acquisition, including the monitoring of subject respiratory and cardiac cycles as well as eye movements. If these signals are available, they can potentially be used in regression models to remove contaminants from the data. Effective characterization and removal of noise is of critical importance in analysis of fMRI time series where the BOLD response to a task represents a signal change of at most a few percent (and sometimes a fraction of a percent).

11.3   Experimental Overview

PET and fMRI experiments usually involve the subject actively or passively performing a behavioral task while functional images are being acquired. The subject lies supine inside the detector array (in PET) or the bore of the magnet (in fMRI). With either method, the subject must remain stationary with as little movement as possible throughout the experiment. In PET studies, radioactive tracer is injected or inhaled one or more times throughout the session. An experiment can last from a few minutes to an hour or more, and is often subdivided into several shorter sessions or *runs*. During a run, the subject is presented with designed stimuli that follow a particular task paradigm or protocol developed by the experimenter.

11.3.1 Experimental Protocols

Various experimental designs can be used in fMRI studies, whereas the options in PET studies are limited by the poor temporal resolution of the technique. The goal of the experimental design is generally to maximize the detection power for effects related to experimental variables while minimizing potential confounds.

Blocked (also sometimes called *epoch-related*) designs partition the temporal duration of the experiment into blocks of time during which a particular stimulus or category of stimulus is presented repeatedly in order to maintain the subject's cognitive state. In PET these blocks often correspond to a single injection of tracer and thus are determined by the half-life of the radioisotope used. Functional MRI offers much greater flexibility, but block designs still form the dominant experimental paradigm in use. In the simplest case of alternating blocks of two different conditions A and B, the design is periodic (ABABAB), with the *stimulus paradigm frequency* determined by the time between onsets of blocks of the same condition. For task blocks with long duration relative to the BOLD response, the signal is expected to saturate after some time, leading to a robust, sustained BOLD response. Blocked designs offer good detection power but also suffer from the possibilities of reduced subject attention, priming or facilitation effects, and adaptation and habituation of responses as a single block of repeated stimuli proceeds.

Event-related designs have also been applied to fMRI. Such designs attempt to measure transient BOLD responses to single stimuli or "events" that can occur at any time point during the experiment rather than the sustained responses to stimulus blocks. Such designs are feasible only for rapidly acquired fMRI sequences and are not an option for PET studies. The temporal spacing of stimulus events is an important variable controlled by the experimenter. If the inter-stimulus interval is large (e.g., ~20 sec or more), then the BOLD response (which is thought to peak ~5–6 sec postonset) to each event can be expected to decay to approximately "baseline" before the onset of the next stimulus. If the inter-stimulus interval is shorter, however, there will be a temporal summation of responses related to the current event and previous events. This summation may be approximately linear over a range of stimulus presentation parameters, but departures from linearity occur when stimuli are presented for brief durations with short inter-stimulus intervals [34, 80, 229].

Traditionally, the experimental designs used in functional imaging have been categorical, in that the independent variables related to a condition take on two levels (e.g., 1 or 0, on or off). An alternative is to manipulate the independent variable (an attribute of the stimulus) continuously. The goal then becomes to detect regions where the measured effect scales (linearly or nonlinearly) with the value of the independent variable (e.g., image contrast in a visual study). Such parametric designs avoid some of the pitfalls of the *cognitive subtraction* assumption built into most categorical analyses, where it is implicitly assumed that the cognitive components of a task do not interact with one another [81].

The experimental protocol chosen by a researcher is of critical importance in estimating the experimental effects. One must be aware of the temporal and spectral properties of the design, as avoiding spectral overlap between the stimulus paradigm and the known noise sources is very beneficial (as is not applying a filter that eliminates the effects of interest!).

11.4   Analysis

11.4.1   Data Conditioning

Motion Correction

A major source of artifacts in fMRI and also in PET is subject head motion. The general approach to correcting for motion is to realign each functional image in the time series to a reference image (e.g., the first image). This can be done by estimating a six-parameter (three rotation angles about and three translations along each axis) rigid-body transformation that minimizes some cost function, usually related to image intensities. Because each voxel is discrete with finite size, proper realignment requires interpolating intensities between voxels using, for example, *sinc* or *spline* methods.

Realignment is always imperfect due to subject-induced field distortions that result in nonrigid changes in the images, within-volume subject motion, and spin excitation history effects. It can be useful, therefore, to explore and remove potentially confounding signal variations that are correlated with the scan-to-scan motion parameters. Registration across modalities (such as aligning a T_2^*-weighted functional image to a T_1-weighted anatomical image, or a PET image to an MR structural image) is a similar problem, but there is no obvious correspondence between voxel intensity values across acquisition protocols. For this problem, a surface-based matching is preferred (for a review of image registration techniques, see [111].

Slice Timing Correction

Related to both space and time is the problem of slice timing correction. Slices in fMRI are acquired sequentially such that the last slice is acquired approximately TR seconds later than the first. Analyses generally assume that all slices in a volume are acquired at the same phase relative to each stimulus, which makes this delay problematic, particularly for event-related designs. The simplest solution is to interpolate the time series and resample such that each slice is sampled at the same point in time. Such interpolation is not accurate, however, for low acquisition rates (high TRs) due to aliasing.

Prewhitening

Numerous studies have shown that fMRI time series contain significant temporal autocorrelation resulting in colored noise caused by, in part, low-frequency physiological fluctuations (e.g., [27, 158, 254]). Such noise spectra lead to problems for analytical frameworks, such as linear models in the time-domain solved by ordinary least squares, that assume the noise components to be independent and identically distributed in time (with a diagonal autocovariance matrix). Serial correlations in fMRI time series can distort inferred P-values and lead to overdetection of false positives [182]. The magnitude of these effects also depends on the specific parameters of the experimental protocol. It should be noted that in PET imaging, because of the slow acquisition rates, each measurement can be considered independent of the next, and thus serial correlations do not pose such a problem. One approach to the problem of serial correlations in fMRI is to prewhiten the time series, using a low-order auto-regressive model, as described in the chapter on time series analysis.

Data Smoothing

The converse to prewhitening is *smoothing* the voxel time series, for example by applying a bandpass filter. The idea here is to remove physiological noise at the higher frequencies, based on the assumption that the signal is localized at the lower frequencies. Inferences have to be corrected by appropriate adjustments of the model's degrees of freedom. This approach is problematic, however, if the signal is expected to contain energy at high frequencies, such as in rapid event-related designs. An alternative to data smoothing is to perform the statistical tests *locally* in the frequency domain using multitaper techniques, which also decorrelate the data and give rise to relatively simple inferential procedures.

Smoothing is sometimes also performed in the spatial domain, usually by convolving each image with a three-dimensional Gaussian with fixed width. Such smoothing, similar to temporal smoothing above, blurs the data and imposes a known spatial covariance structure. This approach makes the data amenable to treatments based on random field theory (see section 11.4.5) and additionally reduces the errors due to misalignment of functionally activated voxels from scan to scan and even more so from subject to subject. Spatial smoothing also, however, degrades image resolution and runs counter to the basic strength of the fMRI technique (higher spatial resolution compared to PET, EEG, and MEG).

Space-Time Singular Value Decomposition

We now discuss how the singular value decomposition (SVD), used in the chapter on EEG and MEG to extract 60-Hz line noise, can also serve to segregate noise from signal in fMRI measurements.

Five hundred and fifty echo planar images were acquired for 110 sec at 5 Hz during binocular stimulation by a pair of flickering red light-emitting diode (LED) patterns [158]. Each image was masked from the set of original 64×64 pixel images. The resulting image had 1877 pixels, and the SVD was performed on a 1877×550 matrix. Figure 11.1 shows the sorted singular values for this example dataset. Note the shape of the singular value plot, with an initial rapid drop, followed by a slower decay. The large singular values correspond to the *signal subspace*, whereas the slowly decaying part corresponds to the *noise subspace* and originates in uncorrelated scanner noise. The theoretical distribution of singular values for a pure noise matrix can be determined analytically and fitted to the "tail" of the computed singular value spectrum [199]. For uncorrelated random noise, the density of singular values is given by [57, 199]

$$\rho(\lambda) = \frac{1}{\pi \lambda \sigma^2} \sqrt{(\lambda_+^2 - \lambda^2)(\lambda^2 - \lambda_-^2)}, \qquad (11.1)$$

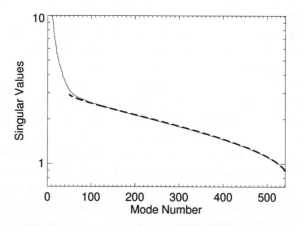

Figure 11.1:   Example of sorted singular values determined by the space-time singular value decomposition. The tail of the singular value spectrum (solid line) is fit by the theoretical density of singular values for a pure noise matrix (dashed line). The range of this plot is truncated to highlight the tail of the spectrum. (Reproduced from [159] with permission of the Biophysical Society.)

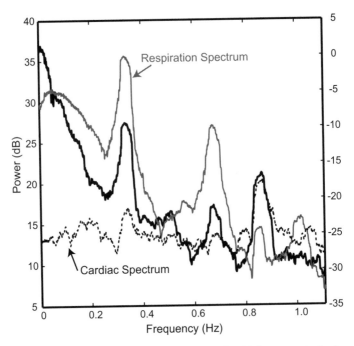

Figure 11.2: Average spectrum computed from the 10 largest principal components (thick line), plotted with the estimated spectra of the monitored respiratory signal (thin line) and cardiac signal (dashed line).

for $\lambda_- < \lambda < \lambda_+$ and zero elsewhere, where $\lambda_\pm = \sqrt{2}\sigma\sqrt{(p+q)/2 \pm \sqrt{pq}}$. The fit in figure 11.1 is of all but the first 50 singular values to this formula. A general formula can also be derived that includes correlations in the noise [199].

In the previous chapter, we identified the temporal mode in the EcoG data that was most affected by the line noise and reconstructed the data using the remaining components. Figure 11.2 shows an example of the frequency spectrum computed from the 10 leading modes for an fMRI data set collected using rapid single-shot gradient-echo Echo Planar Imaging (EPI) at 7 T with a TR of 450 millisec. In this experiment, visual stimuli were presented in 16.2-second blocks with 22-second control periods. Two different visual stimuli were used, and these were presented in alternating blocks (e.g., ABABAB). This resulted in two different stimulus paradigm frequencies: 0.0262 Hz corresponding to the AB frequency and 0.0131 Hz corresponding to the frequency of A or B alone. Respiratory and cardiac signals were collected simultaneously with MR acquisition, and the estimated spectra of those time series are also shown in figure 11.2.

By comparing the average principal component spectrum with the respiration and cardiac spectra, one can visually determine that the spectral peaks at ~ 0.33 Hz and ~ 0.66 Hz are very likely the result of respiratory fluctuations. At frequencies near the stimulus paradigm frequency there appears to be less contribution from the physiological signals, and energy in the principal component spectrum is likely due to stimulus response. This suggests that a frequency-localized analysis could be effective in segregating measured components (see below).

Space-Frequency Singular Value Decomposition

A more refined approach to signal decomposition is obtained by performing the SVD on the cross-spectral matrix of a multivariate dataset. As discussed in chapter 7, this is equivalent to performing an SVD on the tapered fourier transforms and the method has been termed the space-frequency SVD [158, 159]. Thus, if $I(x, t)$ denotes the multivariate dataset, we first Fourier transform this data after multiplying by a family of Slepian functions, $u_k(t)$, $k = 1, \ldots, K$

$$\tilde{I}(x, k; f) = \sum_{t=1}^{n} I(x, t) u_k(t) e^{-2\pi i f t} \tag{11.2}$$

For each frequency this gives an $n_x \times K$ matrix where n_x is the number of spatial channels. When there are multiple trials, say, n_t, one has a $n_x \times n_t K$ matrix. An SVD on this matrix gives

$$\tilde{I}(x, k; f) = \sum_n \lambda_n \tilde{I}_n(x; f) a_n(k; f) \tag{11.3}$$

The reader should note the similarity between this equation and the equation for the space-time SVD discussed in the previous chapter.

Recall from chapter 7 that one can obtain a global estimate of coherence by computing

$$\hat{C}_G(f) = \frac{\lambda_0^2(f)}{\sum_{n=0}^{K-1} \lambda_n^2(f)} \tag{11.4}$$

where $\lambda_n(f)$ are the singular values from the above decomposition. If the space-frequency matrix $\tilde{I}$ is low rank, then the data may be reconstructed using the leading modes. In the degenerate case of all voxels time series being multiples of a single time series, only one singular value is nonzero, and $\hat{C}_G(f) = 1$ for all frequencies.

Reconstruction of data from the truncated space-frequency SVD can be thought of as a spatiotemporal filter, but one that accounts for spatial correlations present in the data that are not necessarily smooth in space. This contrasts with spatial smoothing approaches used frequently in functional image analysis that blur the image data, imposing local spatial correlations regardless of the underlying structure.

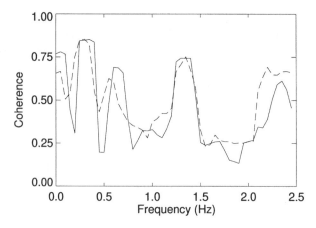

Figure 11.3: Global coherence spectra computed from the space-frequency singular value decomposition of the data set described above. The solid line indicates the spectrum for the data recorded in the presence of visual stimulus and the dashed line in the absence of visual stimulus. (Reproduced from [159] with permission of the Biophysical Society.)

As an example, we consider the visual stimulation experiments used in figure 11.1. The global coherence in the presence and absence of visual stimulation are shown in figure 11.3. The leading spatial eigenmodes for low-center frequencies are shown in figure 11.4. The stimulus response in visual cortex during visual stimulation can be seen in the two lowest frequency spatial modes in figure 11.4.

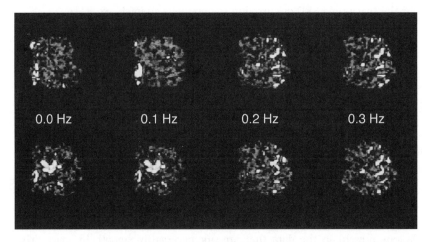

Figure 11.4: Amplitudes of the leading spatial eigenmodes at center frequencies from 0 to 0.3 Hz in 0.1-Hz increments, obtained from a space-frequency singular value decomposition. The top row were obtained from data recorded in the absence of visual stimulus and the bottom row in the presence of visual stimulus. (Reproduced from [159] with permission of the Biophysical Society.)

11.4.2   Harmonic Analysis

In fMRI studies employing periodic blocked designs, the response is localized in frequency. We now show how the multitaper F-test (discussed in chapter 7) can be used to detect such periodic signals. Data were acquired using single-shot gradient-echo EPI at 4 T with a TR of 1 sec. Auditory stimuli were presented in 10-sec intervals with 25-sec control (no stimulation) periods. The fundamental stimulus paradigm frequency was thus $1/35 = 0.0286\,Hz$. The time-half-bandwidth product of the spectral estimates was set to $TW = 4$ and $K = 7$ Slepian sequences were used.

Figure 11.5 shows the computed F-statistics as a function of frequency for a single fMRI time series over the $0 - 0.5\,Hz$ frequency range. Figure 11.5 (bottom) reveals several prominent peaks. At the stimulus paradigm frequency ($\sim0.0286\,Hz$) the corresponding F-value is 14.61, which corresponds to a P-value of ~0.0006 in the $F_{2,2K-2}$ distribution. Another, slightly larger, peak

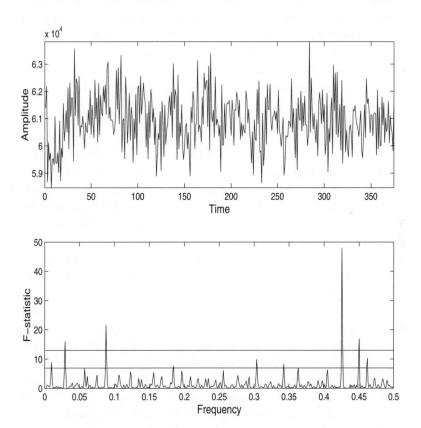

Figure 11.5:   Top: The time series for an individual voxel. Bottom: Multitaper harmonic F-statistic plot as a function of center frequency. Horizontal lines indicate the 99 and 99.9 percentile values in the F-distribution.

occurs at the second harmonic ($f = 0.0857$ Hz). The F-value at this frequency is larger than would be expected in a smooth process such as the BOLD response and may reflect interactions with vasomotor oscillations that have previously been observed at ~ 0.1 Hz [158]. It is also of note that the largest F-statistic is obtained for a frequency of 0.42 Hz, much higher than the stimulus paradigm frequency, and is likely the result of aliasing of cardiac cycle artifacts.

Regression in the multitaper framework guarantees that the autocovariance matrix of the residual error terms will be diagonal because of the orthogonality of the data tapers. This obviates the need for some signal conditioning methods discussed above, including prewhitening of the time series, which are designed to compensate for the off-diagonal covariance terms obtained in time-domain regression models. Unlike the majority of time-domain estimation methods, the multitaper F-test is not sensitive to phase difference in the stimulus response. The least squares solution is complex, containing estimates of both magnitude and phase. Thus, it is possible to construct, for example, a *phase map* for those voxels with significant F-values at the stimulus paradigm frequency. Such a phase map provides details of the temporal organization of responses across cortical space (see, for example, [158]).

The method described in this section can be generalized to nonperiodic, event related designs, as long as the nonperiodic waveform corresponding to the task paradigm has some degree of frequency localization [158].

11.4.3 Statistical Parametric Mapping

Most often functional data from fMRI or PET studies are analyzed using a univariate approach. A test statistic of choice is computed at each voxel to yield a statistical *map* across the set of brain voxels. The majority of currently available software packages for PET and fMRI analysis make use of parametric models, where the probability distributions of the data are assumed to follow well-characterized forms. Following the application of some set of preprocessing and data conditioning procedures, the parameters of the model are estimated to best fit the observed data according to some definition of optimality (e.g., ordinary least squares, maximum likelihood).

The most widely applied procedure in functional neuroimaging for parameter estimation is a linear model of the form $Y = X\beta + \varepsilon$ where the observed response Y is expressed as a linear combination of explanatory variables (the columns in *design matrix X*) plus some residual error. In general the parameters of an identical linear model are estimated for each voxel in the volume. A more detailed description of linear models can be found in chapter 6. In order for this to be a useful framework, the design matrix must contain a well-chosen set of paradigm-related and confounding effects that are expected to combine linearly to capture the majority of the variance in the observed measurements. It should also be noted that various approaches, including computing correlation maps, between the observed response and modeled response [15] fall within the umbrella of the linear model.

In PET studies, the individual measurements are independent of one another and can be arbitrarily ordered in the measurement vector Y. In fMRI, however, it is important to treat the data as bona fide time series. The linear model expressed as a function of time is given by

$$y(t) = \sum_i x_i(t)\beta_i + \varepsilon(t), \quad \varepsilon(t) \sim N(0, \sigma^2 \Sigma) \qquad (11.5)$$

where $x_i(t)$ are now time-domain regressors and β_i are time-invariant model parameters. To model the expected task-related BOLD response, the explanatory variables are usually expressed as a convolution of a function describing the stimulus presentation and a hemodynamic response function (HRf) $h(\tau)$

$$x(t) = s(t)*h(\tau) \qquad (11.6)$$

where $h(\tau)$ is defined over a finite time interval τ and models the BOLD impulse response. Such a formulation assumes that the BOLD response is the output of a linear time-invariant system, which is invalid in certain conditions [34]. The shape of $h(\tau)$ has been modeled in various ways, including the use of a fixed "canonical" HRF or a more flexible linear combination of *temporal basis functions*. In the latter case, a model parameter is estimated for each basis function at each voxel. Thus the *model* remains the same at every voxel, but the shape of the HRF fitted is allowed to change across voxels according to the parameter estimates. Figure 11.6 shows several parameterizations of the HRF that are commonly used in statistical parametric mapping with fMRI.

In blocked designs, the stimulus function $s(t)$ for a particular stimulus condition usually takes the form of a boxcar function with value 1 when that condition is being applied. In event-related designs, individual stimuli are modeled by delta functions at precisely defined times. It should be noted that typically individual regressors are calculated at a higher temporal resolution than that provided by the image sampling rate. This allows the timing of a stimulus onset to be "in between" consecutive scans in the initial computation of the expected response; then, the high resolution regressors are subsampled at the appropriate image acquisition times and entered into the model. This also highlights the importance of slice timing in event related designs, mentioned earlier.

Additional explanatory variables (regressors) can take a variety of forms. For instance, if a behavioral measure (e.g., reaction time) was obtained during trials in the experiment, this time series can also be entered (after mean subtraction) as a column in the design matrix. This models a linear relationship between the observed response and the behavioral correlate. Polynomial expansions of the behavioral vector can also be used to model hypothesized higher order relationships. Additionally, confounding effects such as estimated motion parameters or cardiac time series can be entered into the model in a similar way in order to reduce the residual error.

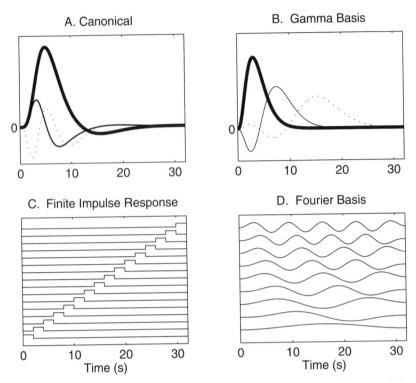

Figure 11.6: Time-domain models of the hemodynamic response function. (A) "Canonical" HRF (thick line) with time (thin line) and dispersion (dotted line) derivatives. (B) HRF modeled with combination of three gamma functions. (C) Finite impulse or deconvolution basis with 16 bins, making no assumptions about the response shape. (D) Fourier basis formed by sine and cosine functions of varying frequency. In C and D the set of temporal basis functions are shown in a "stack" along the y-axis for clarity.

Figure 11.7 shows a sample design matrix for an experiment with two "runs," and with two conditions varied in a periodic block design within each run. The TR is 2 s, and the stimulus function is convolved with a canonical HRF. Also included in the model is a regressor corresponding to a behavioral measure collected during the study (the third and sixth columns in the design matrix), as well as a constant regressor over the duration of each run (the seventh and eighth columns).

Parameter Estimation and Inference

As discussed in chapter 6, when the error terms are uncorrelated zero-mean Gaussians, the maximum likelihood parameter estimate is equivalent to the ordinary least squares estimate given by:

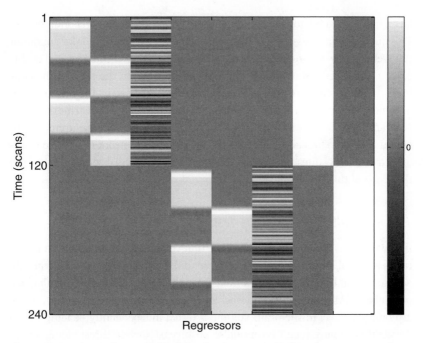

Figure 11.7: A simple example of the design matrix X plotted as an image for a linear model analysis. The large blocks in the image correspond to individual "runs." The x-dimension defines different explanatory variables, for each of which a single β_i value will be estimated. The y-dimension defines time, sampled at the acquisition time of each of 240 scans obtained during the experiment. The first two columns corresponding to each run are the stimulus function convolved with a canonical hemodynamic response function. The third and sixth columns are parametric behavioral measures obtained during the study.

$$\hat{\beta} = (X^{\dagger}X)^{-1}X^{\dagger}y \qquad (11.7)$$

When the errors are Gaussian but with some nondiagonal covariance matrix Σ, the maximum likelihood estimate is given by *weighted least squares*:

$$\hat{\beta} = (X^{\dagger}\Sigma^{-1}X)^{-1}X^{\dagger}\Sigma^{-1}y \qquad (11.8)$$

If X is rank deficient (i.e. if the explanatory variables are linearly dependent), then the inversion of $X^{\dagger}X$ will require additional assumptions. Typically a pseudoinverse technique is employed, which constrains the solution to the minimum-norm solution.

Once the model parameters have been estimated the experimenter is usually interested in testing one or more linear combinations or *contrasts* of the parameters in order to infer effects of interest. In the linear model framework these linear combinations are simply $c^{T}\hat{\beta}$ where c is a column vector of "weights." In terms of the experiment in question, this amounts to asking questions of the form, "what voxels showed a larger effect in condition A than in condition B?" This question is addressed by using a contrast where the regressor for condition A is weighted by $+1$ and the regressor for condition B is weighted by -1. For this case, a one-tailed t-statistic can then be computed from the ratio of the contrast $c^T\hat{\beta}$ to the standard error of that contrast, determined by the residual sum of squared error. This t-value is then compared against the t-distribution with $N - \text{rank}(X)$ degrees of freedom (where N is the number of measurements) to obtain a P-value for each voxel. The linear model framework is suitable to address a number of questions in classical inference, but a full discussion is beyond the scope of this chapter.

11.4.4   Multiple Hypothesis Tests

In the previous chapter, we pointed out that comparison of function estimates raises issues of multiple comparisons. Due to the univariate approach typically adopted in statistical parametric mapping, this is an issue of particular importance in fMRI where the number of voxels are very large. Usually, every gray matter voxel in the brain volume is tested independently, leading to the possibility of many type I errors (false positives). Naively thresholding statistical images consisting of $\sim 10^5$ voxels at a threshold of $\alpha = 5\%$ is, therefore, inappropriate. The multiple testing problem must be addressed with care.

In discussing detection of line noise in a background signal in the previous chapter, the threshold for detection was taken to be α/n where n was the number of hypothesis tests. Note that this Bonferroni correction constrains the total number of false positives, also known as the family-wise error rate (FWER). Thus, to control the FWER at 5% over a 100,000 voxel image, the Bonferroni correction sets α to 5×10^{-7}. The Bonferroni correction is overconservative for large n, particularly in the case when individual tests are not truly independent, as is often in the case in brain imaging due to spatial correlations. A number of methods attempt to correct the Bonferroni procedure while still controlling the FWER. The simplest is the Holm stepdown test [118]. The p-values are sorted in increasing order $P_{(i)}$, where $P_{(1)} < P_{(2)} < \cdots < P_{(n)}$, and thresholds $\alpha_i = \alpha/(n - i + 1)$ are defined. Then, in the stepdown procedure, beginning with $P_{(1)}$, one checks whether $P_{(i)} > \alpha_i$, stopping when this is true and rejecting all previous tests.

An alternative approach is to control the expected ratio of Type I errors to the number of significant tests. This has been termed the *false discovery rate* (FDR) [22, 85]. In other words, this procedure controls the proportion of voxels deemed to be significant that are actually false positives. Although the FDR approach is conceptually different from the FWER schemes discussed above, mathematically it is quite similar. Thus, to implement the FDR correction, the P-values are ordered as in the preceding paragraph. Then, to control the FDR at level α, we find the largest k such that $P_{(k)} \leq \alpha k/n$. The FDR approach is less conservative than FWER approaches, but must be carefully interpreted, because the resulting statistical map will contain a fraction of false detections.

Spatial correlations in brain imaging data can be the result of characteristics of the actual stimulus response, the acquisition method, or of spatial filtering and/or interpolative resampling techniques applied to the data during preprocessing. Any such correlations effectively reduce the number of independent tests being performed in the univariate approach. The discussion in the preceding paragraph did not explicitly account for correlations between voxels. Such correlations can be incorporated in two ways: parametrically using random field theory [251, 252], or nonparametrically using permutation or resampling tests. Random field theory methods model the data as a multivariate Gaussian and use this assumption to infer the distribution of maxima in the images. These methods are related to older ideas in statistics originating in the work of Hotelling [120] and Weyl [242].

11.4.5   Anatomical Considerations

In this chapter we have presented a brief survey of experimental and analysis protocols for functional neuroimaging, with a primary focus on fMRI. In so doing, we have focused on fMRI data as voxel time series. In various methods, spatial correlations are assumed or imposed across voxel space, but spatial organization typically only enters analysis procedures as a final step, in order to correct for the multiple hypothesis tests performed in the univariate analysis. Additionally, the size of a voxel (typically $\sim$2–5 mm in each dimension) is quite small relative to the size of the units for which functional roles are typically hypothesized (e.g., Brodmann's areas or specific gyri). Localizing the effects of interest to particular anatomical regions of interest is a problem in itself.

Cortical Anatomy

Almost all spatial processing in functional imaging proceeds in a voxel space defined by a uniform three-dimensional sampling of the volume. Cortical anatomy, however, does not follow this lattice. Instead, the cortex has the topology of a two-dimensional sheet that is folded in a complex geometry in the three-dimensional space. This implies an alternative to the standard voxel-based approaches, which is to construct cortical surface models in which nearest neighbor *vertices* are in close proximity to one another in the intrinsic cortical space (e.g., [53, 75, 227]). In contrast, in the volumetric grid, a voxel may have a neighbor that lies, for example, across a sulcus and is quite distant along the cortical sheet. This is problematic, particularly for methods that smooth isotropically in the voxel-space, which may result in "smearing" of the response across unrelated areas.

For a single subject, the anatomical localization of an inferred effect of interest is easily performed if an anatomical MR scan has been successfully coregistered to the functional images. The problem is more difficult for localizing responses in multi-subject studies. The usual solution adopted is to *spatially normalize* the brains of each subject in the study, theoretically placing them into a common coordinate system. In volumetric analyses, each brain is *warped* to a reference template using an intensity matching algorithm. With surface-based approaches, each hemisphere can be inflated and the individual folding patterns aligned to an average sulcal template [12, 76]. With any spatial normalization method, however, there is registration error that is difficult to quantify. This is because of the widely acknowledged high degree of variability in individual brain anatomy, which makes a definition of optimality for intersubject registration elusive. This presents another motive for spatial smoothing, which is to *intentionally blur* each estimated response to increase the probability of functional overlap across subjects.

Acknowledgments

This chapter was written mostly by Jason Bohland, who prepared an initial draft of the chapter, including text, figures, and bibliographic entries. The material was selected in consultation with the book authors, who then edited the results.

12

Optical Imaging

12.1   Introduction

Of the experimental techniques discussed in previous chapters, microelectrode recordings have the best spatial and temporal resolutions, but they are most suited for studies of one or a few neurons. Activity in large brain areas and networks can be recorded with electroencephalography/magnetoencepalography or imaged with positron emission tomography/functional magnetic resonance imaging (fMRI) but these modalities have much poorer spatial and temporal resolutions, respectively. In this chapter we discuss analysis of data acquired using optical imaging techniques, which have the potential to combine good spatial and temporal resolution.

12.2   Biophysical Considerations

There are many optical techniques in current use for measuring neural activity. The discussion here focuses on intrinsic optical imaging and imaging using fluorescent indicators. A number of extensive reviews are available, to which the reader is referred for further details [14, 64, 98, 99, 170, 178, 235, 255].

The intrinsic optical imaging signal is closely related to the blood oxygen level dependent signal measured with fMRI techniques [28, 29]. Deoxyhemoglobin has a higher absorbtion coefficient that oxyhemoglobin at wavelengths higher than 600 nm. Consequently, the optical reflectance signal is sensitive to the balance of oxy and deoxyhemoglobin in blood, as well as changes in blood flow and volume. Because the intrinsic optical signal is tied to the vasculature, it is limited to measurements on spatial scales of order the intercapillary distance of about $50\,\mu m$ or so. In practice the scale may be substantially larger, ranging from hundreds of microns to millimeters. The timescale for measurement of a response is ~ 1 sec due to the slow nature of the hemodynamic response. The measured intensity changes are typically small relative to the background reflectance.

Fluorescent indicators, either externally applied or genetically encoded, are molecules that respond to specific alterations in their environment with a conformational change that affects their fluorescence. The most common indicators used to image neural activity respond to changes in calcium concentration or transmembrane voltage. Voltage-sensitive dyes provide direct measures of electrical activity, and in principle have high temporal and spatial resolution, but the signal to noise ratio is poor. Calcium indicators have better signal to noise but poorer temporal resolution, because calcium dynamics is slower than the dynamics of the transmembrane voltage.

12.2.1   Noise Sources

Shot noise due to fluctuations in the number of photons arriving at the detector and "dark noise" due to thermal electron fluctuations in the detector are two limiting sources of instrumental noise. Amplifier noise and other noise sources in the measurement electronics add to these.

Physiological sources of noise are typically larger than instrumental sources, as for fMRI. Because the reflectance of tissue is related to blood oxygenation, changes in oxygenation or blood volume due to cardiac, respiratory, and vasomotor fluctuations also result in changes in light intensity. These are important noise sources both for intrinsic optical imaging, as well as fluorescence measurements in vivo. All of these quasiperiodic changes give rise to reasonably regular changes in the signal that are unrelated to the response to stimulus. In frequency analyses of optical imaging data, these artifacts result in peaks in the frequency spectrum. A final source of noise is physical motion of the object being imaged.

12.3   Analysis

The result of an optical imaging experiment is a series of frames, each frame containing thousands of pixels. In intrinsic optical imaging, sampling rates are around 30 frames/sec. Therefore, for a 640×480 pixel image, sampled at 30 frames/sec, digitized at 12 bits, the data rate is $640 \times 480 \times 12 \times 30 \times 3600 \approx 49$ gigabytes per hour [207]. In voltage-sensitive dye imaging, the data may be sampled at rates exceeding 1 kHz. Thus, like fMRI data, optical imaging time series data are highly multivariate, and the data volumes are large.

12.3.1 Difference and Ratio Maps

Traditional analyses of optical imaging data have focused on averaging the images across a large number of trials or time slices, on a pixel-by-pixel basis [82, 97]. Because the main objective of these experiments is to map stimulus-induced changes in neural activity, the conventional procedure is to normalize the poststimulus images with an estimate of the background. Popular methods for estimating the background include averaging across pre-stimulus images, and the so-called "cocktail average," which uses the average of the response to all the stimuli. Instead of ratios, differences between images may also be used.

Example Data

Figure 12.1 shows examples of spatial maps obtained using the ratio and difference methods. The data set is from cat visual cortex, using a moving grating stimulus. Optical images measuring the cortical reflectance of 605 nm light were acquired at 15 Hz for a duration of $T = 34$ sec, and were subsequently filtered and subsampled at 1.1 Hz. Twenty measurements were taken for each of the six different orientations of the grating. The maps shown are the ratio and difference of the average responses to the horizontal and vertical grating stimuli.

12.3.2 Multivariate Methods

Multivariate data analysis methods have proven useful for optical imaging data [68, 181]. Multivariate spectral estimation techniques have been used to characterize the dynamics of ongoing as well as evoked activity [181], and the response to periodic stimulation paradigms [210–212].

Ratio Estimate   Difference Estimate

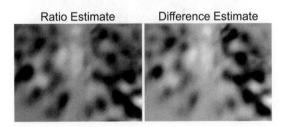

Figure 12.1: The ratio and difference between average response to two stimuli. The first visual stimulus was a horizontally drifting grating, and the second stimulus was a vertically drifting grating. (Left) The ratio of the averaged responses to the horizontal and vertical gratings. (Right) The difference of the averaged responses for the same two stimuli.

Singular Value Decomposition and Harmonic Analysis

Experiments in which the stimulus is presented periodically may be analyzed directly using the Thomson F-test. Stimuli presented repeatedly, but not necessarily periodically, may be rearranged into a periodic pattern that makes them amenable to harmonic analysis (the "periodic stacking method" [210, 212]).

In a typical repeated stimulation experiment, the subject is exposed M times to a set of N stimuli (often in random order). The data can be rearranged to form a periodic sequence such that the stimuli appear in order [210, 212]. For example, a sequence of responses to the stimulus sequence ABCCACBBCABA... is rearranged in the form ABCABCABCABC... Because the stimuli now appear periodically, the rearranged time series can be decomposed into a periodic response with period NT (T is the time of presentation of each stimulus) and noise. Therefore, the spectrum of the rearranged dataset should exhibit peaks at harmonic multiples of the fundamental frequency $f_0 = 1/NT$ that may be subjected to harmonic analysis.

The periodic component is itself composed of a generalized response to any stimulus, called the *nonspecific* response, and responses that are specific to individual stimuli. The nonspecific response is rarely of interest, and it is easy to show it corresponds to the peaks in the spectrum at $Nf_0, 2Nf_0, \ldots$. The peaks at the remaining harmonics constitute the specific response.

Because the data are noisy, it is preferable to apply this procedure to the temporal modes obtained from a singular value decomposition (SVD) rather than the time series of the individual pixel responses. Furthermore, such a procedure reduces the number of time series that have to be subjected to harmonic analysis. Thus, the data $I(t, x)$ are expanded as

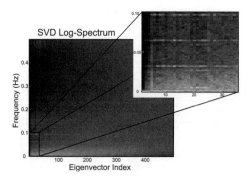

Figure 12.2: The log-spectrum of leading temporal modes, calculated for optical imaging data shown in figure 12.1. The index of the mode is displayed on the x-axis and the frequency in Hz on the y-axis. Lighter shades indicate more spectral power and darker shades indicate less spectral power. Also shown in an enlargement of the low-frequency region. SVD, singular value decomposition.

$$I(t, x) = \sum_i \lambda_i u_i(t) v_i(x) \qquad (12.1)$$

where t denotes time and x denotes the pixels in the image. The spatial modes or eigenimages are given by $v_i(x)$ and the corresponding temporal modes by $u_i(t)$. Figure 12.2 shows the spectra of $u_i(t)$ for the example dataset described above (after application of the "periodic stacking" procedure).

Note that, across many modes, up to an index of 300 or so, there is a sequence of harmonics with a fundamental frequency of around 0.03 Hz. Harmonics are also seen at multiples of a lower fundamental frequency of approximately 0.005 Hz in the range of mode indices from about 20 to 30. Because $N = 6$ and $T = 34$ sec (see above), the fundamental frequency $f_0 = 1/204 \sim 0.005$ Hz. Thus, the peak at 0.005 Hz reflects the periodicity of the N stimulus stack. Because $0.03 = 6*0.005$, the peaks at multiples of 0.03 Hz correspond to the nonspecific response.

The amplitudes and the F-values of the sinusoidal components at $f = nf_0$ for $n \neq N, 2N, \ldots$ can be determined as described in (section 7.3.4). The data are then reconstructed from the statistically significant sinusoids. Thus, if the

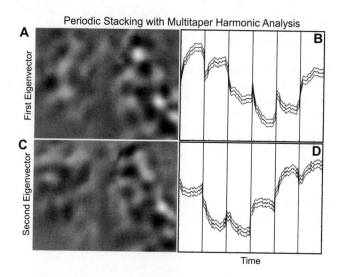

Figure 12.3: Two leading modes in the singular value decomposition of the dataset reconstructed from the statistically significant periodic responses. (A, C) These modes contain 90% of the variance of the extracted signal Spatial modes. These two modes represent basis functions that make up the orientation response in cat primary visual cortex. (B, D) Time courses (black) with one-sigma global confidence bands (gray) for 1 stack of stimuli. The vertical lines (34 sec apart) indicate the separation between responses to different orientation stimuli within a stack. (Adapted from 212].)

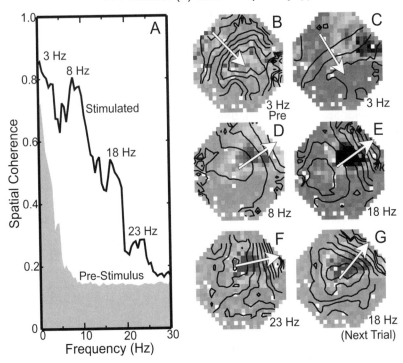

Figure 12.4: Space-frequency singular volume decomposition analysis applied to voltage sensitive dye imaging data from turtle. (A) The coherence averaged over a $T = 3$ sec interval both prior to and subsequent to the onset of visual stimulation. The coherence was estimated at successive frequency bins ($2WT = 3.0$; $K = 7$); a value of $C(f) > 0.14$ is significant. (B) Phase (contour lines) and amplitude of the leading spatial modes corresponding to $f = 3$ Hz, in the period prior to stimulation. Lighter shades indicate larger amplitudes. The phase is overlaid as a contour plot with $\pi/12$ radians per contour. The arrow indicates the direction of the phase gradient, corresponding to a traveling wave. (C–F) Corresponding phases and amplitudes at $f = 3$, 8, 18, and 22 Hz, respectively, during visual stimulation (G) Phase and amplitude at 18 Hz for the next trial with the same animal. (Reproduced from [181].)

F-test for the singular vector $u_i(t)$ is significant at frequencies f_{ij}, the reconstructed data is given by

$$I_R(t, x) = \sum_i \lambda_i v_i(x) \sum_j a_{ij} cos(2\pi f_{ij} t + \phi_{ij}) \tag{12.2}$$

where a_{ij} are the amplitudes and Φ_{ij} are the phases of the significant sinusoids.

Figure 12.3 shows the results of this analysis on the example dataset. To better visualize the response, the figure shows the two leading spatial modes and reconstructed temporal modes retaining the specific response.

Space-Frequency Singular Value Decomposition

In the discussion on space-frequency SVD in chapter 7 we mentioned that the phase gradients of the spatial modes are related to traveling waves. An illustration is provided by the example in figure 12.4. The data are measurements of neural activity in visual areas of turtle imaged using a voltage-sensitive dye [181], before and during presentation of a visual stimulus. As shown in figure 12.4A, prior to the stimulus presentation, there was a small but significant peak in the global coherence at frequencies less than 5 Hz. After stimulus presentation, the coherence increased, and several distinct peaks appeared. Note that the noise level is approximately 0.14. The phase gradient plots indicate the presence of traveling waves at the displayed frequencies.

Acknowledgments

We gratefully acknowledge the contribution of Andrew Sornborger who collaborated with us on this chapter and contributed text, figures, and bibliographic entries.

PART IV

SPECIAL TOPICS

13

Local Regression and Likelihood

Local regression and likelihood methods are nonparametric approaches for fitting regression functions and probability distributions to data. In this chapter we present a brief discussion of the basic ideas behind these methods at a level that is of relevance to the analysis of neural data. A detailed exposition of these methods and the history behind their development may be found in the monograph by Clive Loader [147].

13.1 Local Regression

Given a set of observations $x_1, \ldots, x_n$ of an independent variable x, and corresponding set of values $y_1, \ldots, y_n$ of the dependent variable y, the regression problems of interest to the current discussion have the form

$$y_i = \mu(x_i) + \varepsilon_i, \qquad (13.1)$$

Here $\mu(x)$ is the regression function to be determined from data, and ε_i are i.i.d Gaussian variables that represent noise. In the parametric case, one assumes a parametric form of the function $\mu(x; \theta)$ that specifies the function globally. The parameters in $\mu(x; \theta)$ may be determined by the method of least squares. The Gaussian and cosine tuning curves presented in chapter 8 (see figure 8.5) are instances of this procedure. This presupposes a known functional form. However, in many situations the functional form is not known in advance, and a different procedure is needed.

In local regression, one assumes only that $\mu(x)$ can be described in a local neighborhood of any point x by a low-order polynomial. The coefficients of this polynomial are determined by applying the method of least squares only in that neighborhood. This procedure is usually implemented using a local weighting function, an approach that has been referred to by the acronym LOWESS (locally weighted sum of squares).

Consider a point x and an interval $I(x) = [x - h(x), x + h(x)]$ (figure 13.1) around this point. The function $h(x)$ is known as the bandwidth. Let $x_1, \ldots, x_n$ denote observations of x within $I(x)$ and $y_1, \ldots, y_n$ denote the corresponding values of y. Now, assume that within $I(x)$ the function μ can be approximated by a polynomial of order P, namely for $u \in I(x)$,

$$\mu(u) \simeq \sum_{p=0}^{P} \beta_p(x)(u-x)^p \tag{13.2}$$

Let β be the $P+1$ dimensional vector of coefficients β_i, and let Y and ε be the $n \times 1$ dimensional vectors corresponding to the response variables y_i and the noise ε_i, respectively. The matrix X contains the independent variables,

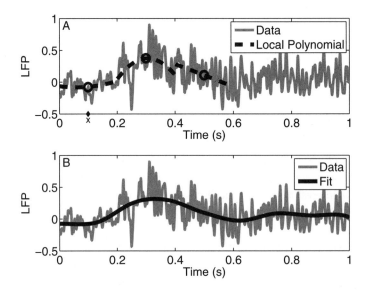

Figure 13.1: Schematic depiction of local regression. The data is a voltage segment recorded from area LIP of macaque. (A) In a window of duration 0.2 s centered on the point x, a second order polynomial is fitted to the data using weighted least squares. The constant term of the polynomial fit centered on at x is taken to be the estimate $\hat{\mu}(x)$. We show local ploynomial fits (degree two) in three windows as examples. As the window slides along the data, a smooth fit is generated. (B) Local regression fit generated by the procedure described above. LFP, local field potential.

and the ith row of X is given by $[1, (x_i - x), \ldots, (x_i - x)^P]$. The regression equation can be written in the standard form for the linear model discussed in chapter 6,

$$Y = X\beta + \varepsilon \qquad (13.3)$$

The simplest local regression procedure would employ equation (13.3) with a sliding window centered at x to determine the coefficients $\beta(x)$. The local regression estimate of $\mu(x)$ according to this procedure is given by

$$\hat{\mu}(x) = \hat{\beta}_0(x) \qquad (13.4)$$

However, in this simple procedure $\hat{\mu}(x)$ changes discontinuously as fitting points enter and leave the window. To obtain a smooth curve, one performs a weighted least squares with a weight function that is peaked at the center of the analysis window and goes to zero at the edges. A common choice is the tricube function defined by

$$w(u) = (1 - |u|^3)^3 \qquad (13.5)$$

The LOWESS is given by

$$SS = \sum_i w_i(x) \left[y_i - \sum_p (x_i - x)^p \beta_p(x) \right]^2 \qquad (13.6)$$

where the weights are given by

$$w_i(x) = w\left(\frac{x_i - x}{h(x)} \right) \qquad (13.7)$$

Defining a diagonal matrix W with diagonal elements given by the weights $w_i(x)$, the weighted sum of squares is given by

$$SS = (Y - X\beta)^\dagger W(Y - X\beta) \qquad (13.8)$$

The sum of squares is minimized to obtain

$$\beta = (X^\dagger W X)^{-1} X^\dagger W Y \qquad (13.9)$$

The local regression estimate of $\mu(x)$, $\hat{\mu}(x)$ is equal to the constant term $\hat{\beta}_0(x)$. The same procedure can be carried out all points x where the function needs to be evaluated. Figure (13.1) illustrates the procedure.

1. For a local constant regression ($P = 0$), it is possible to show that $\hat{\mu}(x)$ is simply the weighted average of $\{y_i\}$ with weights $w_i(x)$.
2. Local constant regression requires small windows, and in addition suffers from bias at the boundaries.
3. For a local linear regression, $\hat{\mu}(x)$ is the weighted average of the observations plus a correction for the local slope of the data.

13.2 Local Likelihood

The regression procedure based on the method of least squares implicitly assumes that the error variables are Gaussian distributed. In local likelihood modeling, the Gaussian assumption is relaxed—the response variables are assumed to arise from other distribution that need not be Gaussian. The *parameters* of this distribution are now modeled locally as low-order polynomials, and the coefficients are determined using the maximum likelihood procedure.

Local regression provides a local version of the linear model. Similarly, local likelihood modeling can be seen as a local version of the generalized linear model (GLM). As with local regression, local likelihood models offer flexibility because parametric forms of the model do not have to be assumed a priori.[1]

As in the previous section, consider independent variables x_i, $i = 1, \ldots, n$ within a window $I(x)$ around x and corresponding response variables y_i. Assuming that the response variables y_i are drawn from a density $f(y, \theta_i)$ where $\theta_i = \theta(x_i)$ is a function of x_i, the weighted log likelihood is defined to be

$$L(x, \theta) = \sum_{i=1}^{n} w_i(x) \log \left[f(y_i, \theta(x_i)) \right] \qquad (13.10)$$

In the regression case, a polynomial form was assumed for the functional dependence of the $\{y_i\}$ on the $\{x_i\}$. Here we assume that $\theta(x)$ can be described as a low-order polynomial within the interval $I(x)$

$$\theta(x) = \sum_{p=0}^{P} \beta_p (x_i - x)^p \qquad (13.11)$$

The coefficients can be determined by differentiating $L(x, \theta)$ with respect to β_i and setting the derivatives to zero. This gives $p + 1$ equations in $p + 1$ unknowns. For the regression case, the solution can be written in closed form (equation 13.9). This is not possible for likelihood models, and a numerical procedure has to be employed. The local likelihood estimate of the parameters is given as before by $\hat{\theta}(x) = \hat{\beta}_0(x)$.

The choice of the density depends on the problem under consideration. For example, if y_i are binary (for example, zero or one, denoting the absence or presence of a point in a binned point process), one can use a binomial likelihood model. If on the other hand, one wants to model spike count data using larger bins containing multiple points, the Poisson likelihood is more appropriate. We now discuss these two cases in more detail. The difference between what follows and the GLM discussion of chapter 6 is just that here we will maximize the weighted likelihood using a sliding window.

---

1. Local regression is equivalent to the local likelihood procedure with a Gaussian likelihood model.

13.2.1 Local Logistic Regression

Let the response variables be a sequence of ones and zeros with probability $\mu(t_i)$ and $1 - \mu(t_i)$, respectively. One application of this model would be to a sequence of binary choices y_i at times t_i, in a situation where the associated probability is time dependent. The local log-likelihood is given by

$$L(t) = \sum_{i=1}^{n} w_i(t)[y_i log(\mu(t_i)) + (1 - y_i)log(1 - \mu(t_i))] \tag{13.12}$$

$$= \sum_{i=1}^{n} w_i(t)\left[y_i log\left(\frac{\mu(t_i)}{1 - \mu(t_i)}\right) + log(1 - \mu(t_i))\right] \tag{13.13}$$

Using the logistic link function discussed in Chapter 6,

$$\theta(t) = log\left(\frac{\mu(t)}{1 - \mu(t)}\right), \tag{13.14}$$

and the log-likelihood can be written as

$$L(t) = \sum_{i=1}^{n} w_i(t)[y_i\theta(t_i) - log(1 + exp(\theta(t_i)))] \tag{13.15}$$

Now expanding $\theta(u) = \sum_{p=0}^{P} \beta_p(u - t)^p$ for $u \in I(t)$, we can solve the resulting maximization problem to get the solution $\hat{\theta}(t)$ as before. The estimate $\hat{\mu}(t)$ is found from $\hat{\theta}(t)$ by inverting equation 13.14

$$\hat{\mu}(t) = \frac{exp(\hat{\theta}(t))}{1 + exp(\hat{\theta}(t))} \tag{13.16}$$

13.2.2 Local Poisson Regression

In this case, we assume that the response variables are counts (typically in a histogram bin) given by a Poisson density. The local log-likelihood is given by

$$L(t) = \sum_{i=1}^{n} w_i(t)[y_i log(\lambda(t_i)) - log(y_i!) - \lambda(t_i)] \tag{13.17}$$

where $\lambda(t_i)$ is the rate at t_i. Because rates are constrained to be positive, we again transform to new parameters $\theta(t) = log(\lambda(t))$ and write the log-likelihood as

$$L(t) = \sum_{i=1}^{n} w_i[y_i\theta(t_i) - exp(\theta(t_i))] \tag{13.18}$$

Expanding $\theta(t)$ as a polynomial and maximizing the log-likelihood gives estimates of the coefficients as before. In the previous equation, we have dropped the $log(y_i!)$ term because it is independent of the parameters. Because $\hat{\theta}(t) = \hat{\beta}_0(t)$, we have $\hat{\lambda}(t) = exp(\hat{\beta}_0(t))$ as an estimate of the rate of the Poisson process.

13.3 Density Estimation

In many instances one is given a set of points x_i and wants to estimate their density $f(x)$. The log-likelihood is given by

$$L(f) = \sum_i \log \left(f(x_i) \right) - n \left(\int_X f(u) du - 1 \right)$$ (13.19)

Here X denotes the domain of x, and the second term enforces the constraint that the density integrates to 1. Note that density estimation is closely related to rate estimation for a finite Poisson process. Recall (from chapter 6) that for an inhomogeneous Poisson process with rate $\lambda(t)$, the log-likehood for a sequence of spike times t_i in a window $[0, T]$ is

$$L(\lambda) = \sum_i \log \left(\lambda(t_i) \right) - \int_0^T \lambda(u) du$$ (13.20)

Thus, the only difference between rate estimation for an inhomogeneous Poisson process and density estimation is that the Poisson rate does not have to integrate to 1.

Restricting the analysis to a window $I(t)$ around point t as before, the local log-likelihood for the rate estimation problem is given by

$$L(t) = \sum_{i=1}^n w_i \log \left(\lambda(t_i) \right) - n \int_{I(t)} w \left(\frac{u-t}{h(t)} \right) \lambda(u) du$$ (13.21)

Expanding $\log(\lambda(u))$ inside $I(t)$ as a low-order polynomial, $\log \left(\lambda(u) \right) = \sum_{p=0}^P \beta_p (u-t)^p$, the solution is again obtained by setting the derivatives of $L(t)$ with respect to the β_i's to zero. The local rate estimate is simply $\exp(\hat{\beta}_0(t))$, also known as the Parzen estimator.

13.4 Model Assessment and Selection

The preceding discussion has shown how local regression and likelihood models may be fit to data. We now discuss how to estimate confidence intervals and fix the two key parameters: (1) degree of the local polynomial fits, and (2) bandwidth.

13.4.1 Degrees of Freedom

As discussed in chapter 6, the degrees of freedom depends on the number of parameters. For global fits, the number of parameters is easy to determine. For example, for a global polynomial fit, the number of parameters is $p + 1$, where p is the polynomial degree. The situation is more complicated for local regression.

The fitted value $\hat{\mu}(x)$ for any x is a linear function of the response variables y_i i.e. $\hat{\mu}(x) = \sum_{i=1}^{n} l_i(x)y_i$. Assuming the independently and identically distributed noise model,

$$E[\hat{\mu}(x)] = \sum_{i=1}^{n} l_i(x)\mu(x_i) \tag{13.22}$$

$$Var[\hat{\mu}(x)] = \sigma^2 \sum_{i=1}^{n} l_i(x)^2 = \sigma^2 ||l(x)||^2 \tag{13.23}$$

where σ^2 is the variance of the y_i's. The functions $l_i(x)$, $i = 1, \ldots, n$ are known as the weight diagrams.

Equation 13.23 show that the variance of the smoothed estimate $\hat{\mu}(x_i)$ is reduced relative to the variance of the y_is by a factor $||l(x)||^2$. If the fit agrees with the data exactly we have, $l_i(x_i) = 1$ and $l_j(x_i) = 0$ for $j \neq i$. If instead, the fit is equal to the mean of the y_i's, we have $l_j(x_i) = \frac{1}{n}$. These observations motivate two definitions of the degrees of freedom that are in common use

$$v_1 = \sum_{i=1}^{n} l_i(x_i) \tag{13.24}$$

$$v_2 = \sum_{i,j=1}^{n} l_j(x_i)^2 \tag{13.25}$$

When the fit is just the sample mean, both v_1 and v_2 are equal to 1. When the fit is perfect, v_1 and v_2 are equal to n, the number of data points, reflecting the intuition that to fit stochastic data perfectly, the degrees of freedom have to equal the number of data points.

13.4.2 Selection of the Bandwidth and Polynomial Degree

The choice of the bandwidth and polynomial degree is a trade-off between bias and variance. A high-order polynomial will fit every data point but will be too variable to be useful. A low-order polynomial will have bias. Similarly, a small bandwidth will lead to a variable fit, and a large bandwidth to a biased fit. In practice, the polynomial is selected to be linear, quadratic, or at most cubic, and the selection criteria discussed below are used primarily for selecting the bandwidth.

The idea behind cross-validation is to leave out one observation, $\{x_i, y_i\}$, and to the compute the regression estimate $\hat{\mu}_{-i}(x_i)$, from the remaining $n-1$ points. One can then compute the squared difference between $\hat{\mu}_{-i}(x_i)$ and y_i, and assess the quality of the estimate by computing the cross-validation score, which provides an estimate of the generalization error

$$CV(\hat{\mu}) = \frac{1}{n}\sum_{i=1}^{n}(y_i - \hat{\mu}_{-i}(x_i))^2 \tag{13.26}$$

A good estimate should have a low cross-validation score. Computing the cross-validation score is computationally expensive because one has to drop each sample in turn and recompute the fit. The generalized cross-validation (GCV) score is an approximation to the cross-validation score, which is easier to compute. It is given by

$$GCV(\hat{\mu}) = n \frac{\sum_{i=1}^{n} (y_i - \hat{\mu}(x_i))^2}{n - v_1} \tag{13.27}$$

The cross-validation and generalized cross-validation scores are estimates of prediction errors. One can also ask how well the estimate $\hat{\mu}(x)$ agrees with the true mean $\mu(x)$ and quantify this using a loss function

$$L(\hat{\mu}, \mu) = \sum_{i=1}^{n} (\hat{\mu}(x_i) - \mu(x_i))^2 \tag{13.28}$$

Of course, we do not know the true mean. However, an unbiased estimate of $L(\hat{\mu}, \mu)$ is provided by the Mallow's CP

$$CP(\hat{\mu}(x)) = \frac{1}{\sigma^2} \sum_{i=1}^{n} (y_i - \hat{\mu}(x_i))^2 - n + 2v_1, \tag{13.29}$$

where σ^2 is typically estimated using equation 13.35 at a small bandwidth.

As mentioned in chapter 6, a generalization of residuals for likelihood models is provided by the deviance,

$$D(y_i, \hat{\theta}(x)) = 2(max_\theta \, l(y_i, \theta(x)) - l(y_i, \hat{\theta}(x))) \tag{13.30}$$

This can be interpreted as the evidence provided by an observation y_i against parameter $\hat{\theta}(x)$, and leads to a generalization of CV known as the likelihood cross-validation criterion

$$LCV(\hat{\theta}) = \sum_{i=1}^{n} D(y_i, \hat{\theta}_{-i}(x_i)) = C - 2 \sum_{i=1}^{n} l(y_i, \hat{\theta}_{-i}(x_i)) \tag{13.31}$$

Here C is a constant that does not depend on the parameters, and $\hat{\theta}_{-i}(x_i)$ is the leave-one-out estimate of θ. The equivalent of the Mallow's CP is the Akaike information criterion, given by

$$AIC(\hat{\theta}) = \sum_{i=1}^{n} D(y_i, \hat{\theta}(x_i)) + 2v_1 \tag{13.32}$$

Given an appropriate scoring procedure, the usual procedure compute the fits with varying bandwidths and to pick the bandwidth that gives the minimum score. However, as mentioned in chapter 6, one does not generally find sharp minima using this procedure. Figure 13.2 shows the GCV score for the data in figure 13.1. Note that it is conventional to plot the score versus the degrees of freedom rather than the bandwidth. The reason for this is that the meaning

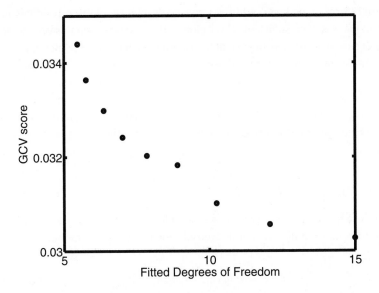

Figure 13.2: GCV score versus degrees of freedom for the data in figure 13.1.

of the bandwidth depends on the smoothing method, and the degrees of freedom is a more unambiguous measure. In our case, using about 12–15 degrees
of freedom seems reasonable. This corresponds to a bandwidth of around 200–
250 samples. Figure 13.1 was computed with a bandwidth of 200 samples.

The previous discussion of bandwidth selection and determination of polynomial degree implicitly assumes that the bandwidth and polynomial degree
are chosen independently of location. There are two ways of using an adaptive
bandwidth that depend on the data. The simplest procedure is to use bandwidth criterion based on a fixed number of neighbors. Instead of choosing a
fixed bandwidth across all locations in the data, the bandwidth is chosen so
that each window includes a fixed fraction of the total number of points. Thus
regions of high density are modeled with small bandwidths, and regions of
low density are modeled with high bandwidths. More sophisticated methods
use local versions of the criteria discussed above. This allows a choice of both
bandwidth and polynomial degree in an adaptive manner. Such schemes may
be appropriate when the data shows rapid changes in scale, but they are more
difficult to assess than the simpler scheme.

13.4.3   Residuals

An important method for assessing the quality of a local regression fit is to
study the residuals

$$\varepsilon_i = y_i - \hat{\mu}(x_i) \tag{13.33}$$

Although formal goodness of fit tests can be developed, plotting residuals in different ways is often sufficient. Thus, plots of the absolute residuals versus the fit are useful to detect dependence of the residual variance on the mean. Plotting quantiles of the residuals vs. those of a normal distribution (Q-Q plots) can help detect departures from normality, and plots of successive residuals ε_i versus ε_{i+1} help detect correlations in the residuals. Note that the definition of the residuals given above is valid for a regression problem. For likelihood models, a number of generalizations are available, including the deviance discussed above.

13.4.4 Confidence Intervals

Given the expression in the preceding section for the variance of the fitted values, approximate confidence bands around a local regression estimate $\hat{\mu}(x)$ are given by

$$(\hat{\mu}(x) - c\hat{\sigma}||l(x)||, \hat{\mu}(x) + c\hat{\sigma}||l(x)||) \tag{13.34}$$

where c is a quantile of the normal distribution ($c = 1.96$ for 95% confidence bands) and $\hat{\sigma}$ is an estimate the variance of the y_i. A commonly used estimate for this variance is

$$\hat{\sigma}^2 = \frac{1}{n - 2v_1 + v_2} \sum_{i=1}^{n} (y_i - \hat{\mu}(x_i))^2 \tag{13.35}$$

This is typically computed using a small bandwidth.

The confidence bands discussed in the previous paragraph are pointwise confidence bands. It is also possible to develop global confidence bands. Such confidence bands describe the distribution of the maximum deviation of the data from the fit. Finally, we note that based on the deviance, confidence bands can also be computed for likelihood models.

14

Entropy and Mutual Information

The most frequent statistic used to characterise the variability of a random variable is its variance. To measure the association between two random variables, the correlation coefficient is widely used. This is consistent with the method of moments, which is the approach we have mainly adopted for purposes of time series analysis in this book. In the neuroscience literature, significant use has been made of entropy as a measure of variability, and mutual information as a measure of association. Part of the attraction of these measures arise from their use in statistical physics and in communication theory. The idea is that they are free of distributional assumptions and have elevated theoretical status [50, 194] compared with second-moment measures that may be associated with Gaussian distributions.

The usage of these quantities as statistical measures is a mixed blessing. It is true that they are theoretically elegant and have desirable invariance properties. However, apart from difficulties of estimation, they are *by construction* not informative about the shape of the distributions or the nature of the functional relationships between variables. In trying to gain an understanding of a neural system, one might want more detailed characterisations of neural time series and the relations between them. Nevertheless, these measures are in use and may on occasion provide useful supplements to other more detailed characterisations of the variability and functional relationships between time series. We therefore include a brief review of the relevant information theoretic approaches, including links to Gaussian processes and inhomogeneous Poisson processes.

14.1 Entropy and Mutual Information for Discrete Random Variables

From the earlier section on probability theory in the chapter on mathematical preliminaries, recall the definition of the Gibbs-Shannon entropy[1] of a discrete valued random variable that takes values labeled by the index i with probability p_i

$$H = -\sum_i p_i \log (p_i) \tag{14.1}$$

The simplest example is that of a Bernoulli distribution, or a binary random variable taking two values with probability p and $1-p$. The corresponding entropy is given by

$$H = -p \log (p) - (1-p) \log (1-p) \tag{14.2}$$

The maximum value is achieved for $p = 1/2$, which is consistent with the "most variable" case. One may alwo write $H = -E[\log(p)]$. Another example to keep in mind is that of the Poisson distribution with parameter λ. The entropy is given in terms of an infinite sum, by

$$H = -E\left[\log\left(\frac{\lambda^n e^{-\lambda}}{n!}\right)\right]$$
$$= \lambda(1 - \log (\lambda)) + \sum_{n=1}^{\infty} \frac{\log (n!)\lambda^n e^{-\lambda}}{n!} \tag{14.3}$$

For large λ, the asymptotic form of this expression is

$$H \approx \frac{1}{2} \log (2\pi e \lambda) \tag{14.4}$$

This can be understood as follows—the Poisson distribution has variance λ and standard deviation $\sqrt{\lambda}$. Assuming the distribution is uniform over a set of integers of size proportional to the standard deviation, one obtains the form of the entropy for large λ, apart from numerical constants.

Other similar measures have been defined. The Renyi entropy [193] of order α is defined as

$$H_\alpha = \frac{\log (\sum_i p_i^\alpha)}{1-\alpha} \tag{14.5}$$

The usual entropy is recovered in the limit $\alpha \to 1$. A slightly different limiting procedure is given by the so called "replica trick" well known in the statistical physics literature,

---

1. We will refer to this quantity as the entropy without further qualification.

$$\log (p) = \lim_{n \to 0} \frac{p^n - 1}{n} \qquad (14.6)$$

The replica trick originates from the observation that $E[z^n]$ is typically easier to compute than $E[\log(z)]$. It follows that[2]

$$H = \lim_{n \to 1} \frac{1 - E[p^{n-1}]}{n-1} \qquad (14.7)$$

These two alternatively defined entropies may be used to bound the Gibbs-Shannon entropy. The Renyi entropy for $\alpha = 2$ provides such a bound. It is the logarithm of the fraction of coincidences, and was investigated by Ma [149] for estimation of entropies from dynamical trajectories.

Recall the definition of the Kullback-Leiber (KL) divergence $D(p\|q)$ (also known as relative entropy), given for discrete probability distributions by

$$D(p\|q) = \sum_i p_i \log (p_i / q_i) \qquad (14.8)$$

We have previously noted that $D(p\|q) \geq 0$. The KL divergence indicates how difficult it would be to determine whether samples drawn from the distribution p, were not actually drawn from the distribution q, and plays a fundamental role in coding theory [138].

The KL divergence between two Poisson distributions with parameters λ_1 and λ_2 has a simpler form

$$D(p_{\lambda_1}\|p_{\lambda_2}) = (\lambda_1 - \lambda_2) - \lambda_1 \log \left(\frac{\lambda_1}{\lambda_2}\right) \qquad (14.9)$$

The mutual information $I(X, Y)$ between two discrete random variables X, Y, with joint probability distribution $p(X_i, Y_j) = p_{ij}$, is defined as the relative entropy between the joint distribution p_{ij} and the product of the marginal distributions $p(X_i) = p_i$ and $p(Y_i) = q_i$

$$I(X, Y) = D(p(X, Y)\|p(X)p(Y)) = \sum_{ij} p_{ij} \log \left(\frac{p_{ij}}{p_i q_j}\right) \qquad (14.10)$$

The mutual information can also be expressed in terms of conditional entropies

$$I(X, Y) = H(Y) - H(Y|X) \qquad (14.11)$$
$$I(X, Y) = H(X) - H(X|Y) \qquad (14.12)$$

The conditional entropy $H(Y|X)$ is defined by first fixing the variable X and computing the entropy of the conditional probability distribution for Y, and then averaging over Y.

---

2. The quantity on the right hand side (of which the limit is taken) has been designated the Tsallis entropy [223].

The mutual information satisfies the *data processing inequality* [50]. If Z is derived from Y, which is itself derived from X, then $I(X, Y) \geq I(X, Z)$. This has the intuitive meaning that any signal processing performed on a variable Y cannot increase the mutual information between the variable Y and an underlying source variable X. Put differently, some signal could be lost (but none added) when performing any signal processing.

This does not mean that signal processing is a bad thing: one may be willing to give up a little bit of signal if a lot of noise can be removed in the process, improving the signal-to-noise ratio. In many applications, the final goal is to make a decision between alternatives, which does entail loss of information. Whether this information is lost in two stages, with a primary signal processing stage, and a secondary decision stage, or a combined decision stage, is an architectural choice. Also, data reduction is essential to making any progress in analysing and visualising large volumes of data.

The concept of mutual information readily generalises to more than two random variables and has been used to formulate indices of redundancy and synergy between multiple variables.

14.2   Continuous Random Variables

The definition of entropy does not naturally generalize to continuous valued random variables described by a probability density function $p(x)$. This can be seen by approximating the continuous variable on a discrete grid x_i with spacing Δx. The probability measure associated with a grid point may be approximated as $p(x_i)\Delta x$. Applying the definition of entropy to this discrete random variable gives

$$
\begin{aligned}
H &= -\sum_i p(x_i)\Delta x \, \log \, (p(x_i)\Delta x) \\
&= -\sum_i p(x_i)\Delta x \, \log \, (p(x_i)) - \log \, (\Delta x)
\end{aligned}
\tag{14.13}
$$

The first term in this sum has a limiting value referred to as the differential entropy

$$
H_{diff} = -\int dx p(x) \, \log \, (p(x))
\tag{14.14}
$$

Unfortunately, the second term does not have a meaningful limit, so that the entropy of the continuous valued random variable is not well defined. This limits the utility of the notion of entropy for a single continuous random variable. The *difference* between the entropies between two random variables on the same domain can be defined as the difference between the corresponding differential entropies.

The KL divergence or *relative* entropy between two continuous distributions does not suffer from these discretisation difficulties and is well defined. It is given by

$$D(p||q) = \int dx p(x) \, \log \, (p(x)/q(x)) \qquad (14.15)$$

Similarly, the mutual information between two continuous random variables is also well defined, and is given by

$$I(X, Y) = \int dx dy p(x, y) \, \log \left(\frac{p(x, y)}{p(x)q(y)} \right) \qquad (14.16)$$

As an example, consider the relative entropy between two Gaussian distributions with variances σ_1^2 and σ_2^2. This is given by

$$D(p_1||p_2) = \frac{1}{2} \log \left(\frac{\sigma_2^2}{\sigma_1^2} \right) + \frac{\sigma_1^2}{\sigma_2^2} - 1 \qquad (14.17)$$

As an example of a mutual information computation, consider two Gaussian variables with equal variances σ^2 and correlation coefficient ρ. The mutual information is then given by

$$H = -\frac{1}{2} \log \, (1 - \rho^2) \qquad (14.18)$$

It should be noted that the mutual information in this case is simply a transform of the correlation coefficient ρ.

14.3   Discrete-Valued Discrete-Time Stochastic Processes

A finite segment of a discrete-valued, discrete-time stochastic process corresponds to a discrete-valued random variable itself, and the entropy can be defined as earlier. For most stochastic processes of interest (such as stationary processes), the entropy and the mutual information are extensive quantities,[3] so that for long time intervals they become proportional to the length of the time interval. One may therefore define entropy rates

$$H_{rate}(X) = \lim_{T \to \infty} \frac{1}{T} H_T(X) \qquad (14.19)$$

If the discrete-valued random variable is uncorrelated from one time point to the next, then the entropy rate is simply the entropy of the variable at a single time point. A simple example of a correlated process for which entropies

---

3. This terminology is borrowed from statistical physics, where the thermodynamic quantities are said to be extensive if they are proportional to the volume, in the large volume limit. The Renyi entropy is also extensive, but the Tsallis entropy is not.

can be calculated analytically is that of a Markov chain. In a Markov chain, the conditional probability of a variable (conditioned on the past) depends only on the value at the previous time point

$$p(x_t|x_{t-1}, x_{t-2}, \ldots) = p(x_t|x_{t-1}) \qquad (14.20)$$

The Markov chain is fully specified in terms of the on-site probability p_i and the transition probability $\pi_{j|i}$. In terms of these two quantities, the entropy rate of the Markov process is given by

$$H_{rate} = -\sum_{ij} p_i \pi_{j|i} \log (\pi_{j|i}) \qquad (14.21)$$

14.4   Continuous-Valued Discrete-Time Stochastic Processes

The difficulties with defining entropies for continuous random variables carry over to stochastic processes, and additional difficulties may appear due to the difficulties of defining stochastic processes measures as discussed earlier in the book. We therefore focus on relative entropies and mutual information, because these are well defined. We confine ourselves to discrete-time or bandlimited continuous processes to avoid divergences coming from infinitely high frequencies. For two Gaussian stochastic processes, the role of the variances is played by the corresponding power spectra $S_1(f)$ and $S_2(f)$. Further, different frequencies are independent, and the corresponding relative entropies add. The relative entropy rate of two processes is then given by

$$D_{rate} = -\int_{-1/2}^{1/2} df \left(\frac{1}{2} \log \left(\frac{S_2(f)}{S_1(f)} \right) + \frac{S_1(f)}{S_2(f)} - 1 \right) \qquad (14.22)$$

The mutual information rate between two Gaussian processes is given in terms of the cross-coherence between the two processes

$$I_{rate} = -\frac{1}{2} \int_{-1/2}^{1/2} df \log (1 - |C(f)|^2) \qquad (14.23)$$

The mutual information for the bivariate Gaussian process is the source of a useful inequality. Consider the pair (X_G, Y) where X_G has a Gaussian distribution, but that the distribution of Y is not necessarily Gaussian. Consider a second pair (X_G, Y_G), where both X_G and Y_G are Gaussian distributed, and the second-order statistics of the pair (X_G, Y_G) are matched with the corresponding statistics of the pair (X_G, Y). In other words, (X_G, Y_G) has the same covariance matrix or cross-spectral matrix as the pair (X_G, Y). Then it can be shown that [160]

$$I(X_G, Y) \geq I(X_G, Y_G) \qquad (14.24)$$

The utility of this Gaussian lower bound lies in the fact that the cross-covariance or the cross-spectral matrix of X_G (which could be thought of as a noise stimulus input to a sensory modality), and Y (which could be a measure of the neural response) can be estimated with relative ease, using the methods described earlier in the book. The mutual information rate formula for a bivariate Gaussian process can then be used to estimate a lower bound to the true mutual information between the inputs and the outputs. In case it is legitimate to think of the corresponding input output relationship as a communication channel, along with the corresponding encoder and decoder, this Gaussian lower bound then also provides a lower bound for the channel capacity for fixed input power.

The relative entropy rates or mutual information rates cannot in general be computed analytically for non-Gaussian processes, with rare exceptions, and Monte Carlo methods have to be employed to estimate these quantities.

14.5 Point Processes

A finite point process (which has a finite number of points with probability one) is specified in terms of a family of density functions $p(t_1, t_2, \ldots, t_n; n)$. The relative entropy between two such processes can be defined as earlier

$$D(p\|q) = -\sum_n \int dt_1 dt_2 \ldots dt_n p(t_1, t_2, \ldots, t_n; n) \log \left(\frac{p(t_1, t_2, \ldots, t_n; n)}{q(t_1, t_2, \ldots, t_n; n)} \right)$$
$$(14.25)$$

For two Poisson processes on a finite interval T, this equation yields

$$D(\lambda_1 \| \lambda_2) = T \left[\lambda_1 - \lambda_2 - \lambda_1 \log \left(\frac{\lambda_1}{\lambda_2} \right) \right] \qquad (14.26)$$

The coefficient of T is the relative entropy rate. Although the entropy rate of a Poisson process is not well defined [150], the relative entropy rate is, and one may adopt a unit rate process as a standard to compute relative entropies.

The entropy of an inhomogeneous Poisson process with intensity $\lambda(t)$ on a given time interval $[0\ T]$ with respect to a constant rate Poisson process λ_0 is given by

$$\int_0^T dt \left[\lambda(t) - \lambda_0 - \lambda(t) \log \left(\frac{\lambda(t)}{\lambda_0} \right) \right] \qquad (14.27)$$

As for continuous valued processes, the relative entropy rates or mutual information rates cannot be computed analytically for most point process models of interest. There is an extensive literature in physics applying Monte Carlo methods to models of point particles with Gibbs probability distributions. Entropy densities are one of the thermodynamic quantities that may be evaluated in these models, and these numerical methods apply to point processes as well.

14.6 Estimation Methods

Consider the simplest Bernoulli case of a binary random variable taking the two values $(0, 1)$ with $p(1) = p$. Consider a sample of size n from which the probability p can be estimated using the relative fraction $f = n_1/n$. Now f is an unbiased estimator of p, because $E[f] = p$. However, the simple substitution of f for p in the formula for entropy

$$\hat{H} = -f \log (f) - (1-f) \log (1-f) \tag{14.28}$$

leads to a biased estimate. This can be seen by noting that the entropy function $H(x)$ is strictly convex, with $H(\alpha x + (1 - \alpha)x) > H(x)$, which implies that

$$E[\hat{H}] = E[H(f)] < H(E[f]) = H(p) \tag{14.29}$$

Thus, the simple estimator obtained by substitution is biased downward. This bias does go to zero for large sample size. For large sample sizes, the bias has a simple asymptotic form, depending only on the number of samples n and the number of bins k (or values of the discrete variable) [154]. However, one is typically not in the asymptotic regime $k/n \ll 1$, because one is normally interested in high dimensional distributions corresponding to discretized stochastic processes. In the undersampled regime, the asymptotic corrections are not useful.

There is a significant literature on the estimation of entropies and mutual information in the context of neural spike trains. We will not cover these methods in any detail here, but will note some of the basic ideas. Many of these have been recently reviewed [231]. One way to proceed is to estimate the density function of the stochastic process using an appropriate model and then calculate the entropy rates or mutual information for the model. In particular, the Gaussian bound provides a useful route for continuous stochastic processes when one of the processes has a Gaussian distribution. Model-based approaches can also be used for spike trains that have been been discretized into symbol sequences [135].

Much of the interest in this area has been for computing mutual entropies between spike trains and input stimuli. The stimuli may belong to a discrete set or may consist of continuous stochastic processes themselves. One may attempt to directly discretize the space of spike trains by binning time, and consider appropriate limiting procedures where the binsize is taken to zero and the length of the time interval subjected to such binning allowed to grow large. Such time binning introduces significant bias, because the number of bins (the number of possible discretized words) grows exponentially as time resolution is refined. Better bias correction methods may provide some help in this circumstance [161, 174].

An alternative is to avoid binning altogether by embedding segments of point processes into a vector space [232] or a metric space [233]. In the former case, nearest neighbor distances provide an asymptotically unbiased estimate of entropy [137]; in the latter case, a lower bound for mutual information between the spike train and the stimuli can be estimated by comparing the distances within a stimulus cluster, and between stimulus clusters.

Acknowledgments

We gratefully acknowledge the contributions of Jonathan Victor for an initial draft from which material for this chapter was drawn in the form of ideas, text, and bibliographic entries.

Appendix A
The Bandwagon
C. E. Shannon

Information theory has, in the last few years, become something of a scientific bandwagon. Starting as a technical tool for the communication engineer, it has received an extraordinary amount of publicity in the popular as well as the scientific press. In part, this has been due to connections with such fashionable fields as computing machines, cybernetics, and automation; and in part, to the novelty of its subject matter. As a consequence, it has perhaps been ballooned to an importance beyond its actual accomplishments. Our fellow scientists in many different fields, attracted by the fanfare and by the new avenues opened to scientific analysis, are using these ideas in their own problems. Applications are being made to biology, psychology, linguistics, fundamental physics, economics, the theory of organization, and many others. In short, information theory is currently partaking of a somewhat heady draught of general popularity.

Although this wave of popularity is certainly pleasant and exciting for those of us working in the field, it carries at the same time an element of danger. While we feel that information theory is indeed a valuable tool in providing fundamental insights into the nature of communication problems and will continue to grow in importance, it is certainly no panacea for the communication engineer or, a fortiori, for anyone else. Seldom do more than a few of nature's secrets give way at one time. It will be all too easy for our somewhat artificial prosperity to collapse overnight when it is realized that the use of a few exciting words like *information, entropy, redundancy,* do not solve all our problems.

What can be done to inject a note of moderation in this situation? In the first place, workers in other fields should realize that the basic results of the subject

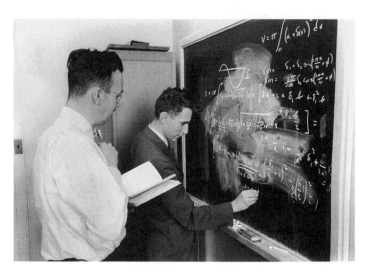

Figure 1: Claude Shannon, the originator of information theory, and Dave Hagelbarger work out some equations at the board at Bell Laboratories. The photo is dated 1955.

are aimed in a very specific direction, a direction that is not necessarily relevant to such fields as psychology, economics, and other social sciences. Indeed, the hard core of information theory is, essentially, a branch of mathematics, a strictly deductive system. A thorough understanding of the mathematical foundation and its communication application is surely a prerequisite to other applications. I personally believe that many of the concepts of information theory will prove useful in these other fields—and, indeed, some results are already quite promising—but the establishing of such applications is not a trivial matter of translating words to a new domain, but rather the slow tedious process of hypothesis and experimental verification. If, for example, the human being acts in some situations like an ideal decoder, this is an experimental and not a mathematical fact, and as such must be tested under a wide variety of experimental situations.

Secondly, we must keep our own house in first class order. The subject of information theory has certainly been sold, if not oversold. We should now turn our attention to the business of research and development at the highest scientific plane we can maintain. Research rather than exposition is the keynote, and our critical thresholds should be raised. Authors should submit only their best efforts, and these only after careful criticism by themselves and their colleagues. A few first rate research papers are preferable to a large number that are poorly conceived or half finished. The latter are no credit to their writers and a waste of time to their readers. Only by maintaining a thoroughly scientific attitude can we achieve real progress in communication theory and consolidate our present position.

Appendix B
Two Famous Papers

Peter Elias

It is common in editorials to discuss matters of general policy and not specific research. But the two papers I would like to describe have been written so often, by so many different authors under so many different titles, that they have earned editorial consideration.

The first paper has the generic title "Information Theory, Photosynthesis and Religion" (title courtesy of D. A. Huffman), and is written by an engineer or physicist. It discusses the surprisingly close relationship between the vocabulary and conceptual framework of information theory and that of psychology (or genetics, or linguistics, or psychiatry, or business organization). It is pointed out that the concepts of structure, pattern, entropy, noise, transmitter, receiver, and code are (when properly interpreted) central to both. Having placed the discipline of psychology for the first time on a sound scientific base, the author modestly leaves the filling in of the outline to the psychologists. He has, of course, read up on the field in preparation for writing the paper, and has a firm grasp of the essentials, but he has been anxious not to clutter his mind with such details as the state of knowledge in the field, what the central problems are, how they are being attacked, et cetera, et cetera, et cetera.

There is a constructive alternative for the author of this paper. If he is willing to give up larceny for a life of honest toil, he can find a competent psychologist and spend several years at intensive mutual education, leading to productive joint research. But this has some disadvantages from his point of view. First, psychology would not be placed on a sound scientific base for several extra years. Second, he might find himself, as so many have, diverted from the broader questions, wasting his time on problems whose only merit is that they are vitally important, unsolved, and in need of interdisciplinary effort. In fact, he might spend so much time solving such problems that psychology never *would* be placed on a sound scientific base.

The second paper is typically called "The Optimum Linear Mean Square Filter for Separating Sinusoidally modulated Triangular Signals from Randomly Sampled Stationary Gaussian Noise, with Applications to a Problem in Radar." The details vary from version to version, but the initial physical problem has as its major interest its obvious nonlinearity. An effective discussion of this problem would require some really new thinking of a difficult sort, so the author quickly substitutes an unrelated linear problem which is more amenable to analysis. He treats this irrelevant linear problem in a very general way, and by a triumph of analytical technique is able to present its solution, not quite in closed form, but as the solution to an integral equation whose kernel is the solution to another, bivariate integral equation. He notes that the problem is now in a form in which standard numerical analysis techniques, and one of the micromicrosecond computers which people are now beginning to discuss, can provide detailed answers to specific questions. Many authors might rest here (in fact many do), but ours wants real insight into the character of the results. By carefully taking limits and investigating asymptotic behavior he succeeds in showing that in a few very special cases (which include all those which have any conceivable application or offer any significant insight) the results of this analysis agree with the results of the Wiener-Lee-Zadeh-Raggazzini theory—the very results, indeed, which Wiener, Lee, Zadeh, and Raggazzini obtained years before.

These two papers have been written—and even published—often enough by now.

I suggest that we stop writing them, and release a large supply of manpower to work on the exciting and important problems which need investigation.

Photograph Credits

Cara Allen collected the photographs that appear in this book and secured permission for their reproduction. She is grateful to Douglas Atkins at the National Library of Medicine (Bethesda, MD); Bernard Horrocks and Susanna Brown at the National Portrait Gallery (London); Clare Clark at Cold Spring Harbor Laboratory (Cold Spring Harbor, NY); Alicja Kawecki, Ed Eckert, Henry Landau, and Adriaan De Lind Van Wijngaarden of Alcatel-Lucent/Bell Laboratories (Murray Hill, NJ); and Frank Conahan at the MIT Museum (Cambridge, MA), for their kind assistance.

1. Cover image: Detail of the Mona Lisa, c. 1503–6 (panel) (see 3179) by Vinci, Leonardo da (1452–1519); Louvre, Paris, France; The Bridgeman Art Library. Cover design: Cara Allen.
2. Fig. 1.3, Norbert Wiener. Courtesy MIT Museum.
3. Fig. 2.2, Sir Charles Scott Sherrington. Courtesy of the National Library of Medicine.
4. Fig. 2.5, Hermann Ludwig Ferdinand von Helmholtz. Courtesy of the National Library of Medicine.
5. Fig. 3.3, Claude Shannon. Courtesy MIT Museum.
6. Fig. 3.5, Alan Turing. Life Magazine/Time & Life Pictures/Getty Images.
7. Fig. 4.3, Sir Francis Bacon. Courtesy of the National Library of Medicine.
8. Fig. 4.4 Illustration by Sir John Tenniel, from Alice's Adventures in Wonderland by Lewis Carroll (1865).
9. Fig. 5.2, Jean Baptiste Joseph Fourier. From "Portraits et Histoire des Hommes Utiles, Collection de Cinquante Portraits," Societe Montyon et Franklin, 1839–1840. Reproduced in accord with Creative Commons ShareAlike License v. 3.0.
10. Fig. 6.1 Ronald Aylmer Fisher. Photograph by A. Barrington Brown, courtesy of the Fisher Memorial Trust.

11. Fig. 6.2, John W. Tukey. Reprinted with permission of Alcatel-Lucent.
12. Fig. 8.1, James D Watson and Alan Lloyd Hodkin. Courtesy of Cold Spring Harbor Laboratory Archives.
13. Fig. 8.2, Andrew Fielding Huxley, Photograph by Walter Bird, 1963, reproduced with kind permission of Mrs. A. M. Bird. Courtesy of the National Library of Medicine.
14. Fig. 8.6, Cat LGN. Reprinted with permission from Blackwell Publishing.
15. Appendix 1, Claude Shannon and Dave Hagelbarger, reprinted with permission of Alcatel-Lucent.

.

References

[1] M. Abeles, M.H. Goldstein. Multispike train analysis. *Proc IEEE.* 65(5):762–773, 1977.

[2] W.R. Adey, D.O. Walter, C.E. Hendrix. Computer techniques in correlation and spectral analyses of cerebral slow waves during discriminative behavior. *Exp Neurol.* 3:501–524, 1961.

[3] E.D. Adrian. Electrical activity of the nervous system. *Arch Neurol Psychiat.* 32:1125–1136, 1932.

[4] E.D. Adrian. The impulses produced by sensory nerve endings. Part 1. *J Physiol.* 61:49–72, 1926.

[5] E.D. Adrian, B.H.C. Matthews. The Berger rhythm: potential changes from the occipital lobes in man. *Brain.* 57:355–385, 1934.

[6] E.D. Adrian, Y. Zotterman. The impulses produced by sensory nerve endings: Part 2. The response of a single end-organ. *J Physiol.* 61:151–171, 1926.

[7] E.D. Adrian, Y. Zotterman. The impulses produced by sensory nerve endings. Part 3. Impulses produced by touch and pressure. *J Physiol.* 61:465–483, 1926.

[8] O. Aftab, P. Cheung, A. Kim, S. Thakkar, N. Yeddanapudi. Information theory and the digital revolution. Project history MIT 6:933, 1–27, 2001.

[9] I.A. Ahmad. Multisample jackknife statistics. *Survey Research Methods Section of the American Statistical Assoc.* Page 318–322, 1981.

[10] K.F. Ahrens, H. Levine, H. Suhl, D. Kleinfeld. Spectral mixing of rhythmic neuronal signals in sensory cortex. *Proc Natl Acad Sci U S A.* 99(23):15176–15181, 2002.

[11] J. Arvesen. Jackknifing U-Statistics. *Ann of Math Statistics.* 40(6):2076, 1969.

[12] J. Ashburner, J.L. Andersson, K.J. Friston. High-dimensional image registration using symmetric priors. *Neuroimage.* 9(6 Pt 1):619–628, 1999.

[13] S. Baillet, J.C. Mosher, R.M. Leahy. Electromagnetic brain mapping. *IEEE Signal Processing Magazine.* 18(6):14–30, 2001.

[14] B.J. Baker, E.K. Kosmidis, D. Vucinic, et al. Imaging brain activity with voltage- and calcium-sensitive dyes. *Cell Mol Neurobiol.* 25(2):245–282, 2005.

[15] P.A. Bandettini, A. Jesmanowicz, E.C. Wong, J.S. Hyde. Processing strategies for time-course data sets in functional MRI of the human brain. *Magn Reson Med.* 30(2):161–173, 1993.

[16] R. Barbieri, L.M. Frank, M.C. Quirk, M.A. Wilson, E.N. Brown. Diagnostic methods for statistical models of place cell spiking activity. *Neurocomputing.* 38:1087–1093, 2001.

[17] J.S. Barlow. EMG artifact minimization during clinical EEG recordings by special analog filtering. *Electroencephalogr Clin Neurophysiol.* 58(2):161–174, 1984.

[18] J.S. Barlow. The early history of EEG data-processing at the Massachusetts Institute of Technology and the Massachusetts General Hospital. *Int J Psychophysiol.* 26(1–3):443–454, 1997.

[19] J.S. Barlow, M.A. Brazier. A note on a correlator for electroencephalographic work. *Electroencephalogr Clin Neurophysiol Suppl.* 6(2):321–325, 1954.

[20] M.F. Bear, B.W. Connors, M.A. Paradiso. *Neuroscience: Exploring the Brain.* 3rd ed. Philadelphia, PA: Lippincott Williams & Wilkins; 2007.

[21] S. Behseta, R.E. Kass. Testing equality of two functions using bars. *Stat Med.* 24(22):3523–3534, 2005.

[22] Y. Benjamini, Y. Hochberg. Controlling the false discovery rate—a practical and powerful approach to multiple testing. *J Roy Statistical Society Series B–Methodological.* 57(1):289–300, 1995.

[23] M.R. Bennett, P.M.S. Hacker. *Philosophical Foundations of Neuroscience.* Oxford, England: Blackwell; 2003.

[24] H. Berger. Uber das electroenzephalorgamm des menschen. *Archiv fur Psychiatrie und Nervenkrankheiten.* 87:527–570, 1929.

[25] T. Berger. Living information theory. *IEEE Information Theory Society Newsletter.* 53(1):1, 2003.

[26] R.M. Birn, P.A. Bandettini, R.W. Cox, A. Jesmanowicz, R. Shaker. Magnetic field changes in the human brain due to swallowing or speaking. *Magn Reson Med.* 40(1):55–60, 1998.

[27] B. Biswal, F.Z. Yetkin, V.M. Haughton, J.S. Hyde. Functional connectivity in the motor cortex of resting human brain using echo-planar MRI. *Magn Reson Med.* 34(4):537–541, 1995.

[28] G.G. Blasdel. Differential imaging of ocular dominance and orientation selectivity in monkey striate cortex. *J Neurosci.* 12(8):3115–3138, 1992.

[29] G.G. Blasdel. Orientation selectivity, preference, and continuity in monkey striate cortex. *J Neurosci.* 12(8):3139–3161, 1992.

[30] L. Blum, F. Cucker, M. Shub, S. Smale. *Complexity and Real Computation.* New York, NY: Springer; 1998.

[31] R. de Boer, P. Kuyper. Triggered correlation. *IEEE Trans Biomed Eng.* 15(3): 169–179, 1968.

[32] H. Bokil, K. Purpura, J.M. Schoffelen, D. Thomson, P. Mitra. Comparing spectra and coherences for groups of unequal size. *J Neurosci Methods.* 159(2): 337–345, 2007.

[33] H.S. Bokil, B. Pesaran, R.A. Andersen, P.P. Mitra. A method for detection and classification of events in neural activity. *IEEE Trans Biomed Eng.* 53(8): 1678–1687, 2006.

[34] G.M. Boynton, S.A. Engel, G.H. Glover, D.J. Heeger. Linear systems analysis of functional magnetic resonance imaging in human V1. *J Neurosci.* 16(13): 4207–4221, 1996.

[35] M.A. Brazier. Electroencephalography. *Prog Neurol Psychiatry*. 11:119–144, 1956.

[36] M.A. Brazier, J.U. Casby. Cross-correlation and autocorrelation studies of electroencephalographic potentials. *Electroencephalogr Clin Neurophysiol Suppl.* 4(2):201–211, 1952.

[37] D.R. Brillinger. The 1983 Wald memorial lectures—some statistical-methods for random process data from seismology and neurophysiology. *Ann. Statistics.* 16(1):1–54, 1988.

[38] D.R. Brillinger, H.L. Bryant, J.P. Segundo. Identification of synaptic interactions. *Biol Cybernetics.* 22(4):213–228, 1976.

[39] D.R. Brillinger, J.P. Segundo. Empirical-examination of the threshold-model of neuron firing. *Biol Cybernetics.* 35(4):213–220, 1979.

[41] E.N. Brown. Theory of point processes for neural systems. In: C. Chow, B. Gutkin, D. Hansel, C. Meunier, J. Dalibard, eds. *Methods and Models in Neurophysics, Session LXXX*, Elsevier, 2003: 862.

[42] E.N. Brown, L.M. Frank, D.D. Tang, M.C. Quirk, M.A. Wilson. A statistical paradigm for neural spike train decoding applied to position prediction from ensemble firing patterns of rat hippocampal place cells. *J Neurosci.* 18(18): 7411–7425, 1998.

[43] E.N. Brown, R.E. Kass, P.P. Mitra. Multiple neural spike train data analysis: state-of-the-art and future challenges. *Nature Neurosci.* 7(5):456–461, 2004.

[44] E.N. Brown, D.P. Nguyen, L.M. Frank, M.A. Wilson, V. Solo. An analysis of neural receptive field plasticity by point process adaptive filtering. *Proc Natl Acad Sci U S A.* 98(21):12261–12266, 2001.

[44] G. Buzsaki. Large-scale recording of neuronal ensembles. *Nature Neurosci.* 7(5):446–451, 2004.

[45] J.M. Carmena, M.A. Lebedev, R.E. Crist, et al. Learning to control a brain-machine interface for reaching and grasping by primates. *PLoS Biol.* 1(2): 193–208, 2003.

[46] W.S. Cleveland. *Visualizing Data.* AT & T Bell Laboratories. Murray Hill, Summit, NJ: Hobart Press; 1993.

[47] D. Cohen. Magnetoencephalography: detection of the brain's electrical activity with a superconducting magnetometer. *Science.* 175(22):664–666, 1972.

[48] D. Cohen. Magnetoencephalography: evidence of magnetic fields produced by alpha-rhythm currents. *Science.* 161(843):784–786, 1968.

[49] D. Cohen, E. Halgren. Magnetoencephalography (neuromagnetism). In G. Adelman, B.H. Smith, eds. *Encyclopedia of Neuroscience.* Amsterdam, Netherlands: Elsevier BV; 2004.

[50] T.M. Cover, J.A. Thomas. *Elements of Information Theory.* Wiley Series in Telecommunications. New York, NY: Wiley; 1991.

[51] R.J. Croft, R.J. Barry. Removal of ocular artifact from the EEG: a review. *Neurophysiol Clin.* 30(1):5–19, 2000.

[52] R.J. Croft, J.S. Chandler, R.J. Barry, N.R. Cooper, A.R. Clarke. EOG correction: a comparison of four methods. *Psychophysiology.* 42(1):16–24, 2005.

[53] A.M. Dale. Optimal experimental design for event-related fMRI. *Hum Brain Mapp.* 8(2–3):109–114, 1999.

[54] D.J. Daley, D. Vere-Jones. *An Introduction to the Theory of Point Processes.* New York, NY: Springer; 2003.

[55] G.D. Dawson. Autocorrelation and automatic integration. *Electroencephalography Clinical Neurophysiology.* Supplement 4:26–37, 1954.

[56] P. Dayan, L.F. Abbott. *Theoretical neuroscience: computational and mathematical modeling of neural systems.* Computational neuroscience. Cambridge, MA: MIT Press; 2001.

[57] L. Denby, C.L. Mallows. Computing sciences and statistics. Proceedings of the 23rd Symposium on the Interface. Fairfax Station, VA: Interface Foundation; 1991: 54–57.

[58] G. Dietsch. Fourier-analyse von elektrenkephalogrammen des menschen. *Pflger's Arch. Ges. Physiol.* 230:106–112, 1932.

[59] I. DiMatteo, C.R. Genovese, R.E. Kass. Bayesian curve-fitting with free-knot splines. *Biometrika.* 88(4):1055–1071, 2001.

[60] A.G. Dimitrov, J.P. Miller, T. Gedeon, Z. Aldworth, A.E. Parker. Analysis of neural coding through quantization with an information-based distortion measure. *Network-Computation in Neural Systems.* 14(1):151–176, 2003.

[61] J.P. Donoghue. Connecting cortex to machines: recent advances in brain interfaces. *Nature Neurosci.* 5:1085–1088, 2002.

[62] J.C. Doyle, B.A. Francis, A. Tannenbaum. *Feedback Control Theory.* Macmillan Pub. Co. New York, 1992.

[63] R.O. Duda, P.E. Hart, D.G. Stork. *Pattern Classification.* 2nd ed. New York, NY: Wiley; 2001.

[64] T.J. Ebner, G. Chen. Use of voltage-sensitive dyes and optical recordings in the central nervous system. *Prog Neurobiol.* 46(5):463–506, 1995.

[65] B. Efron. *The jackknife, the bootstrap, and other resampling plans.* CBMS-NSF Regional Conference Series in Applied Mathematics; 38. Society for Industrial and Applied Mathematics, Philadelphia, PA, 1982.

[66] B. Efron, R. Tibshirani. *An Introduction to the Bootstrap.* Monographs on Statistics and Applied Probability; 57. New York, NY: Chapman & Hall; 1993.

[67] R. Elul. Gaussian behavior of the electroencephalogram: changes during performance of mental task. *Science.* 164(877):328–331, 1969.

[68] R. Everson, B.W. Knight, L. Sirovich. Separating spatially distributed response to stimulation from background.1. optical imaging. *Biol. Cybernetics.* 77(6): 407–417, 1997.

[69] U. Fano. Ionization yield of rations. 2. The fluctuations of the number of ions. *Physical Review.* 72:26–29, 1947.

[70] M. Fatourechi, A. Bashashati, R.K. Ward, G.E. Birch. EMG and EOG artifacts in brain computer interface systems: a survey. *Clin Neurophysiol.* 118(3):480–494, 2007.

[71] M.S. Fee, P.P. Mitra, D. Kleinfeld. Automatic sorting of multiple unit neuronal signals in the presence of anisotropic and non-gaussian variability. *J Neurosci Methods.* 69(2):175–188, 1996.

[72] M.S. Fee, P.P. Mitra and D. Kleinfeld. Variability of extracellular spike waveforms of cortical neurons. *J Neurophysiol.* 76(6):3823–3833, 1996.

[73] Paul Feyerabend. *Against Method.* 3rd ed. Verso, London; 1993.

[74] R.P. Feynman, A.J.G. Hey, R.W. Allen. *Feynman Lectures on Computation.* Cambridge, MA: Perseus Books; 1999.

[75] B. Fischl, M.I. Sereno, A.M. Dale. Cortical surface-based analysis. 2: Inflation, flattening, and a surface-based coordinate system. *Neuroimage.* 9(2):195–207, 1999.

[76] B. Fischl, M.I. Sereno, R.B. Tootell, A.M. Dale. High-resolution intersubject averaging and a coordinate system for the cortical surface. *Hum Brain Mapp.* 8(4):272–284, 1999.

[77] R.S.J. Frackowiak. *Human Brain Function.* 2nd ed. Amsterdam, The Netherlands: Elsevier Academic Press; 2004.

[78] G.F. Franklin, J.D. Powell, A. Emami-Naeini. *Feedback Control of Dynamic Systems.* 5th ed. Upper Saddle River, N J; Pearson Prentice Hall; 2006.

[79] B. Friedland. *Control System Design: An Introduction to State-Space Methods.* Mineola, NY: Dover Publications; 2005.

[80] K.J. Friston, P. Fletcher, O. Josephs, A. Holmes, M. D. Rugg, and R. Turner. Event-related fMRI: characterizing differential responses. *Neuroimage.* 7(1): 30–40, 1998.

[81] K.J. Friston, S. Williams, R. Howard, R.S. Frackowiak, R. Turner. Movement-related effects in fmri time-series. *Magn Reson Med.* 35:346–355, 1996.

[82] R.D. Frostig, Z. Frostig, R.M. Harper. Recurring discharge patterns in multiple spike trains. 1. Detection. *Biol. Cybernetics,* 62(6):487–493, 1990.

[83] T. Gasser, L. Sroka, J. Mocks. The transfer of EOG activity into the EEG for eyes open and closed. *Electroencephalogr Clin Neurophysiol.* 61(2):181–193, 1985.

[84] T.H. Gasser, P. Ziegler, W.F. Gattaz. The deletricious effects of ocular artefacts on the quantitative eeg, and a remedy. *Eur Arch Psychiatry Neurosci.* 241: 352–356, 1992.

[85] C.R. Genovese, N.A. Lazar, T. Nichols. Thresholding of statistical maps in functional neuroimaging using the false discovery rate. *Neuroimage.* 15(4): 870–8, 2002.

[86] A.P. Georgopoulos, J.F. Kalaska, R. Caminiti, J.T. Massey. On the relations between the direction of two-dimensional arm movements and cell discharge in primate motor cortex. *J Neurosci.* 2(11):1527–1537, 1982.

[87] A.P. Georgopoulos, A.B. Schwartz, R.E. Kettner. Neuronal population coding of movement direction. *Science.* 233(4771):1416–1419, 1986.

[88] W. Gersch, G.V. Goddard. Epileptic focus location: spectral analysis method. *Science.* 169(946):701–702, 1970.

[89] E.D. Gershon, M.C. Wiener, P.E. Latham, B.J. Richmond. Coding strategies in monkey V1 and inferior temporal cortices. *J Neurophysiol.* 79(3):1135–1144, 1998.

[90] G.L. Gerstein, N.Y. Kiang. An approach to the quantitative analysis of electrophysiological data from single neurons. *Biophys J.* 1:15–28, 1960.

[91] G.L. Gerstein, B. Mandelbrot. Random Walk Models for the Spike Activity of a single neuron. *Biophysical Journal,* 4, 41–68, 1964.

[92] G. L. Gerstein, D. H. Perkel. Simultaneously recorded trains of action potentials: analysis and functional interpretation. *Science.* 164(3881):828–830, 1969.

[93] G. L. Gerstein, D. H. Perkel. Mutual temporal relationships among neuronal spike trains—statistical techniques for display and analysis. *Biophys J.* 12(5): 453, 1972.

[94] J. Gotman, D.R. Skuce, C.J. Thompson, P. Gloor, J.R. Ives, W.F. Ray. Clinical applications of spectral analysis and extraction of features from electroencephalograms with slow waves in adult patients. *Electroencephalogr Clin Neurophysiol.* 35(3):225–235, 1973.

[95] A. M. Grass, F.A. Gibbs. A Fourier transform of the electroencephalogram. *J Neurophysiol.* 1(6):521–526, 1938.

[96] C.M. Gray, P.E. Maldonado, M. Wilson, B. McNaughton. Tetrodes markedly improve the reliability and yield of multiple single-unit isolation from

multi-unit recordings in cat striate cortex. *J Neuroscience Methods*, 63(1–2):43–54, 1995.

[97] A. Grinvald, R.D. Frostig, R.M. Siegel, E. Bartfeld. High-resolution optical imaging of functional brain architecture in the awake monkey. *Proc Nat Acad Sci U S A*. 88(24):11559–11563, 1991.

[98] A. Grinvald, R. Hildesheim. VSDI: a new era in functional imaging of cortical dynamics. *Nat Rev Neurosci*. 5(11):874–885, 2004.

[99] A. Grinvald, D. Shoham, A. Shmuel, et al. In-vivo optical imaging of cortical architecture and dynamics. In: U. Windhorst, H. Johansson, eds. *Modern Techniques in Neuroscience Research*. Springer Verlag, New York, NY, 1999.

[100] M. Gur, A. Beylin, D.M. Snodderly. Response variability of neurons in primary visual cortex (v1) of alert monkeys. *J Neurosci*. 17(8):2914–2920, 1997.

[101] A.A. Gydikov, N.A. Trayanova. Extracellular potentials of single active muscle fibres: effects of finite fibre length. *Biol Cybern*. 53(6):363–372, 1986.

[102] M.S. Hamalainen. Magnetoencephalography: a tool for functional brain imaging. *Brain Topogr*. 5(2):95–102, 1992.

[103] J.P. Hansen, I.R. McDonald. 3rd ed. *Theory of Simple Liquids*. Boston, MA: Elsevier; 2006.

[104] K.D. Harris, D.A. Henze, J. Csicsvari, H. Hirase, G. Buzsaki. Accuracy of tetrode spike separation as determined by simultaneous intracellular and extracellular measurements. *J Neurophysiol*. 84(1):401–414, 2000.

[105] H.K. Hartline. The receptive fields of optic nerve fibres. *Am J Physiol*. 130:690–699, 1940.

[106] H.K. Hartline. The response of single optic nerve fibers of the vertebrate eye to illumination of the retina. *Am J Physiol*. 121:400–415, 1938.

[107] T. Hastie, R. Tibshirani, J.H. Friedman. *The Elements of Statistical Learning: Data Mining, Inference, and Prediction: With 200 Full-Color Illustrations*. Springer series in statistics. New York, NY: Springer; 2002.

[108] M. Hausser. The Hodgkin-Huxley theory of the action potential. *Nat Neurosci*. 3 Suppl:1165, 2000.

[109] G.H. Henry, P.O. Bishop, B. Dreher. Orientation, axis and direction as stimulus parameters for striate cells. *Vision Research*. 14(9):767–777, 1974.

[110] D.A. Henze, Z. Borhegyi, J. Csicsvari, A. Mamiya, K.D. Harris, G. Buzsaki. Intracellular features predicted by extracellular recordings in the hippocampus in vivo. *J Neurophysiol*. 84(1):390–400, 2000.

[111] D.L. Hill, P. G. Batchelor, M. Holden, D.J. Hawkes. Medical image registration. *Phys Med Biol*. 46(3):R1–45, 2001.

[112] D.V. Hinkley. Improving jackknife with special reference to correlation estimation. *Biometrika*. 65(1):13–21, 1978.

[113] A.L. Hodgkin, A.F. Huxley. A quantitative description of membrane current and its application to conduction and excitation in nerve. *J Physiol*. 117(4):500–544, 1952.

[114] A.L. Hodgkin, A.F. Huxley. Currents carried by sodium and potassium ions through the membrane of the giant axon of loligo. *J Physiol*. 116(4):449–472, 1952.

[115] A.L. Hodgkin, A.F. Huxley. The components of membrane conductance in the giant axon of loligo. *J Physiol*. 116(4):473–496, 1952.

[116] A.L. Hodgkin, A.F. Huxley. The dual effect of membrane potential on sodium conductance in the giant axon of loligo. *J Physiol*. 116(4):497–506, 1952.

[117] A.L. Hodgkin, A.F. Huxley, B. Katz. Measurement of current-voltage relations in the membrane of the giant axon of loligo. *J Physiol.* 116(4):424–448, 1952.

[118] S. Holm. A simple sequentially rejective multiple test proceedure. *Scandinavian Journal of Statistics.* 6:65–70, 1979.

[119] N. Hoogenboom, J.M. Schoffelen, R. Oostenveld, L.M. Parkes, P. Fries. Localizing human visual gamma-band activity in frequency, time and space. *Neuroimage.* 29(3):764–773, 2006.

[120] H. Hotelling. Tubes and spheres in n-spaces, and a class of statistical problems. *American Journal of Mathematics.* 61:440–460, 1939.

[121] D.A. Howard. Albert Einstein as a philosopher of science. *Physics Today.* page 34, December, 2005.

[122] K. Huang. *Statistical Mechanics.* 2nd ed. New York, NY: Wiley; 1987.

[123] K. Imahori, K. Suhara. On the statistical method in brain wave study. Part I. *Fol. Psychiat. Neurol. Jap.* 3:137–155, 1949.

[124] J.R. Ives, D.L. Schomer. A 6-pole filter for improving the readability of muscle contaminated eegs. *Electroencephalogr Clin Neurophysiol.* 69(5):486–490, 1988.

[125] M.R. Jarvis, P.P. Mitra. Sampling properties of the spectrum and coherency of sequences of action potentials. *Neural Computation.* 13(4):717–749, 2001.

[126] H. Jasper. Progress and problems in brain research. *J Mt Sinai Hosp N Y,* 25(3):244–253, 1958.

[127] J. Johnson. Thermal agitation of electricity in conductors. *Physical Review,* 32:97, 1928.

[128] D. Johnston, S. Miao-sin Wu. *Foundations of Cellular Neurophysiology.* Cambridge, MA: MIT Press; 1995.

[129] J.P. Jones, L.A. Palmer. An evaluation of the two-dimensional gabor filter model of simple receptive fields in cat striate cortex. *J Neurophysiol.* 58(6): 1233–1258, 1987.

[130] J.P. Jones, L.A. Palmer. The two-dimensional spatial structure of simple receptive fields in cat striate cortex. *J Neurophysiol.* 58(6):1187–1211, 1987.

[131] M.W. Jung, Y. Qin, D. Lee, I. Mook-Jung. Relationship among discharges of neighboring neurons in the rat prefrontal cortex during spatial working memory tasks. *J Neurosci.* 20(16):6166–6172, 2000.

[132] T.P. Jung, S. Makeig, M.J. McKeown, A.J. Bell, T.W. Lee, T.J. Sejnowski. Imaging brain dynamics using independent component analysis. *Proc IEEE,* 89(7):1107–1122, 2001.

[133] E. Kandel. *Principles of Neural Science.* New York, NY: McGraw-Hill; 2000.

[134] P. Kara, P. Reinagel, R.C. Reid. Low response variability in simultaneously recorded retinal, thalamic, and cortical neurons. *Neuron.* 27(3):635–646, 2000.

[135] M.B. Kennel, J. Shlens, H.D.I. Abarbanel, E.J. Chichilnisky. Estimating entropy rates with bayesian confidence intervals. *Neural Computation.* 17(7): 1531–1576, 2005.

[136] D. Kleinfeld, R.N. Sachdev, L.M. Merchant, M.R. Jarvis, F.F. Ebner. Adaptive filtering of vibrissa input in motor cortex of rat. *Neuron.* 34(6):1021–34, 2002.

[137] L.F. Kozachenko, N.N. Leonenko. Sample estimate of the entropy of a random vector. *Problemy Peredachi Informatsii*, 23(2):9–16, 1987.

[138] S. Kullback, R.A Leibler. On Information and Sufficiency. *Ann Mathematical Statistics*. 22(1):79–86, 1951.

[139] M.W. Kwakkelstein. *Leonardo da Vinci as a Physiognomist: Theory and Drawing Practice*. Leiden, Primavera Pers; 1994.

[140] T.D. Lagerlund, F.W. Sharbrough, N.E. Busacker. Spatial filtering of multichannel electroencephalographic recordings through principal component analysis by singular value decomposition. *J Clin Neurophysiol*. 14(1):73–82, 1997.

[141] J.L. Lebowitz. Statistical mechanics: a selective review of two central issues. *Rev Mod Phys*. 71(2):S346–S357, 1999.

[142] A.K. Lee, I.D. Manns, B. Sakmann, M. Brecht. Whole-cell recordings in freely moving rats. *Neuron*. 51(4):399–407, 2006.

[143] M.S. Lewicki. A review of methods for spike sorting: the detection and classification of neural action potentials. *Network*. 9(4):R53–78, 1998.

[144] O.G. Lins, T.W. Picton, P. Berg, M. Scherg. Ocular artifacts in EEG and event-related potentials. I: Scalp topography. *Brain Topogr*. 6(1):51–63, 1993.

[145] O.G. Lins, T.W. Picton, P. Berg, M. Scherg. Ocular artifacts in recording EEGs and event-related potentials. II: Source dipoles and source components. *Brain Topogr*. 6(1):65–78, 1993.

[146] R.R. Llinas, U. Ribary, D. Jeanmonod, E. Kronberg, P. P. Mitra. Thalamocortical dysrhythmia: a neurological and neuropsychiatric syndrome characterized by magnetoencephalography. *Proc Natl Acad Sci U S A*. 96(26): 15222–15227, 1999.

[147] C. Loader. *Local regression and Likelihood*. New York, NY: Springer; 1999.

[148] S.J. Luck. *An Introduction to the Event-related Potential Technique*. Cognitive Neuroscience. Cambridge, MA; MIT Press; 2005.

[149] S. Ma. Calculation of entropy from Data of motion. *J Statistical Physics*. 26(2):221–240, 1981.

[150] J.A. McFadden. The entropy of a point process. *J Soc Industrial Applied Mathematics*. 13(4):988–994, 1965.

[151] B.L. McNaughton, J. O'Keefe, C.A. Barnes. The stereotrode: a new technique for simultaneous isolation of several single units in the central nervous system from multiple unit records. *J Neurosci Methods*. 8(4):391–7, 1983.

[152] C. Mehring, J. Rickert, E. Vaadia, Oliveira S. Cardosa de, A. Aertsen, S. Rotter. Inference of hand movements from local field potentials in monkey motor cortex. *Nat. Neurosci*. 6(12):1253, 2003.

[153] C.M Michel, M.N. Murray, G. Lantz, S. Gonzalez, L. Spinelli, and R.G. de Peralta. EEG source imaging. *Clinical Neurophysiol*. 115(10):2195–2222, 2004.

[154] G.A. Miller. Note on the bias of information estimates. *Information Theory in Psychology: Problems and Methods*. II(B):95–100, 1955.

[155] R.G. Miller Jr. A trustworthy jackknife. *Mathematical Statistics*. 35(4):1594–1605, 1964.

[156] R.G. Miller Jr. Jackknifing variances. *Ann Mathematical Statistics*. 39(2):567–582, 1968.

[157] R.G. Miller, Jr. The jackknife—a review. *Biometrika*. 61(1):1–15, 1974.

[158] P.P. Mitra, S. Ogawa, X.P. Hu, K. Ugurbil. The nature of spatiotemporal changes in cerebral hemodynamics as manifested in functional magnetic resonance imaging. *Magn Res Med*. 37(4):511–518, 1997.

[159] P.P. Mitra, B. Pesaran. Analysis of dynamic brain imaging data. *Biophys J,* 76(2):691–708, 1999.

[160] P.P. Mitra, J.B. Stark. Nonlinear limits to the information capacity of optical fibre communications. *Nature.* 411(6841):1027–1030, 2001.

[161] I. Nemenman, W. Bialek, R.D. van Steveninck. Entropy and information in neural spike trains: progress on the sampling problem. *Phys Rev E.* 69(5), 2004.

[162] D.P. Nguyen, L.M. Frank, E.N. Brown. An application of reversible-jump markov chain Monte Carlo to spike classification of multi-unit extracellular recordings. *Network.* 14(1):61–82, 2003.

[163] J.G. Nicholls, J. G. Nicholls. *From Neuron to Brain.* 4th ed. Sinauer Associates; MA: Sunderland, 2001.

[164] M.A. Nicolelis. Actions from thoughts. *Nature.* 409(6818):403, 2001.

[165] M.A. Nicolelis. Brain-machine interfaces to restore motor function and probe neural circuits. *Nat Rev Neurosci.* 4(5):417, 2003.

[166] M.A. Nicolelis, J.K. Chapin. Controlling robots with the mind. *Sci Am.* 287(4):46, 2002.

[167] P.L. Nunez, R. Srinivasan. *Electric Fields of the Brain: The Neurophysics of EEG.* 2nd ed. Oxford, England: Oxford University Press; 2006.

[168] H. Nyquist. Thermal agitation of electricity in conductors. *Physical Review.* 32:110, 1928.

[169] I. Obeid, P.D. Wolf. Evaluation of spike-detection algorithms for a brain-machine interface application. *IEEE Trans on Biomed Eng.* 51(6):905–911, 2004.

[170] H. Obrig, A. Villringer. Beyond the visible—imaging the human brain with light. *J Cerebral Blood Flow Metabo.* 23(1):1–18, 2003.

[171] S. Ogawa, T.W. Lee, A.S. Nayak, P. Glynn. Oxygenation-sensitive contrast In magnetic resonance image of rodent brain at high magnetic fields. *Magn Reson Med.* 14:69–78, 1990.

[172] J.G. O'Leary, N.G. Hatsopoulos. Early visuomotor representations revealed from evoked local field potentials in motor and premotor cortical areas. *J Neurophysiol.* 96(3):1492–506, 2006.

[173] M.W. Oram, M.C. Wiener, R. Lestienne, B.J. Richmond. Stochastic nature of precisely timed spike patterns in visual system neuronal responses. *J Neurophysiol.* 81(6):3021–3033, 1999.

[174] L. Paninski. Estimating entropy on m bins given fewer than m samples. *IEEE Trans Information Theory.* 50(9):2200–2203, 2004.

[175] D.H. Perkel, G.L. Gerstein, G.P. Moore. Neuronal spike trains and stochastic point processes. 2. Simultaneous spike trains. *Biophysical J.* 7(4):419, 1967.

[176] B. Pesaran, J.S. Pezaris, M. Sahani, P.P. Mitra, R.A. Andersen. Temporal structure in neuronal activity during working memory in macaque parietal cortex. *Nat Neurosci.* 5(8):805–811, 2002.

[177] M. Plischke, B. Bergersen. *Equilibrium Statistical Physics.* 3rd ed. Hackensack, NJ: World Scientific; 2006.

[178] N. Pouratian, S.A. Sheth, N.A. Martin, A.W. Toga. Shedding light on brain mapping: advances in human optical imaging. *Trends Neurosci.* 26(5):277–282, 2003.

[179] C. Pouzat, M. Delescluse, P. Viot, J. Diebolt. Improved spike-sorting by modeling firing statistics and burst-dependent spike amplitude attenuation: a

Markov chain Monte Carlo approach. *J Neurophysiol.* 91(6):2910–2928, 2004.

[180] C. Pouzat, O. Mazor, G. Laurent. Using noise signature to optimize spike-sorting and to assess neuronal classification quality. *J Neuroscience Methods.* 122(1):43–57, 2002.

[181] J.C. Prechtl, L.B. Cohen, B. Pesaran, P.P. Mitra, D. Kleinfeld. Visual stimuli induce waves of electrical activity in turtle cortex. *Proc Natl Acad Sci U S A.* 94(14):7621–7626, 1997.

[182] P.L. Purdon, R.M. Weisskoff. Effect of temporal autocorrelation due to physiological noise and stimulus paradigm on voxel-level false-positive rates in fMRI. *Hum Brain Mapp.* 6(4):239–249, 1998.

[183] D. Purves. *Neuroscience.* 3rd ed. Sunderland, MA: Sinauer Associates; 2004.

[184] M.H. Quenouille. Approximate tests for correlation in time-series. *J Roy Statistical Soc, Series B.* 11:68–84, 1949.

[185] M.H. Quenouille. Notes on bias in estimation. *Biometrika.* 43:353–360, 1956.

[186] P.M. Quilter, B.B. McGillivray, D.G. Wadbrook. The removal of eye movement artifact from the EEG signals using correlation techniques. In *Random Signal Analysis*, volume 159. IEEE Conference Publication, 1977: 93–100.

[187] R.Q. Quiroga, Z. Nadasdy, Y. Ben-Shaul. Unsupervised spike detection and sorting with wavelets and superparamagnetic clustering. *Neural Computation.* 16(8):1661–1687, 2004.

[188] S. Raghavachari, M.J. Kahana, D.S. Rizzuto, et al. Gating of human theta oscillations by a working memory task. *J Neuroscience.* 21(9):3175–3183, 2001.

[189] Santiago Ramon y Cajal. *Advice for a Young Investigator.* Cambridge, MA: MIT Press; 1999.

[190] D. Regan. An apparatus for the correlation of evoked potentials and repetitive stimuli. *Med Biol Eng.* 4(2):169–177, 1966.

[191] D. Regan. An effect of stimulus colour on average steady-state potentials evoked in man. *Nature.* 210(40):1056–1057, 1966.

[192] D. Regan. *Human Brain Electrophysiology: Evoked Potentials and Evoked Magnetic Fields in Science and Medicine.* New York, NY: Elsevier; 1989.

[193] A. Renyi. *Probability Theory.* Amsterdam; North-Holland Pub. Co.; 1970.

[194] F. Rieke, D. Warland, R. de Ruyter van Steveninck, W. Bialek. *Spikes: Exploring the Neural Code.* Cambridge, MA: MIT Press; 1997.

[195] B.D. Ripley. *Pattern Recognition and Neural Networks.* Cambridge, England; Cambridge University Press; 1996.

[196] S. Rosen. *The Examined Life: Readings From Western Philosophy From Plato to Kant.* New York, NY: Random House; 2000.

[197] E. Schechtman, S.J. Wang. Jackknifing two-sample statistics. *J Statistical Planning and Inference.* 119(2):329–340, 2004.

[198] H. Scherberger, M.R. Jarvis, R.A. Andersen. Cortical local field potential encodes movement intentions in the posterior parietal cortex. *Neuron.* 46(2): 347–354, 2005.

[199] A.M. Sengupta, P.P. Mitra. Distributions of singular values for some random matrices. *Physical Review E.* 60(3):3389–3392, 1999.

[200] M. Serruya, N. Hatsopoulos, M. Fellows, L. Paninski, J. Donoghue. Robustness of neuroprosthetic decoding algorithms. *Biol Cybernetics.* 88(3):219–228, 2003.

[201] M.D. Serruya, N.G. Hatsopoulos, L. Paninski, M.R. Fellows, J.P. Donoghue. Instant neural control of a movement signal. *Nature.* 416(6877):141, 2002.

[202] M.N. Shadlen, W.T. Newsome. The variable discharge of cortical neurons: implications for connectivity, computation, and information coding. *J Neurosci.* 18(10):3870–96, 1998.

[203] C.E. Shannon, N.J.A. Sloane, A.D. Wyner and IEEE Information Theory Society. *Claude Elwood Shannon: Collected Papers.* New York, NY: IEEE Press; 1993.

[204] S.D. Silvey. *Statistical Inference.* Monographs on Statistical Subjects. Wiley, London, New York, reprinted with corrections. edition, 1975.

[205] N.C. Singh, F.E. Theunissen. Modulation spectra of natural sounds and ethological theories of auditory processing. *J. Acoust Soc Am.* 114 (6 Pt. 1) 3394–3411, 2003.

[206] M. Sipser. *Introduction to the Theory of Computation.* 2nd ed. Boston, MA: Thomson Course Technology; 2006.

[207] L. Sirovich, E. Kaplan. Analysis methods for optical imaging. In R.D. Frostig, ed., *Optical Imaging: CRC Reviews.* Boca Raton, FL: CRC Press; 2002.

[208] D.L. Snyder, M.I. Miller, D.L. Snyder. *Random Point Processes in Time and Space.* 2nd ed. New York, NY: Springer-Verlag; 1991.

[209] W.R. Softky, C. Koch. The highly irregular firing of cortical-cells is inconsistent with temporal integration of random epsps. *J Neurosci.* 13(1):334–350, 1993.

[210] A. Sornborger, C. Sailstad, E. Kaplan, L. Sirovich. Spatiotemporal analysis of optical imaging data. *Neuroimage.* 18(3):610–621, 2003.

[211] A. Sornborger, T. Yokoo. A multitaper approach to detection of harmonic response in multivariate data, submitted 2007.

[212] A. Sornborger, T. Yokoo, A. Delorme, C. Sailstad, L. Sirovich. Extraction of the average and differential dynamical response in stimulus-locked experimental data. *J Neurosci Methods.* 141(2):223–9, 2005.

[213] M. Steinbach, L. Ertoz, V. Kumar. The challenges of clustering high dimensional data. In: L.T. Wille, ed. *New Directions in Statistical Physics.* New York, NY: Springer-Verlag; 2004.

[214] Mircea Steriade. *The Intact and Sliced Brain.* Cambridge, MA: MIT Press, 2001.

[215] B.E. Swartz, E.S. Goldensohn. Timeline of the history of EEG and associated fields. *Electroencephalogr Clin Neurophysiol.* 106(2):173–176, 1998.

[216] D.M. Taylor, S.I. Tillery, A.B. Schwartz. Direct cortical control of 3-d neuroprosthetic devices. *Science.* 296(5574):1829–1832, 2002.

[217] B.R. Tharp, W. Gersch. Spectral analysis of seizures in humans. *Comput Biomed Res.* 8(6):503–521, 1975.

[218] D.J. Thomson. Multitaper analysis of nonstationary and nonlinear time series data. In: W.J. Fitzgerald, R.L. Smith, A.T. Walden, P.C. Young, ed. *Nonlinear and Nonstationary Signal Processing.* Cambridge, England Cambridge University Press; 2004.

[219] D.J. Thomson. Spectrum estimation and harmonic-analysis. *Proc IEEE,* 70(9):1055–1096, 1982.

[220] D.J. Thomson. Quadratic-inverse spectrum estimates—applications to paleoclimatology. *Philosophical Trans Roy Soc London Series A—Mathematical Physical and Engineering Sciences.* 332(1627):539–597, 1990.

[221] D.J. Thomson, A.D. Chave. Jackknifed error estimates for spectra, coherences, and transfer functions. In: S. Haykin, ed. *Advances in Spectrum Estimation.* Prentice Hall, 1991: 58–113.

[222] D.J. Tolhurst, J.A. Movshon, A.F. Dean. The statistical reliability of signals in single neurons in cat and monkey visual-cortex. *Vision Research.* 23(8): 775–785, 1983.

[223] C. Tsallis. Possible generalization of Boltzmann-Gibbs statistics. *J Statistical Physics.* 52(1–2):479–487, 1988.

[224] H. C. Tuckwell. *Introduction to Theoretical Neurobiology Volume 2: Nonlinear and Statistical Theories,* New York, NY: Cambridge University Press; 1988.

[225] A.M. Turing, B.J. Copeland. *The Essential Turing: Seminal writings in Computing, Logic, Philosophy, artificial intelligence, and artificial Life, plus the Secrets of Enigma.* Oxford University Press; New York, 2004.

[226] V.J. Uzzell, E.J. Chichilnisky. Precision of spike trains in primate retinal ganglion cells. *J Neurophysiol.* 92(2):780–789, 2004.

[227] B.D. Van Veen, W. Van Drongelen, M. Yuchtman, A. Suzuki. Localization of brain electrical activity via linearly constrained minimum variance spatial filtering. *IEEE Trans Biomed Eng.* 44(9):867–880, 1997.

[228] V.N. Vapnik. *Statistical Learning Theory.* New York, NY: Wiley, 1998.

[229] A.L. Vazquez, D.C. Noll. Nonlinear aspects of the bold response in functional mri. *Neuroimage.* 7(2):108–118, 1998.

[230] S. Verdu, S.W. McLaughlin, IEEE Information Theory Society. *Information Theory: 50 Years of Discovery.* New York, NY: IEEE Press; 2000.

[231] J.D. Victor. Approaches to information theoretic analysis of neural activity. *Biol Theory.* 1:302–316, 2006.

[232] J.D. Victor, Binless strategies for estimation of information from neural data. *Physical Review E.* 66(5), 2002.

[233] J.D. Victor, K.P. Purpura. Metric-space analysis of spike trains: theory, algorithms and application. *Network-Computation in Neural Systems.* 8(2): 127–164, 1997.

[234] R. Vigario, J. Sarela, V. Jousmaki, M. Hamalainen, E. Oja. Independent component approach to the analysis of EEG and MEG recordings. *IEEE Trans Biomed Eng.* 47(5):589–93, 2000.

[235] A. Villringer, B. Chance. Non-invasive optical spectroscopy and imaging of human brain function. *Trends Neurosciences.* 20(10):435–442, 1997.

[236] D.O. Walter, W.R. Adey. Analysis of brain-wave generators as multiple statistical time series. *IEEE Trans Biomed Eng.* 12:8–13, 1965.

[237] D.O. Walter, W.R. Adey. Spectral analysis of electroencephalograms recorded during learning in the cat, before and after subthalamic lesions. *Exp Neurol.* 7:481–501, 1963.

[238] W.G. Walter. An automatic low frequency analyzer. *Electron. Eng.* 16:3–13, 1943.

[239] W.G. Walter. An improved low frequency analyzer. *Electron. Eng.* 16:236–240, 1943.

[240] D.K. Warland, P. Reinagel, M. Meister. Decoding visual information from a population of retinal ganglion cells. *J Neurophysiology.* 78(5):2336–2350, 1997.

[241] J. Wessberg, M.A.L. Nicolelis. Optimizing a linear algorithm for real-time robotic control using chronic cortical ensemble recordings in monkeys. *J Cognitive Neurosci.* 16(6):1022–1035, 2004.

[242] H. Weyl. On the volume of tubes. *Am J Mathematics.* 61:461–472, 1939.

[243] N. Wiener. *Cybernetics; or, Control and communications in the animal and the machine.* John Wiley & Sons and Hermann et Cie, New York, Paris, 1948.

[244] N. Wiener. *Cybernetics: or Control and communication in the animal and the machine.* 2nd ed. Cambridge, MA: MIT Press; 1973.

[245] N. Wiener. *Extrapolation, interpolation, and smoothing of stationary time series, with engineering applications.* Cambridge, MA: Technology Press of the Massachusetts Institute of Technology; 1949.

[246] N. Wiener M.A.B. Brazier. Discussion of correlation analysis. *Electroencephalography Clinical Neurophysiology.* Supplement 4:41–44, 1954.

[247] L.C. Diamond Editor, *Wittgenstein's Lectures on the Foundations of Mathematics, Cambridge, 1939: From the Notes of R. G. Bosanquet, Norman Malcolm, Rush Rhees and Yorick Smythies.* Hassocks: Harvester Press; 1976.

[248] J.C. Woestenburg, M.N. Verbaten, J.L. Slangen. The removal of the eye-movement artifact from the EEG by regression analysis in the frequency domain. *Biol Psychol.* 16(1–2):127–147, 1983.

[249] J.R. Wolpaw, N. Birbaumer, D.J. McFarland, G. Pfurtscheller, T.M. Vaughan. Brain-computer interfaces for communication and control. *Clin Neurophysiol.* 113(6):767–791, 2002.

[250] T. Womelsdorf, P. Fries, P.P. Mitra, R. Desimone. Gamma-band synchronization in visual cortex predicts speed of change detection. *Nature.* 439(7077):733–736, 2006.

[251] K.J. Worsley, A.C. Evans, S. Marrett, P. Neelin. A three-dimensional statistical analysis for CBF activation studies in human brain. *J Cereb Blood Flow Metab.* 12(6):900–18, 1992.

[252] K.J. Worsley, S. Marrett, P. Neelin, A.C. Vandal, K.J. Friston, A.C. Evans. A unified statistical approach for determining significant signals in images of cerebral activation. *Human Brain Mapping.* 4(1):58–73, 1996.

[253] A. Zador. Impact of synaptic unreliability on the information transmitted by spiking neurons. *J Neurophysiol.* 79(3):1219–1229, 1998.

[254] E. Zarahn, G.K. Aguirre, M. D'Esposito. Empirical analyses of bold fMRI statistics. I. Spatially unsmoothed data collected under null-hypothesis conditions. *Neuroimage.* 5(3):179–197, 1997.

[255] A. Zepeda, C. Arias, F. Sengpiel. Optical imaging of intrinsic signals: recent developments in the methodology and its applications. *J Neurosci Methods.* 136(1):1–21, 2004.

Index

Page numbers followed by an *f* or *t* indicate figures and tables. Page numbers followed by an "n" and another number indicate notes.

chi-square test, hypothesis testing,
177–178
Cholesky factorization, matrix
technique, 68
Chomsky hierarchy, languages, 38–39
circulant matrices, class, 65
clustering, spike sorting, 266–268
cognitive neuroscience, space of
theories, 16*f*
coherence. *See also* cross-coherence
between spike trains, 246, 247*f*
comparison of spectra and, 286–288
coherency, cross-spectral estimate,
208–209
communication theory
encoding and decoding process,
32–33
founder Claude Shannon, 32, 33*f*
introduction of time delays, 35*f*
multiuser, 34
mutual information as statistical
measure, 36
neuroscience and, 34–35
signal to noise ratio (SNR), 35
single-user, 33
compensator process, conditional
intensity process, 140–141
complex numbers, scalars, 52–53
complexity, simplicity and, of nervous
system, 21–22
computation, concepts, 27
computation theory, mathematics,
36–39
computer, view of brain, 5
computer science, founder Alan Turing,
37*f*
conceptual clarity
importance, 41*f*
valid reasoning and, 41–42
conditional intensity process, point
process, 135–137
confidence
bands, global, 288–290
interval estimation, 171–172
intervals for spectrum, 285–286
confidence intervals, local regression
and likelihood, 332
confusion
nervous system, 14–15
neuroscientists, 40

consciousness, transient and reversible
loss, 3
consequence, conceptual clarity and
valid reasoning, 42
conservation of energy, Hermann
Helmholtz, 23*f*
continuous movements, prediction,
255–256
continuous processes, class of
stochastic processes, 113
continuous random variables, entropy
and mutual information,
336–337
controlled experiments, empirical and,
43–44
controlled vocabulary, nomenclature,
42
control system design, classical and
modern views, 32*f*
control theory
feedback control, 31–32
nervous system, 29
convergence
Fourier expansions on interval,
81–82
Fourier series examples, 78*f*, 79*f*, 80*f*,
81*f*
notions, 76
topological vector spaces, 75
convergent evolution, problem-solution
pair, 30–31
correlations
causation and, 46–48
spectral power at different
frequencies, 216
spike trains, 238–239
cortical anatomy, functional magnetic
resonance imaging (fMRI) and
positron emission tomography
(PET), 311
counting measures, point processes as,
125–126
Cramer–Rao bound, point estimation,
156–157
critical region, binary hypotheses, 173
cross-coherence
between spikes and local field
potential, 243–244
bivariate spectral analysis, 208–209
hybrid multivariate processes, 215

engineering theories (*continued*)
comparative animal physiology, 30
computation, 36–39
control theory, 31–32
convergent evolution, 30–31
disconnect between, 38–39
introduction of time delays, 35*f*
mutual information as statistical
measure, 36
nervous system, 27–29
entropy
Boltzmann, 11
Gibbs-Shannon, 11–12
reversible and irreversible dynamics,
9–12
statistical measure, 36
Wiener, 111
entropy and mutual information
continuous random variables,
336–337
continuous-valued discrete-time
stochastic processes, 338–339
discrete random variables, 334–336
discrete-valued discrete-time
stochastic processes, 337–338
estimation methods, 340–341
point processes, 339–340
ergodicity, stochastic processes,
117–118
errors
method of least squares, 165–166
type I and II, in hypothesis testing,
174, 175*f*
estimation
asymptotic normality of MLE,
159–160
asymptotic properties of maximum
likelihood estimator (MLE),
158–159
bias, 155
classical statistics, 153
Cramer-Rao bound, 156–157
difficulties for small sample sizes,
160–161
entropy and mutual information,
340–341
estimator: bias and variance,
154–156
Fisher information matrix, 160
identifiability, 159

interval, 171–172
method of maximum likelihood,
157–158
point, 154–161
sufficient statistics, 156
estimation variance
jackknife method for, 195–196
multitaper estimator, 195
estimator variance, method of least
squares, 162–164
ethology, space of theories, 16*f*
Euclidean geometry, vector in higher
dimensional space, 58–60
events, probability theory, 100–102
evoked potentials
term, 188n.2
time series analysis, 187–188
evolution, biological phenomena, 30
evolutionary psychology, space of
theories, 16*f*
experimental methods, empirical and
controlled, 43–44
experimental psychology, space of
theories, 16*f*
experimental techniques,
spatiotemporal resolutions, 220*t*
exploratory data analysis, approaches,
151–152
exponential functions, scalars, 54–55
exponentials
Fourier series, 77–81
functions of matrices, 66–67
extracellular potentials, neuronal
biophysics, 223
eye movement, denoising in EEG/MEG,
279

factorial moments, product densities or,
142–143
Fano factor, spike train analysis, 234,
235*f*
fast Fourier transform (FFT)
algorithm, 86–89
spectral estimation, 190, 213
feature vectors, prediction, 253–254
feedback, control theory, 31–32
Fejer kernel, time frequency analysis,
93
Fisher, Sir Ronald Aylmer, modern
statistics founder, 151

jackknife method
  comparing spectra and coherences,
    286–288
  confidence intervals for spectrum and
    coherence estimates, 285–286
  estimation variance, 195–196
  global confidence bands, 288–290
  permutation tests, 288–290
  single group, 283–284
  two groups, 284–285
joint occurrence density
  conditional intensity, 138–139
  inhomogeneous Poisson, 137
  point process, 128
joint peristimulus time histogram,
    measure, 244–245
Jordan normal form, matrices, 69

Kolmogorov's axioms, probability
    theory, 101
Kolmogorov's formalism, probability
    theory, 98, 99
Kolmogorov Smirnov test,
    nonparametric test, 178–179
Krogh's principle, comparative animal
    physiology, 30
Kullback-Leiber (KL) divergence,
    probability theory, 105
kurtosis, probability distribution, 104

languages
  Chomsky hierarchy, 38–39
  syntax, 41–42
  Tower of Babel, 8f
law of averages, probability theory,
    111–112
law of large numbers, probability
    theory, 111–112
laws of motion
  biological arrow of time, 12–13
  deterministic vs. random, 12
layering, engineering, 18
least squares method
  estimator variance and model
    assessment, 162–164
  generalization error, 165–166
  linear model, 161–167
  mean squared error (MSE), 162
  model selection, 166–167
  multivariate case, 164–165

statistical protocol example,
    150–151
  training error, 165–166
levels of organization
  bridging across levels, 19–21
  nervous system, 17–22
  physics and engineering, 18
  space of theories, 16f
likelihood, nonparametric approach,
    326–327
likelihood ratio test, hypothesis testing,
    174–176
linear algebra
  angles, distances, and volumes,
    58–60
  basis expansions, 56
  classes of matrices, 64–66
  classical matrix factorization
    techniques, 67–70
  functions of matrices, 66–67
  linear independence and basis sets,
    61–62
  linear transformations of vectors,
    63–64
  matrices, 63–64
  pseudospectra, 70–72
  subspaces and projections, 62–63
  vectors and matrices, 56–72
  vectors as points in high-dimensional
    space, 57–58
linear dependence, generalization, 61
linear independence, linear algebra,
    61–62
linear model. See also least squares
    method
  method of least squares, 161–167
linear prediction, continuous
    movements, 256
link function, generalized linear model,
    169–170
local field potential (LFP)
  cross-coherence between spikes and,
    243–244
  data analysis, 239–242
  evoked, for preferred and
    antipreferred directions, 240,
    241f
  neuronal biophysics, 223
  separation from raw voltage, 226f
  tuning curve, 240, 242f

multitaper estimates
  bispectrum, 215
  quadratic estimates as, 193
multitaper spectral estimator, using
    Slepians, 194
multiuser communication, theory, 34
multivariate case, method of least
    squares, 164–165
multivariate spectral analysis
  decomposition of cross spectral
      matrix, 209–211
  optical imaging, 315–319
  traveling waves, 210–211
muscle discharges, denoising in
    EEG/MEG, 279
mutual information. *See also* entropy
    and mutual information
  statistical measure, 36

narrowband bias
  periodogram estimate, 191
  time frequency analysis, 90–94
nervous system. *See also* engineering
    theories
  active perspective, 5–6
  biological function, 23
  bridging across levels, 19–21
  complex engineering systems, 19, 20*f*
  complexity, 14–15
  conservation of energy in biological
      processes, 22, 23*f*
  direction of causal explanations, 22–24
  emergent phenomena, 19
  instrumental approach, 24–25
  level of organization, 17–22
  levels of organization in physics and
      engineering, 18
  method of controlled experiments,
      24–25
  parable of blind men and elephant,
      14, 15*f*
  partial views of brain, 25*f*
  simplicity and complexity, 21–22
  symmetry principles, 20–21
  vs. scale, 17–18
neural activity, predicting behavior
    from, 251, 253–256
neural code
  statistical analysis, 148–149
  time series analysis, 186

neural signals
  evoked potentials, 187–188
  experimental methods, 219
  probability distribution of stochastic
      process, 186
  stochastic processes for analysis,
      113–114
neuroanatomy, well-formed state-
    ments, 42
neurobiology, second moments, 189
neuronal code, stimulus-response,
    220
neurons
  action potentials and synaptic
      potentials, 221, 223
  biophysics of, 221–223
  example from hippocampus of rat,
      250–251
neurophysiology, space of theories,
    16*f*
neuroscience
  communication theory and, 34–35
  data analysis goals, 149–150
  dynamics, 7
  experimental approaches, 220–221
  periodic stimuli in experiments, 246,
      247*f*, 248
  role of Fourier analysis, 72–73
  Tower of Babel, 7, 8*f*
Newtonian dynamics
  deterministic vs. random motion, 12
  laws of motion, 12–13
  physical systems, 7, 9
Nobel Prize, Huxley, Hodgkin, and
    Eccles, 222*f*
noise, electroencephalography and
    magnetoencephalography, 275
noise sources
  functional magnetic resonance
      imaging (fMRI), 296–297
  optical imaging, 314
  positron emission tomography (PET),
      296–297
  recordings, 225
non-Gaussian processes
  Markovian, 123–124
  stochastic process, 123–124
nonparametric quadratic estimates
  data taper, 191
  estimation variance, 195